19 55

CHRISTIAN BENNINGER

Epileptic seizures – behaviour – pain

Epileptic seizures – behaviour – pain

Edited by W. Birkmayer, Vienna

University Park Press
Baltimore London Tokyo

An international symposium
St. Moritz, 6th–7th January 1975

Manuscripts coordinated and translated under the supervision of:

Dr. C. ADAMS
Mr. I. C. W. BIGLAND, M. A.
Prof. W. GRÜTER
Dr. W. JOCHUM
Dr. H. KARRER
Mr. H. D. PHILPS, M. A.
Dr. G. ROTHWEILER

Library of Congress Cataloging in Publication Data

Main entry under title:
Epileptic seizures – behaviour – pain

   Includes index.
1. Epilepsy – Congresses. 2. Carbamazepine – Congresses. 3. Problem children – Congresses. 4. Psychopharmacology – Congresses. 5. Neuralgia, Trigeminal – Congresses. I. Birkmayer, Walther, 1910 [DNLM: 1. Epilepsy–Drug therapy. 2. Anticonvulsants – Therapeutic use. 3. Behaviour – Drug effects. 4. Social behavior disorders – In infancy and childhood. 5. Social behavior disorders – Drug effects. 6. Pain – Drug therapy. WL385 B646]

Published in North and South America by
University Park Press

RC372.E673 616.8'53 76-16096

ISBN 0-8391-0938-5

Contents

List of speakers

Prof. L. BARRAQUER-BORDAS, Director del Servicio de Neurología, Hospital de la Santa Cruz y San Pablo, Facultad de Medicina, Universidad Autónoma, Provenza 285, Barcelona, Spain

Prof. H. J. BEIN, Meisenstrasse 11, CH–4104 Oberwil, Switzerland

Prof. W. BIRKMAYER, Leiter des Ludwig-Boltzmann-Instituts für Neurochemie, Versorgungsheimplatz 1, A–1130 Vienna, Austria

Dr. S. BLOM, M.D., Department of Clinical Neurophysiology, University Hospital, S–901 85 Umeå, Sweden

Prof. M. BONDUELLE, Service de Neurologie, Hôpital Saint-Joseph, 1 rue Pierre-Larousse, F–75674 Paris Cedex 14, France

Prof. J. CAMBIER, Clinique neurologique de la Faculté Xavier Bichat, Hôpital Beaujon, 100 boulevard du Général Leclerc, F–92110 Clichy, France

Prof. R. DREYER, Nervenfacharzt, Bethelweg 22, D–4813 Bielefeld-Bethel, German Federal Republic

Dr. J. W. FAIGLE, Research Department, Pharmaceuticals Division, CIBA-GEIGY LIMITED, Klybeckstrasse 141, CH–4002 Basle, Switzerland

Dr. A. R. GAGNEUX, Research Department, Pharmaceuticals Division, CIBA-GEIGY LIMITED, Klybeckstrasse 141, CH–4002 Basle, Switzerland

Prof. INGRID GAMSTORP, Department of Paediatrics, University Hospital, S–750 14 Uppsala, Sweden

Dr. R. H. E. GRANT, M.B., B.S., D.C.H., Director of The David Lewis Centre for Epilepsy, near Alderley Edge, Cheshire SK9 7UD, England

Dr. C. GROH, Allgemeines Krankenhaus der Stadt Wien, Universitäts-Kinderklinik, Spitalgasse 23, A–1100 Vienna, Austria

Prof. W. GRÜTER, Head of the Medical and Pharmaceutical Information Service, CIBA-GEIGY LIMITED, Klybeckstrasse 141, CH–4002 Basle, Switzerland

Prof. B. HAGBERG, Department of Paediatrics, University of Gothenburg, Östra Sjukhuset, Smörslottsgatan 1, S–416 85 Gothenburg, Sweden

Prof. H. HEIMANN, Direktor der Universitäts-Nervenklinik, Osianderstrasse 22, D–74 Tübingen, German Federal Republic

Prof. H. HELMCHEN, Direktor der Psychiatrischen Klinik der Freien Universität Berlin, Nussbaumallee 36, D–1 Berlin 19

Dr. J. HIRTZ, Centre de Recherche Biopharmaceutique CIBA-GEIGY, B. P. 130, F–92505 Rueil Malmaison, France

Prof. D. Janz, Leiter der Abteilung für Neurologie im Klinikum Charlottenburg der Freien Universität Berlin, Spandauer Damm 130, D–1 Berlin

Prof. P. Kielholz, Direktor der Psychiatrischen Universitätsklinik, Wilhelm-Klein-Strasse 27, CH–4056 Basle, Switzerland

Prof. W. P. Koella, Research Department, Pharmaceuticals Division, CIBA-GEIGY LIMITED, Klybeckstrasse 141, CH–4002 Basle, Switzerland

Prof. R. Kuhn, Direktor der Kantonalen Psychiatrischen Klinik, CH–8596 Münsterlingen, Switzerland

Dr. Verena Kuhn-Gebhart, Leitende Ärztin, Kantonale Psychiatrische Klinik, CH–8596 Münsterlingen, Switzerland

Dr. L. Marques-Assis, Assistant Professor of Neurology, Medical School, University of São Paulo, São Paulo, Brazil

Dr. P. Martinelli, Clinica delle Malattie Nervose e Mentali dell'Università di Bologna, Via Ugo Foscolo 7, I–40123 Bologna, Italy

Dr. F. Monaco, Clinica delle Malattie Nervose e Mentali dell'Università di Torino, Via Cherasco 15, I–10126 Turin, Italy

Dr. P. L. Morselli, Laboratorio di Farmacologia Clinica, Istituto di Ricerche Farmacologiche "M. Negri", Via Eritrea 62, I–20157 Milan, Italy

Prof. M. Mumenthaler, Direktor der Neurologischen Universitätsklinik, Freiburgstrasse 12, CH–3008 Berne, Switzerland

Prof. G. Nissen, Ärztlicher Direktor der Städtischen Klinik für Kinder- und Jugendpsychiatrie Wiesengrund, Frohnauer Strasse 74–80, D–1 Berlin 28

Prof. R. Oberholzer, Head of the Medical Department, CIBA-GEIGY LIMITED, Klybeckstrasse 141, CH–4002 Basle, Switzerland

Prof. J. Obiols Vié, Catedrático de Psiquiatría y Psicología Médica de la Facultad de Medicina de Barcelona, Via Augusta 20, Barcelona, Spain

Dr. L. Oller-Daurella, Director del Centro de Lucha Antiepiléptica de Sanidad de Barcelona, Escuelas Pías 89, Barcelona, Spain

Dr. L. Oller Ferrer-Vidal, Médico del Centro Antiepiléptico de PENEPA, Neurofisiólogo del Instituto Neurológico de Barcelona, Manila 57, Barcelona, Spain

Dr. M. Parsonage, F.R.C.P., Senior Consultant Physician, Neurological Department, The General Infirmary, Leeds LS1 3EX, England

Dr. J. Kiffin Penry, M.D., Chief, Applied Neurologic Research Branch, Collaborative and Field Research, National Institute of Neurological and Communicative Disorders and Stroke, National Institutes of Health, Bethesda, Maryland 20014, U.S.A.

Prof. H. Petsche, Vorstand des Neurophysiologischen Instituts der Universität Wien, Währinger Strasse 17, A–1090 Vienna, Austria

Dr. Rosa María Puente, Profesor Titular de Clinicopatología de Sistema Nervioso, Escuela Superior de Medicina del Instituto Politécnico Nacional, Bonampak 96, Mexico 13 D.F., Mexico

Prof. H. Reisner, Vorstand der Neurologischen Universitätsklinik, Lazarett-gasse 14, A–1097 Vienna, Austria

Prof. H. Remschmidt, Klinik für Kinder- und Jugendpsychiatrie der Univer-sität Marburg-Lahn, Hans-Sachs-Strasse 4/6, D–355 Marburg-Lahn, German Federal Republic

Prof. A. Rett, Abteilung für entwicklungsgestörte Kinder, Neurologisches Krankenhaus der Stadt Wien-Rosenhügel, A–1130 Vienna, Austria

Dr. P. Schmidlin, Medical Department, CIBA-GEIGY LIMITED, Klybeckstrasse 141, CH–4002 Basle, Switzerland

Address of chief coordinator:
Dr. C. Adams, c/o CIBA-GEIGY LIMITED, Klybeckstrasse 141, CH–4002 Basle, Switzerland

Pathophysiological aspects of epileptic seizures

by H. Petsche*

The discovery of a method by which the electrical phenomena accompanying an epileptic seizure can be recorded has greatly extended our knowledge of the mechanisms that produce and maintain such seizures. Following the prophetic assumption made by Jackson (1834–1911) that a seizure is akin to a thunderstorm in the brain, it may have seemed only a short step to the first electro-encephalographic recordings of seizures, which appeared to confirm his assumption; but this short step was not taken until half a century later. On the other hand, in the 30 years that have elapsed since these pioneering days of electro-encephalography, countless fragments of knowledge have been collected and fitted together to form a complex mosaic – a mosaic, however, in which some of the pieces still refuse to take up their allotted positions. Nevertheless, this mosaic, or working model of epilepsy, already reveals one important fact, namely, that an epileptic seizure is anything but a chaotic discharge of all the nerve cells in the brain; far from resembling an avalanche that sweeps all before it in utter confusion, it is a highly organised process made up of individual events which interlock with one another in a variety of ways, even though their exact interrelationship may still sometimes be obscure. This highly organised pathophysiological process takes place predominantly in the cerebral cortex, an extremely complex formation whose structural layout has become more puzzling than ever, instead of clearer, as the result of the in-. creasingly sophisticated techniques now being employed in electron microscopy.

Under these circumstances, any attempt to depict the essential features of the epileptic seizure must obviously be subject to considerable limitations. Let us therefore begin by defining our terms of reference.

In principle, the electrophysiological processes involved in an experimentally induced epileptic seizure can be investigated from various points of view: on a macroscopic level, the interaction between fairly extensive areas of cortical substance can be studied by using the relatively large electrodes employed in conventional clinical electro-encephalography; in such studies, processes with a frequency of less than about 1 cycle per second (D.C. potentials) are generally recorded separately from shifts in potential within the electro-encephalographic frequency range, because they call for the use of different amplifiers. On the other hand, with the aid of micro-electrodes the processes can be studied at a cellular level, in order to find out what contribution individual cells are

* Neurophysiologisches Institut der Universität Wien und Hirnforschungsinstitut der Österreichischen Akademie der Wissenschaften, Vienna, Austria.

making to the seizure. Whereas a relatively large body of information about these cellular processes is already available today (cf. the review published by CREUTZFELDT[3]), very little is yet known about the interactions of more extensive regions of the brain, i.e. about the question of synchronisation; the physiological reasons why a seizure discharge should quickly spread to wide areas of the cortex, and why it should be so uniform irrespective of its localisation, are still for the most part obscure and, what is more, had until recently received scant attention. It is with this aspect of the subject that the present paper is chiefly concerned.

The term "synchronisation" originates from clinical electro-encephalography and was coined because, at the slow speed at which E.E.G. tracings are usually recorded (3 cm./sec.), seizure discharges appear synchronously over various regions of the brain. This term is not quite accurate, however, inasmuch as recordings from different sites invariably display phase differences even though the wave forms seem to be identical. These differences become even more pronounced when the records are taken not from the scalp but directly from the exposed cerebral cortex, because the layers of tissue separating the generator zones of electrical activity in the cerebral cortex from the electrodes affixed to the skull possess differing electrical properties and thus have the effect of blurring the wave forms and of reducing their amplitude. In the case of recordings made direct from the cerebral cortex, clear-cut differences in frequency and phase – which can be detected by spectrometric methods – are encountered even where the electrodes are placed only 1 mm. apart[16]. Amplitude distribution, too, is completely unpredictable, and unexpectedly steep potential gradients of up to 2 mV./mm. are often seen at the cerebral cortex[19]. These observations demonstrate that the cerebral cortex is by no means such a good electrical conductor as might perhaps be supposed on the basis of E.E.G. records taken from the scalp, in which the wave forms over different regions often become largely identical owing to passive conduction; E.E.G.s recorded from the scalp represent, in fact, the summated activity of a number of complex generators coupled to one another. In this connection, the importance of the influence exerted by structural peculiarities of the cerebral cortex is revealed by the close relationships existing between wave form during an epileptic attack and cellular architecture: the greater the structural differences between neighbouring cortical zones, the larger the differences recorded in the E.E.G. during a seizure.

Upon what morphological units is the occurrence of an epileptic attack dependent? This problem has not yet been fully elucidated. True, the nerve cells – and presumably also their dendrites – are known to play a decisive role as generators; but how many nerve cells have to be coupled together to produce a seizure? In other words, the question as to how large the "critical mass" of nerve substance must be for a self-sustained after-discharge to occur, and how these cells must be linked together, is one that has yet to be answered. It is known that epileptic activity can be induced by stimulating isolated areas of the cortex; this is, indeed, a commonly employed model for the study of self-sustained activity[11]. Even in tissue cultures, as CRAIN and BORNSTEIN[2] have demonstrated in experiments with embryonic nerve tissue, oscillations can be induced by electrical stimulation as early as one to two weeks after explantation; the explant also reacts to epileptogenic substances in the same way as an intact brain. Particularly worth mentioning in this context are observations concerning the mutual influence exerted on each other by two explants: when explants of embryonic brainstem and spinal-cord tissue were cultured together, tissue bridges developed, across which oscillations induced electrically in the one explant stimulated the other to the same activity. These studies, however, likewise fail to indicate what is the smallest possible number of interconnected nerve cells in which repetitive activity can occur.

Considerable light has been shed on this problem by investigations carried out by SPECKMANN and CASPERS[26] on individual neurones of the visceral ganglia in the edible snail. In these investigations the addition of pentetrazole, a potent epileptogenic substance, to the rinsing liquid led first of all to an increase in the spontaneous discharge frequency of the neurone and eventually to the occurrence of paroxysmal depolarisations of increasing duration. During these D.C. shifts the neurone discharged a burst of high-frequency spikes of decreasing amplitude. Paroxysmal depolarisations of this kind are a typical finding in cells located in experimentally produced epileptogenic foci, irrespective of whether these foci have been induced by cold, by penicillin, by strychnine, or by alumina cream. Nowadays, these complex discharges are generally referred to as "paroxysmal depolarisation shifts" (P.D.S.) and would seem to represent a basic discharge pattern of the nerve cell in an epileptogenic zone. The above-mentioned studies on the edible snail show that this basic discharge pattern is encountered even in such simple aggregates of neurones as the snail's visceral ganglion, which is made up of only a few neurones.

An epileptogenic focus in the intact brain also contains numerous cells which, instead of being activated, are inhibited during a P.D.S.

D.C. recordings made from an epileptogenic focus with electrodes of normal size usually also reveal a negative shift in the D.C. potential. In recent years, evidence has been accumulating to suggest that glial cells are probably responsible for this D.C. shift[23]. If, during a seizure, recordings are made from cells which, in the light of their behaviour – i.e. absence of injury discharge, high membrane potential, and absence of synaptic or action potentials – seem in all probability to be glial cells, these cells will be found to display the same D.C. shift during a seizure as is observed in records taken from the surface of the cortex. The same D.C. shifts are also encountered in the glial cells of penicillin-induced foci. This D.C. shift occurring during a seizure is accompanied by an increase in the extracellular potassium concentration from 3 mM. to 15 mM.[23], a fact that may also possibly have a bearing on the termination of the seizure[7].

In connection with the pathogenesis of neuronal hyperexcitability, WESTRUM et al.[30] have reported one observation that is of considerable interest from the standpoint of human pathology. In studies on Golgi preparations, these authors found that non-degenerated neurones in the vicinity of epileptogenic scars had strikingly few spines. They concluded that the functional, partial deafferentation caused by this loss of spines gives rise to cellular hyperactivity. Also consonant with this view are the observations made by Purpura[22] in the brains of mentally defective children with pathological E.E.G.s and a marked tendency to seizures: although these brains were of normal macroscopic appearance, Purpura found in Golgi-Cox preparations of the cerebral cortex that the spines of the dendrites exhibited conspicuous changes, which corresponded in severity to the clinical picture.

To sum up, therefore, it can be said that in an epileptogenic focus there is an increased incidence of paroxysmal depolarisation shifts in cells whose membrane potential is reduced and in which repolarisation is defective. In the vicinity of these cells one finds a negative D.C. shift, probably induced in part by glial cells. Deafferentation of the cells presumably plays a role in the pathogenesis of this hyperexcitability.

Now let us consider how these cells act together in order to generate the discharges referred to in E.E.G. jargon as "spikes".

To produce a model of these spikes and of the resultant seizure, recourse is usually had nowadays to penicillin applied locally. Penicillin is believed to act on the sodium-potassium pump by inhibiting membrane sodium-potassium adenosine triphosphatase, thereby reducing membrane potential. One of the most important epileptogenic factors stemming from the action of penicillin would seem to be, as in the case of strychnine, suppression of recurrent inhibition[4]. Intracellular studies performed by Prince and Wilder[20] on penicillin-induced foci have shown that the proportions of activated and inhibited cells during a P.D.S. are not the same and are dependent on the distance of the cell from the centre of the site at which the penicillin has been applied: whereas in the centre of the focus the overwhelming majority of the cells are activated, the opposite is the case in the less immediate vicinity of the focus; more than three times as many cells are in fact inhibited during the P.D.S. as are activated. The authors interpret this as a mechanism designed to limit the excitation and to prevent it from becoming generalised.

The spatio-temporal organisation of the spikes induced by topical application of penicillin is simple in the vertical dimension of the cortex, but extremely variable in the horizontal plane. Figure 1 shows the amplitude and latency of 20 successive spikes induced by locally applied penicillin and measured vertically to the surface of the cortex. The measurements were carried out with the aid of a semimicro-electrode from which intracortical recordings were made at different depths 200 μ apart. The spikes attained their maximum amplitude (7 mV.) approximately in the layer of the large pyramidal cells, and then decreased abruptly in amplitude in the recordings made closer to the surface of the cortex (Figure 1A). The time relationship between these intracortical spikes and the spikes in the surface record (Figure 1B) shows a displacement of about 16 msec., which means that between the site of their highest amplitude in the deep cortical layers and the surface of the cortex the penicillin-induced spikes had spread out at the rate of about 5 cm./sec. It should be noted that these spikes represent, not isolated discharges, but extracellularly recorded field potentials produced by the interaction of many individual cells (the tip of the

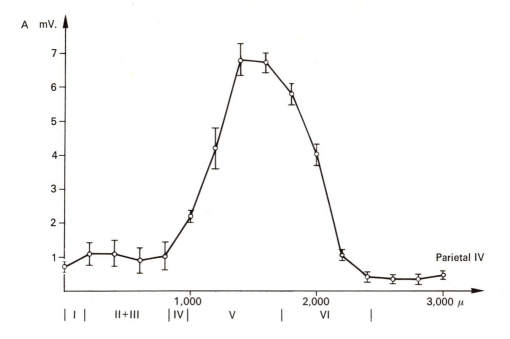

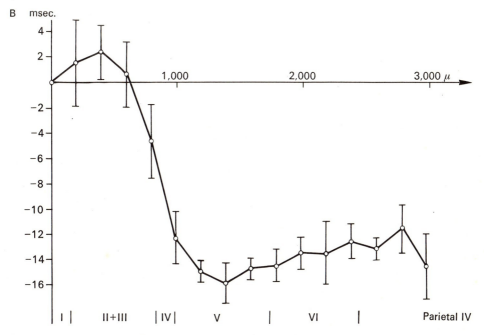

Fig. 1. Intracortical distribution (mean values ± S.D.) of the amplitude (A) and latency (B) of 20 successive spikes induced by the application of penicillin to the parietal region of the rabbit cortex.

The amplitude reaches a maximum in the layer of deep pyramidal cells; the time course of the intracortical spike in relation to that of the spike recorded from the surface of the cortex (B) is marked by a steep latency curve between the second and fifth laminae, the spike spreading corticopetally at a rate of 5 cm./sec. Abscissa: intracortical depth in microns; ordinate: millivolts (A) and milliseconds (B).

micro-electrode measured 5–10 μ in diameter). Also worth pointing out is the fact that the same corticopetal spreading of fast processes in the E.E.G. ("short transients") has likewise been observed in seizures induced by electrical stimulation or by pentetrazole[18].

In the horizontal plane the spatio-temporal organisation of penicillin-induced spikes is much more complicated and variable. Simultaneous recording of the spikes from a grid of 16 equidistant electrodes reveals that, even where the electrodes are only 1 mm. apart, the spikes do not appear simultaneously everywhere, and that the potential field giving rise to the spike is deformed and its peak displaced. In Figure 2 this has been illustrated spatially in several stages, each based on the multiple spike reproduced at the right-hand side of the figure. The grid of electrodes (4×4 electrodes 1 mm. apart), positioned over the striate area, is symbolised by the three squares in the centre of the figure. In these squares the path traced by the positive peak of the multiple spike is depicted in blocks, each of 4 msec. duration (to make the figure easier to understand, the squares have been placed one behind the other and the path projected on to them). The Roman numerals I to IX refer to the configurations of the potential fields (illustrated on the left and right of the three squares) extending from the origin of the spike to the point where it disappears. The Arabic numerals are indices of amplitude.

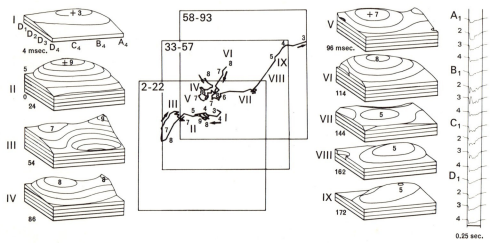

Fig. 2. Spatio-temporal analysis of a penicillin-induced spike *(extreme right)* recorded from a quadratic grid of 16 electrodes positioned 1 mm. apart in the striate area of the rabbit cortex (cf. Figure 4). The paths traced by the positive peaks of the potential fields are illustrated for 186 msec.

The three squares in the middle of the figure represent these paths, projected on to the grid of electrodes, in successive segments of 40 (designated "2–22"), 44 ("33–57"), and 70 ("58–93") msec. To simplify matters, the total path traced by the positive maximum has been divided up among these three intervals.

The three-dimensional representations of the penicillin-induced spike in the grid of electrodes at times I–IX are laterocaudal projections.

The behaviour of penicillin-induced spikes and of their field configuration (potential distribution) is extremely variable, in contrast to the behaviour of a fully developed seizure.

This figure shows that the potential fields built up during the passage of this penicillin-induced spike across the striate area are anything but uniform; they vary so much, in fact, as to create the impression that a plurality of different excitatory processes are constantly interacting with just as many inhibitory processes. In complete contrast to this irregular and unpredictable behaviour of the potential fields during the "spike" period, the situation becomes much simpler as soon as the seizure begins and a self-sustained activity develops.

The longer the time elapsing since the application of the penicillin, the more frequently do single spikes become replaced by double or multiple spikes, until finally, immediately following a spike, the seizure begins with a regular sequence of high-frequency discharges which usually become slower and higher ("tonic" stage); subsequently, the discharges occur in groups separated by intervals ("clonic" stage). The time sequence of the tonic and clonic stages, however, is not rigid; illustrated in Figure 9, for example, is a seizure in which the clonic stage occurred first. The wave forms during the seizure are extremely variable and largely depend, according to SPECKMANN et al.[27], on the regional D.C. potential.

A decisive role in the maintenance of the seizure itself would seem to be played by the facilitatory phenomena which have been observed experimentally following tetanic electrical stimulation and which have been referred to as "post-tetanic potentiation". This post-tetanic potentiation facilitates synaptic transmission, as can be measured experimentally by reference to the increasing amplitude of induced excitatory post-synaptic potentials; this facilitation lasts considerably longer than the stimulation itself. ECCLES[5] interprets this phenomenon as being due to a prolonged after-hyperpolarisation of pre-synaptic fibres, which causes the pre-synaptic spikes to become correspondingly larger. An increase in the supply of transmitter substance may perhaps also be involved. One of the main properties of the hydantoins, for example, is known to be their ability to inhibit post-tetanic potentiation[6].

Let us now consider the phenomenology of the E.E.G. correlatives in an experimentally induced seizure from two points of view – firstly, in the horizontal dimension, i.e. by reference to E.E.G. tracings recorded from surface electrodes, and, secondly, in the vertical dimension, i.e. by reference to intracortical recordings.

Reproduced in Figure 3 is a segment from a regular seizure pattern recorded from the striate area with the aid of a grid of 16 electrodes. The electrical activity is conspicuous for the fact that its frequency is twice as high at the lateral electrodes (D 1–4) as at the medial ones (A 1–4). In the upper part of the figure the first 208 msec. of the seizure discharge are portrayed at 8 msec. intervals in the form of a sequence of equipotential maps. Each of these square maps, which should be read continuously from top left to bottom right, shows the momentary potential distribution below the grid of electrodes. The changes in the configuration of the field, and also the displacement of the positive and negative peaks, are clearly visible. Underneath this sequence of maps, the paths traced by the maximum and minimum values for the E.E.G. half-waves 1–4, as well as the iso-electric lines, have been reproduced. These paths reveal that

17

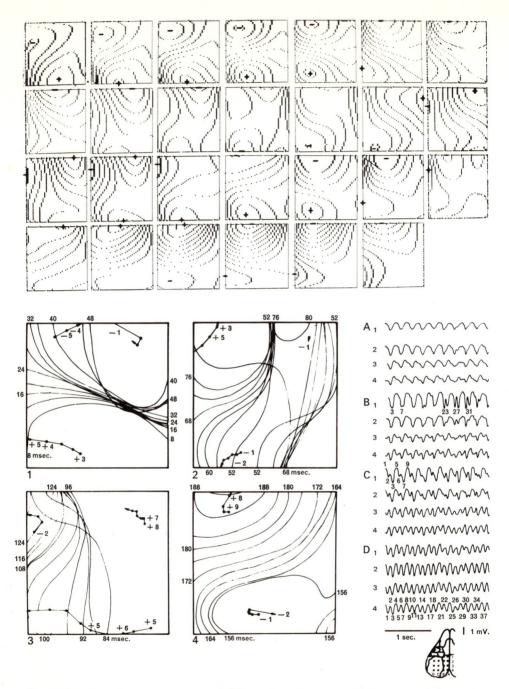

Fig. 3. Regular seizure pattern recorded from the striate area, the frequency being twice as high laterally as medially.

Above: potential fields of the first 208 msec. of the segment of the seizure illustrated. The time interval between one field and the next is 8 msec., and the fields should be read from top left to bottom right.

Below: paths traced by the positive and negative maxima of the first four half-waves in the E.E.G. pattern, illustrated in blocks of 8 msec. and projected on to the quadratic grid of electrodes, as well as the appurtenant iso-electric lines.

the two positive half-waves 1 and 3 display the most marked displacement –
a lateral one, incidentally – but that the rate of displacement is not the same
in both instances. This tendency to spread persists throughout the entire segment of the seizure illustrated here.

Generally speaking, there is a correlation between the regularity with which
the potential fields spread across the cortex and the regularity of the pattern
recorded in the E.E.G. Although this simple method of following the path
traced by the maximum values is no longer adequate for a spatio-temporal
analysis of more irregular forms of seizure, for which mathematical procedures
have had to be developed instead[16], it nevertheless helped to provide a new
insight into the essential nature of synchronisation, as can be seen from the
example given in Figure 4 which illustrates a very regular, tonic seizure discharge. This seizure, induced by the local application of penicillin, was recorded from the visual cortex of the rabbit with the aid of electrodes positioned

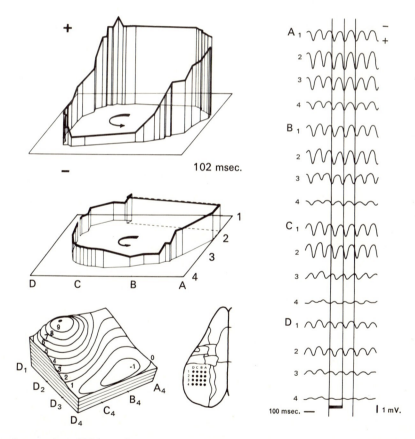

Fig. 4. Tonic, regular, 10/sec. seizure pattern following the application of penicillin;
electrodes positioned 1 mm. apart. The paths traced by the positive and negative
amplitude maxima have been portrayed in perspective in a laterocaudal projection.
Both maxima rotate within the grid of electrodes in a counterclockwise direction and
at a frequency of 10 c.p.s., the positive maximum changing its amplitude periodically.
Below, left: representation in perspective of the field distribution at the time when
the positive maximum was at electrode C 2.

19

1 mm. apart. When recorded under the usual conditions, this seizure discharge seems to appear simultaneously at all electrodes, but as soon as the recording speed is increased (the E.E.G. segment shown in Figure 4 was recorded at a speed of 12 cm./sec.), phase differences can be seen; these phase differences, however, do not seem to conform to any recognisable pattern. Not until the potential fields are analysed does it become clear that the field maxima and minima rotate counterclockwise within the grid of electrodes at a frequency of about 10 c.p.s., i.e. at the same frequency as that of the E.E.G. In the bottom left-hand corner of Figure 4 the positive maximum of the field is portrayed in a three-dimensional drawing at the moment when it is at electrode C 2. During this rotatory movement, it is only the positive maximum which periodically changes its amplitude, and not the negative maximum.

In Figure 5 an attempt has been made to indicate the sites of the positive and negative maxima simultaneously for two such revolutions. The figure shows that the two maxima rotate about each other roughly in the form of a double helix, remaining longer over certain sites and spreading rapidly again over others. It can be seen from these observations that, even in so apparently simple a pattern as a tonic seizure discharge, the behaviour of the cortical potential fields is extremely highly organised.

These findings shed an entirely fresh light on the question of the existence of a morphologically definable pacemaker, particularly since the same regular processes can also be observed in isolated regions of the cortex which have been separated from the thalamus. In other words, it is at best only in a functional sense that the term "pacemaker" can be applied to a fully developed epileptic seizure; in such a context, it can be used merely to denote the site of origin of a potential field, a site which, however, in no way remains constant.

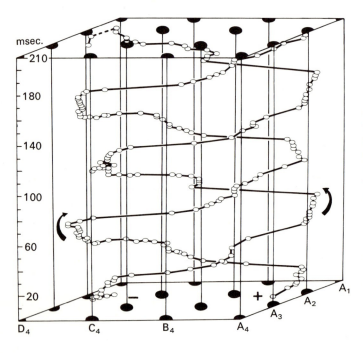

Fig. 5. Paths traced by the positive and negative maxima in the E.E.G. segment shown in Figure 4. Vertical scale: time in milliseconds. The positive and the negative potential maximum rotate about each other roughly in the shape of a double helix. Spreading does not occur at a uniform speed.

20

Another question arising in this connection is that of the morphological substrate underlying the spread of the potential fields within the cortex. As already pointed out, the thalamus is not absolutely necessary to this spreading process; in fact, it is in neuronally isolated hemispheres that the most regular and longest seizures have been seen[17].

At this point, it is essential to consider very carefully the concept of the "centrencephalic system"[14] and the bearing it has on the development of generalised seizures. Although the first studies on the origin of spike-and-wave activity conducted by JASPER and DROOGLEEVER-FORTUYN[12] provided support for the assumption that generalised seizures are centrally controlled, it was subsequently found on repeated occasions that the cortex alone is also capable of producing generalised seizures and even the spike-and-wave pattern[9]. Particularly the experience acquired in the meantime with intracortical recordings in man[1] has shown that so-called primarily generalised epileptic seizures invariably start from a focus and that even spike-and-wave activity can arise in various regions without the thalamus being implicated. In this connection, mention should also be made of an investigation in which WILLIAMS[31] studied the incidence of seizures in cerebral tumour patients with particular reference to the site of the tumour. He found that, the greater the extent to which the tumour involved the cerebral cortex, the higher was the incidence of seizures. Similarly, GLOOR et al.[10], by analysing the E.E.G. records of patients with degenerative systemic diseases, likewise demonstrated the primary role played by the cortex in the development and maintenance of seizures.

Incidentally, it should be emphasised that regular 3/sec. spike-and-wave activity is an extremely widespread epileptic phenomenon, which even occurs in

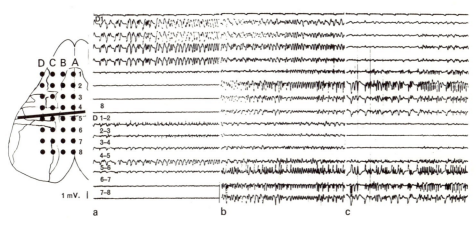

Fig. 6. Longitudinal records of seizure discharges occurring after transverse section of the cortex. The records were taken from a series of electrodes D 1–8 via unipolar and bipolar leads. Ouabain (3^{-10} molar g-strophanthin) was applied to the surface of the cortex and the electrodes were positioned 2 mm. apart.
The seizures developed either in front of the incision (a) or behind it (c), or on both sides of it (b), but independently of one another.
These observations underline the important role played by the cortex in maintaining synchronisation during a seizure.

21

frogs and lizards[25], although the cerebral cortex of these animals is entirely different in structure from that of man and consists of only two layers. Circumscribed intracortical spike-and-wave discharges have also been reported[28].

Consequently, the cerebral cortex appears to be of cardinal importance for synchronisation, and thus also for the spread of the excitation during the seizure. In view of this, the next question to be considered is that of the anatomical substrate implicated in this spread of excitation within the cerebral cortex. If the assumption is correct that intracortical and not thalamocortical connections are responsible for the phenomenon of synchronisation, then it should also be possible, by making vertical incisions into the cortex, to alter the pattern of the seizure in such a way that two regions displaying the same discharge pattern prior to incision discharge differently afterwards. As Figure 6 shows, this is in fact the case. Following a transverse incision, the previously uniform activity disintegrates and seizures now originate either in front of or behind the incision. In cases where seizures develop on both sides of the incision, their patterns differ. The postulate that there must be intracortical connections, or U-shaped fibres, which maintain this synchronisation, is also reinforced by the following observations: if it is desired to split up the uniform pattern of the seizure into two independent patterns by means of an incision, then this incision must extend laterally and medially to a certain distance beyond the region from which the record is being taken. If only short transverse incisions are made, the interactions of the surrounding cortical areas are apparently still sufficient to maintain symmorphism on both sides of the incision[17].

Attention has also been paid to the question of the depth of the cortical layer responsible for maintaining synchronisation. Since synchronisation is interrupted only by incisions extending at least as far as the stratum of large pyramidal cells, horizontal spread of the excitation is probably ensured by, in particular, the horizontal connections between the fifth and sixth laminae, U-shaped fibres[29], and perhaps also basilar dendrite bundles[24].

Having now briefly explained the organisation of the electrical activity occurring in the brain in a horizontal dimension during a seizure, let us now pass on to a laminar analysis of the seizure.

When a fully developed seizure is recorded from deep down in the cortex, instead of from the cortical surface, the principal differences are that the intracortical record shows higher amplitudes and a greater content of fairly high frequencies. A comparison of superficial with intracortical records, each taken from two electrodes the same distance apart, reveals that the two seizure curves recorded intracortically resemble each other much less closely than do the two seizure curves recorded at the surface (cf. Figure 7). One gains the impression, in fact, that the surface E.E.G. has been recorded at a relatively long distance from the actual site of origin of the potential and has been conducted through a low-pass filter. In addition, the activity recorded at the surface may often resemble a phase reversal of the intracortical activity, though it is never a genuine mirror-image of the latter.

These observations on the degree of similarity between the curves, backed up by spectrometric measurements[18, 19], led to the hypothesis that the lower regions

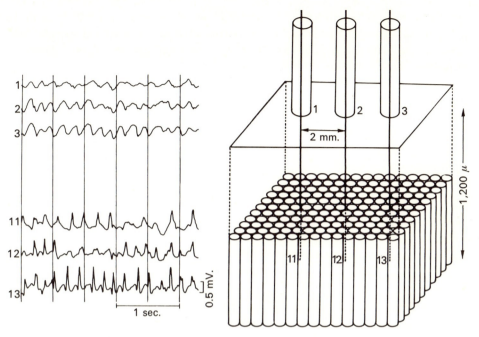

Fig. 7. *Left:* records taken simultaneously from three surface electrodes (1–3) and three intracortical electrodes (11–13) during a pentetrazole-induced seizure in the rabbit. The intracortical activity is higher, less coherent, and has a greater proportion of higher frequencies. The surface activity looks as if it had been conducted through a low-pass filter. These findings have given rise to the hypothesis that the deeper layers of the cortex have a palisade-like structure *(right)*.

of the cortex – i.e. up to a point about 200 μ beneath the surface – might have a palisade-like structure (Figure 7, right). The diameters of the individual columns are in the region of 50 μ. The histological substrate of this structure is no doubt the bundling of apical dendrites which was discovered in the same year, but independently of one another, by FLEISCHHAUER et al.[8] and by PETERS and WALSH[15]. Electron-microscopic studies[13] have shown that the dendrites in these bundles abut one another over about 20% of their surface, being separated merely by the extracellular space, with the result that the individual apical dendrites very probably exert an ephaptic (electrotonic) influence on one another, particularly during a seizure when the potentials that can be measured in this layer are more than ten times higher than under normal conditions. All observations suggest that the spikes induced by penicillin, pentetrazole, or electrical stimulation, which originate in the stratum of the large pyramidal cells and are conducted corticopetally, are in fact antidromic discharges from bundles of apical dendrites. It is known that, under the pathological conditions of a seizure, dendrites can behave like axons and conduct impulses antidromically (for references, see PURPURA[21]). The spatial arrangement of the apical dendrites – i.e. the fact that they are grouped together in bundles – probably promotes the synchronisation of these discharges.

23

On the other hand, dendrite bundles probably do not have the same importance for the slow components of the E.E.G. during a seizure. It has already been pointed out that comparison of the cortical surface record with tracings obtained from deeper layers of the cortex seldom reveals the presence of a clearcut phase reversal. Even in these cases, however, determination of coherence function showed that surface activity and intracortical activity are completely independent of each other, and that they therefore do not have a common

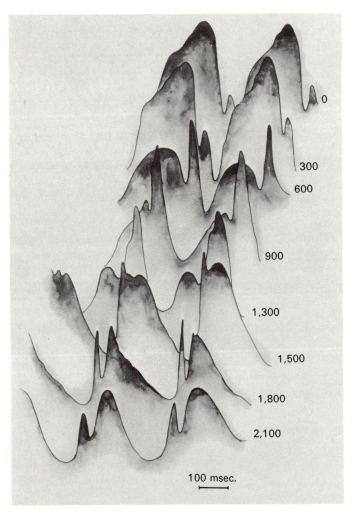

Fig. 8. Spike-and-wave activity in the rabbit, induced by contralateral electrical stimulation and recorded from various intracortical levels. The spike-and-wave groups have been so arranged along an oblique straight line that they lie in an accurate time relation to the surface activity.

The "wave" is in phase with the surface activity for a distance of about 900 μ, after which phase reversal occurs. In the case of the "spike" on the other hand, the greater the depth at which the recording is made, the closer the spike comes to the top of the wave – i.e., as it moves from the deeper layers of the cortex towards the surface, it spreads in the cm./sec. range.

generator. The oft cited hypothesis that the seizure waves might conceivably originate from a vertical intracortical dipole is therefore not tenable. The occasional similarity in form between surface and intracortical activity is no doubt due to the fact that both would seem to be secondary phenomena, i.e. responses of different cell populations to discharges from the pyramidal cells.

That the slow and fast components of the E.E.G. during an epileptic seizure are produced by different generators can be particularly impressively demonstrated by reference to spike-and-wave activity. This type of pattern, produced by electrical stimulation of the contralateral hemisphere and recorded from varying depths in the cortex, is illustrated in Figure 8. Comparison of this activity with the activity at the surface shows that, with increasing depth, a phase displacement occurs between the spike and the wave, inasmuch as the spike approaches steadily closer to the top of the wave. The reason for this is that the spike, being the summation of field potentials derived from a fairly large number of discharges from pyramidal cells and dendrites, spreads in synchronised fashion via the dendrite bundles towards the surface of the cortex, whereas the wave does not spread in this way. This observation also explains why the spike-and-wave pattern recorded from the surface of the brain may occasionally lack a spike but never a wave: on its way through the apical dendrites the spike often fails to travel as far as the surface of the cortex. The surface wave, on the other hand, being the response of nerve cells in the vicinity of the surface to the primary discharge in the fifth lamina, is always present.

It is also apparent from Figure 8 that the spike displays multiple irregularities, from which one can conclude that it must represent not a uniform process but a summation of several events. This observation raises the question as to what is the smallest volume of cortical tissue capable of producing a uniform discharge during a seizure. The volume of a single cell is of course the smallest possible unit involved in a discharge, but there is a considerable body of evidence to suggest that, in an epileptic attack, the smallest elements capable of producing synchronised activity are dendrite bundles.

Figure 9 illustrates how the size of these zones of uniform discharge ("generator zones") can be determined. In the experiment depicted here, records were taken from the surface of the cortex and from two intracortical micro-electrodes 300μ apart, situated at the same depth $(1,500 \mu)$. The fourth curve is a bipolar recording from M 1 and M 2. The reason for including this recording in the experiment was as follows: since the activity at M 1 and M 2 is approximately the same, a bipolar recording could be expected to produce an isoelectric line, unless the activities at the two micro-electrodes were out of phase, a phenomenon which cannot be detected with the naked eye. This was in fact the case: in the clonic stage of the seizure (upper half of the figure) some of the bipolar spikes point upwards and others downwards, whereas those in the two unipolar records are apparently the same. This means that in the case of the upward-pointing spikes the discharge begins at M 1 and in the case of the downward-pointing ones it begins at M 2; in other words, at this depth the volume of cortical tissue in which electrical activity is uniform must be smaller in diameter than the distance between the electrodes. Still more informative

25

is the tonic pattern (lower half of Figure 9). Here, three different stages are shown: in the first, the bipolar recording yields what is virtually an iso-electric line, i.e. the two recording electrodes are within a zone which is discharging uniformly and which must therefore be larger than 300 μ. In the second stage, larger and smaller spikes alternate at both micro-electrodes, while in the bipolar record an upward-pointing spike alternates with an iso-electric line; this means that now the discharge from a small generator zone (M 1 leading) is alternating with that of a large zone (embracing M 1 and M 2). Finally, in the last few seconds of the seizure the generator zones become smaller again and M 1 now regularly takes the lead.

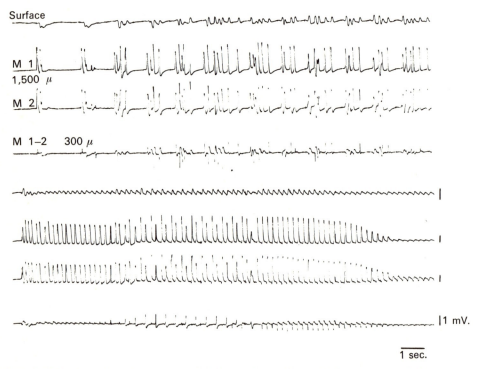

Fig. 9. Clonic-tonic seizure, recorded from the surface of the cortex and from two semimicro-electrodes arranged horizontally 300 μ apart at a depth of 1,500 μ below the surface. The bipolar record taken from M 1 and M 2 displays spikes of varying polarity, i.e. the discharge does not appear simultaneously at M 1 and M 2 and its origin likewise differs (generator zones smaller than the distance of 300 μ between electrodes).

The subsequent tonic pattern consists of three segments: in the first (virtually no activity in the bipolar record), the activity at M 1 and M 2 is almost synchronous, i.e. the generator zones have a diameter larger than 300 μ; in the second segment, the bipolar record reveals a negative peak alternating with an iso-electric line, i.e. smaller and larger generator zones alternate; in the third segment, the bipolar record shows a positive spike throughout, indicating that two generator zones with a diameter of less than 300 μ are present and that the generator zone in which M 1 lies invariably discharges first.

This pattern clearly illustrates the high degree of organisation in the processes taking place during an epileptic seizure.

These observations on the size of the intracortical generator zones are summarised in diagrammatic form in Figure 10. As regards the seizure waves in the superficial and deepest layers of the cortex, in which low-pass effects play an additional role, the zones of uniform electrical activity are relatively broad and can spread out, largely independently of one another, in various directions. In the layer of the apical dendrites, on the other hand, the generator zones are very narrow and can spread only corticopetally.

Let me conclude this paper on a few selected aspects of the pathophysiology of epileptic seizures by pointing out that some of the phenomena I have discussed can be used to analyse the mode of action of anti-epileptic drugs. In order to test the way in which drugs affect the processes taking place during a seizure, it is in fact essential, first of all, to have a detailed knowledge of these processes. In addition, however, the changes they display following the administration of drugs shed new light on physiological problems; hence, this interaction between physiology and pharmacology can be of considerable benefit to the

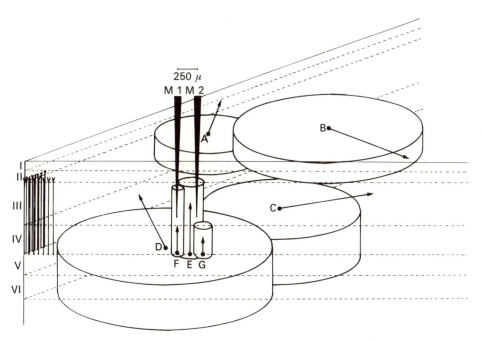

Fig. 10. Diagrammatic representation of a section through the rabbit cortex showing the generator zones (i.e. the volumes of cortical tissue displaying synchronous activity during a seizure), which are symbolised by the cylinders A–G. At the surface (A, B) and in the deep layers (C, D) the generator zones responsible for the slow waves in the seizure are extensive and spread horizontally in various directions (arrows). In the region of the apical dendrites the generator zones are narrow (E, F, G) and spread only corticopetally; they are responsible for the spike components in the seizure record. The vertical lines between the second and fifth laminae represent dendrite bundles, the distance between which has been drawn true to scale. M 1 and M 2: micro-electrodes positioned 250 μ apart.

patient. Analysis of the extent to which a seizure E.E.G. becomes regularised following small doses of diazepam is an example in point: in response to this medication, the rate of spread of the potential fields increases and the generator zones become larger, two effects which can probably be attributed to a decrease in the active elements involved in the seizure.

References

 1 BANCAUD, J., TALAIRACH, J., GEIER, S., SCARABIN, J.-M.: E.E.G. et S.E.E.G. dans les tumeurs cérébrales et l'épilepsie (Edifor, Paris 1973)
 2 CRAIN, S.M., BORNSTEIN, M.B.: Bioelectric activity of neonatal mouse cerebral cortex during growth and differentiation in tissue culture. Exp. Neurol. *10*, 425 (1964)
 3 CREUTZFELDT, O. (Editor): The neuronal generation of the EEG. In Rémond, A. (Editor-in-Chief): Handbook of electroencephalography and clinical neurophysiology, Vol. II, Part C (Elsevier, Amsterdam 1974)
 4 DUIJN, H. VAN, SCHWARTZKROIN, P.A., PRINCE, D.A.: Action of penicillin on inhibitory processes in the cat's cortex. Brain Res. *53*, 470 (1973)
 5 ECCLES, J.C.: The physiology of synapses (Springer, Berlin/Göttingen/Heidelberg 1964)
 6 ESPLIN, D.W.: Effects of diphenylhydantoin on synaptic transmission in cat spinal cord and stellate ganglion. J. Pharmacol. exp. Ther. *120*, 301 (1957)
 7 FERTZIGER, A.P., BRANCK, J.B., Jr.: Potassium accumulation in interstitial space during epileptiform seizures. Exp. Neurol. *26*, 571 (1970)
 8 FLEISCHHAUER, K., PETSCHE, H., WITTKOWSKI, W.: Vertical bundles of dendrites in the neocortex. Z. Anat. Entwickl.-Gesch. *136*, 213 (1972)
 9 GLOOR, P.: Generalized spike and wave discharges: a consideration of cortical and subcortical mechanisms of their genesis and synchronization. In Petsche, H., Brazier, M.A.B. (Editors): Synchronization of EEG activity in epilepsies, Symp., Vienna, Austria, p. 382 (Springer, Vienna/New York 1972)
10 GLOOR, P., KALABAY, O., GIARD, N.: The electroencephalogram in diffuse encephalopathies: electroencephalographic correlates of grey and white matter lesions. Brain *91*, 779 (1968)
11 HALPERN, L.M.: Chronically isolated aggregates of mammalian cerebral cortical neurons studied in situ. In Purpura, D., et al.: Experimental models of epilepsy – a manual for the laboratory worker, p. 197 (Raven Press, New York 1972)
12 JASPER, H.H., DROOGLEEVER-FORTUYN, J.: Experimental studies on the functional anatomy of petit mal epilepsy. Res. Publ. Ass. nerv. ment. Dis. *26*, 272 (1947)
13 MASSING, W., FLEISCHHAUER, K.: Further observations of vertical bundles of dendrites in the cerebral cortex of the rabbit. Z. Anat. Entwickl.-Gesch. *141*, 115 (1973)
14 PENFIELD, W., JASPER, H.: Epilepsy and the functional anatomy of the human brain (Little, Brown, Boston 1954)
15 PETERS, A., WALSH, T.M.: A study of the organization of apical dendrites in the somatic sensory cortex of the rat. J. comp. Neurol. *144*, 253 (1972)
16 PETSCHE, H., NÁGYPAL, T., PROHASKA, O., VOLLMER, R.: Approaches to the spatio-temporal analysis of seizure patterns. In Dolce, G., Künkel, H. (Editors): CEAN – computerised EEG analysis, Int. Working Conf., Kronberg/Taunus 1974 (Fischer, Stuttgart 1975)
17 PETSCHE, H., RAPPELSBERGER, P.: Influence of cortical incisions on synchronization pattern and travelling waves. Electroenceph. clin. Neurophysiol. *28*, 592 (1970)
18 PETSCHE, H., RAPPELSBERGER, P.: The problem of synchronization in the spread of epileptic discharges leading to seizures in man. In Brazier, M.A.B. (Editor): Epilepsy – its phenomena in man, p. 121 (Academic Press, New York/London 1973)

19 PETSCHE, H., RAPPELSBERGER, P., FREY, Z.: Intracortical aspects of the synchronization of self-sustained bioelectrical activities, loc. cit.[9], p. 263

20 PRINCE, D.A., WILDER, B.J.: Control mechanisms in cortical epileptogenic foci. Arch. Neurol. (Chic.) *16*, 194 (1967)

21 PURPURA, D.P.: Dendrites: heterogeneity in form and function. In Rémond, A. (Editor-in-Chief): Handbook of electroencephalography and clinical neurophysiology, Vol. I, Part B, p. 3 (Elsevier, Amsterdam 1971)

22 PURPURA, D.P.: Dendritic differentiation in human cerebral cortex: normal and aberrant developmental patterns. In: Int. Symp. Physiol. Path. Dendrites, Munich 1974 (Raven Press, New York, printing)

23 RANSOM, B.R.: The behavior of presumed glial cells during seizure discharge in cat cerebral cortex. Brain Res. *69*, 83 (1974)

24 SCHEIBEL, M.E., DAVIES, T.L., LINDSAY, R.D., SCHEIBEL, A.B.: Basilar dendrite bundles of giant pyramidal cells. Exp. Neurol. *42*, 307 (1974)

25 SERVÍT, Z.: Comparative physiology of the paroxysmal EEG. Pattern and frequency of paroxysmal activity on different levels of brain phylogeny. In Servít, Z. (Editor): Comparative and cellular pathophysiology of epilepsy, Proc. Symp., Liblice near Prague 1965, p. 103 (Czechoslovak Academy of Sciences, Prague/Int. Congr. Ser. No. 124; Excerpta Medica, Amsterdam etc. 1966)

26 SPECKMANN, E.-J., CASPERS, H.: Paroxysmal depolarization and changes in action potentials induced by pentylenetetrazol in isolated neurons of Helix pomatia. Epilepsia (Amst.) *14*, 397 (1973)

27 SPECKMANN, E.-J., CASPERS, H., JANZEN, R.W.: Relations between cortical DC shifts and membrane potential changes of cortical neurons associated with seizure activity, loc. cit.[9], p. 93

28 STERIADE, M.: Interneuronal epileptic discharges related to spike-and-wave cortical seizures in behaving monkeys. Electroenceph. clin. Neurophysiol. *37*, 247 (1974)

29 TÖMBÖL, T.: A Golgi analysis of the sensory-motor cortex in the rabbit, loc. cit.[9], p. 25

30 WESTRUM, L.E., WHITE, L.E., Jr., WARD, A.A., Jr.: Morphology of the experimental epileptic focus. J. Neurosurg. *21*, 1033 (1964)

31 WILLIAMS, D.: The thalamus and epilepsy. Brain *88*, 539 (1965)

Discussion

W. Birkmayer: Thank you very much for your contribution, Dr. Petsche. Before opening the discussion, I should like to point out that we deliberately decided to begin this symposium with a paper on the pathophysiological background to epilepsy, because papers of this kind not only provide us with up-to-date information extending far beyond the scope of our clinical knowledge, but at the same time also help to dispose of certain notions that we may have grown unduly fond of! I now declare the discussion open.

R. Dreyer: Just one brief question, Dr. Petsche. I expect you will have noticed that in the German literature the term *hypersynchrone Aktivität* ("hypersynchronous activity") is now being employed very frequently. May I ask whether you approve of this expression and also whether you think that in future we ought to avoid using such terms as "spikes-and-waves", "epileptic grapho-elements", and "seizure discharges"?

H. Petsche: That's an important question, Dr. Dreyer, but a difficult one to answer. When I discovered in the course of my experiments that not even so-called synchronous activity is really synchronous, I became even more reluctant to employ the word "hypersynchronous", which is of course a pleonasm. We shall definitely have to introduce new terms in order to designate more accurately those phenomena which in routine electro-encephalograms are observed to begin simultaneously and end simultaneously. So far as I am concerned, much the same also applies to the adjective "epileptic". For years now, I have been resisting the use of expressions such as "epileptic waves" or "seizure discharges". We all know how much confusion expressions of this kind have caused; some doctors, for example, who are not used to interpreting E.E.G. recordings, have mistakenly concluded that the occurrence of seizure discharges is in itself proof of epilepsy. The term "epileptic neurone" is another misnomer to which I have always been opposed. On the other hand, I must confess that I have so far been unable to coin a suitable term with which to designate succinctly but accurately the type of phenomenon occurring when a neurone begins to fire paroxysmally and continues to discharge to the point of exhaustion, i.e. when it simulates precisely what happens in an epileptic seizure. Should we describe it as a "neurone showing a tendency to periods of hypermaximal discharge resulting in self-exhaustion"? We must, I suggest, try to decide upon a new definition for this phenomenon, a definition in which the adjective "epileptic" could perhaps still be employed, because – as I am sure we would all agree – the term "epilepsy" nowadays no longer has the same connotations as it had when first introduced in the 19th century. Meanwhile, I prefer to adopt a wait-and-see attitude towards the term "hypersynchronous activity".

G. Nissen: I should like to ask, Dr. Petsche, whether the synchronous or non-synchronous E.E.G. discharges observed in your animal experiments were also accompanied by behavioural anomalies without the occurrence of actual seizures.

H. Petsche: I am afraid I cannot answer that question, Dr. Nissen, because in our animal experiments we specifically studied the electrical activity of the brain and did not at the same time investigate the behaviour of the animals, which in fact were not able to move about freely. E.E.G. findings obtained in man, however, do shed light on the point you have raised: we all know that in man generalised forms of pathological activity may occur which are unaccompanied by any – or at least by any appreciable – behavioural disturbances; this, incidentally, is further evidence suggesting that in the presence of such generalised activity by no means all the cortical cells are discharging, but, as I believe, only a very small proportion of them.

R. Oberholzer: A technical question, Dr. Petsche: could you tell us how thick the electrodes were that you used in your experiments? What interested me in particular was your remark to the effect that a certain bundling of electrical activity would seem to occur as a result of ephaptic influences.

H. Petsche: The surface electrodes were chloridised silver electrodes measuring 300 μ in diameter. The intracortical electrodes were semimicro-electrodes, the tips of which varied in diameter from 5 to 10 μ; in other words, they were just large enough to record not only individual cell activity but also field potentials.

W. P. Koella: In the course of your presentation, Dr. Petsche, you showed us a very interesting diagram of dendrite bundles which was not included in the written version of your paper. May I ask whether these bundles – which, for want of a better term, we can perhaps call "epileptic" bundles – have any functional connections with the "sensory" cortical bundles as described, for example, by Mountcastle.

H. Petsche: In the light of studies such as those of Mountcastle* and of Hubel and Wiesel**, it has become increasingly clear that in many respects the cortex has a columnar structure. The diagram (Figure 1) to which you have just referred, Dr. Koella, was taken from a paper by Fleischhauer. Working in Bonn, Fleisch-hauer has examined the architectural distribution of the bundles in the cortex and has shown that their ramification patterns differ markedly in the sensory as compared with the motor cortex. So pronounced is the difference that the motor and sensory cortex can be distinguished from each other more clearly on the basis of their bundle structure than, for example, in material stained by Nissl's method. We believe that these ramification patterns do indeed have some functional significance.

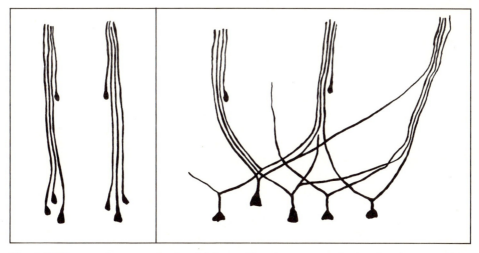

Fig. 1. Differences between the dendritic ramification patterns in the visual cortex *(left)* and sensorimotor cortex *(right)* of the cat. Pyramidal cells in the fifth lamina. [Reproduced, by kind permission of the author and publishers, from Fleischhauer, K.: On different patterns of dendritic bundling in the cerebral cortex of the cat. Z. Anat. Entwickl.-Gesch. *143*, 115 (1974)]

---

* Mountcastle, V. B.: Modality and topographic properties of single neurons of cat's somatic sensory cortex. J. Neurophysiol. *20*, 408 (1957)
** Hubel, T. H., Wiesel, T. N.: Receptive fields, binocular interaction and functional architecture in the cat's visual cortex. J. Physiol. (Lond.) *160*, 106 (1962)

The pharmacology of carbamazepine and some other anti-epileptic drugs

by W. P. KOELLA, P. LEVIN, and V. BALTZER *

1. Introduction

When carbamazepine (®Tegretol) was introduced as an anticonvulsant in 1963, its advent added another important agent to the armamentarium of the epileptologist. It was the first, and has so far remained the only, anti-epileptic substance with a tricyclic structure. This unique structure seems to have endowed carbamazepine with important features in addition to its well-established anticonvulsive properties: for example, it is less sedative than most anticonvulsive drugs; it exhibits certain beneficial psychotropic effects; and, finally, it has an excellent influence on such non-convulsive conditions as trigeminal neuralgia.

In view of this clinical profile it is perhaps worthwhile to re-examine the animal pharmacology of the compound.

For the pharmacologist interested in convulsive disorders and anticonvulsants, it is fortunate that a large number of models are available for animal experimentation.

Physical means (electric current, mechanical insult, and freezing), as well as chemical substances (acetylcholine, alumina cream, bicuculline, cobalt, nicotine, penicillin, pentetrazole, picrotoxin, semicarbazide, strychnine, and thiosemicarbazide), have been, and still are, used in a variety of animal species to induce seizures, which often correspond more or less closely to various clinical types of epileptic attack. Systematically administered convulsive chemicals, or gross transcerebral flow of pulsed or alternating electric current, are followed by ictal episodes that are of a generalised nature. Depending on the agent used, these ictal episodes fall into distinct subtypes, which differ not only in their time course and appearance but also in their responsiveness to various antagonists.

On the other hand, topically and discretely applied chemical and physical agents tend, at least initially, to induce local discharges and thus produce many of the features of the focal type of epilepsy, followed possibly by generalisation into a "grand mal" seizure. These "local" techniques also provide useful information on such interesting phenomena as the "mirror focus"[18] and the "kindling phenomenon"[6].

Finally, nature has provided us with some genetic "mistakes", such as the audiogenic seizures encountered in mice and the photomyoclonic epileptoid

* Research Department, Pharmaceuticals Division, CIBA-GEIGY LIMITED, Basle, Switzerland.

response in the Senegal baboon[13], which serve as welcome and valuable additional epilepsy models.

In this paper, we shall describe the pharmacology of carbamazepine as it developed from investigations in several such models in our laboratories. The anticonvulsive "profile" of carbamazepine emerging from our standard test battery will then be compared with that of a number of other anticonvulsants of proven clinical value. Findings from other laboratories, in which more complex procedures have been used to study the actions of carbamazepine, will also be described and, where possible, again compared with those obtained with other anti-epileptic drugs. Finally, certain further effects of carbamazepine, not directly related to its anticonvulsive action, will be discussed and compared with similar effects of the reference compounds.

2. The profile of carbamazepine in our laboratory tests

2.1. Seizures induced in *rats* by means of an *alternating current* (50–100 volts, 50 c.p.s., for 0.63 sec. applied through corneal electrodes) are inhibited by carbamazepine. The oral ED_{50} for suppression of tonic convulsions of the hind-limbs is 10 mg./kg. A dose-response curve is depicted in Figure 1. This ED_{50}

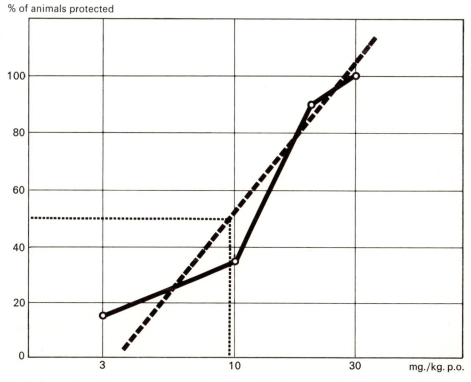

Fig. 1. Dose-response curve plotting the effect of various oral doses of carbamazepine on electroshock-induced seizures in the rat. Abscissa: doses in mg./kg. (log. scale); ordinate: percentage of animals (N = 10) protected from tonic extension seizures of the hind-legs.

and the data presented in Figure 1 refer to the findings obtained when carbamazepine was administered one hour prior to the electric shock.

Figure 2 shows the time course of the anticonvulsive activity displayed by three drugs in this test. It is evident that carbamazepine is maximally effective for at least four hours. Eight hours after its administration the seizure-inhibiting effect is less marked; and, after 16 hours, doses as high as 30 mg./kg. are ineffective.

2.2. In *mice*, the *electroshock* test procedure is similar to that used in the rat. The oral ED_{50} of carbamazepine in this test was found to be about 12 mg./kg.

2.3. In *mice*, carbamazepine inhibits convulsions induced by *pentetrazole* (80 mg. per kg. i.p.); the ED_{50} is about 40 mg./kg. The percentage of mice protected, however, does not increase to any appreciable extent with larger doses.

2.4. In *mice* challenged with *picrotoxin* in intraperitoneal doses of 12 or 9 mg./kg., carbamazepine in oral doses as high as 300 mg./kg. is ineffective. If only 6 mg. of the convulsant is injected per kg. body weight, carbamazepine in an oral dose of 60 mg./kg. brings about a 30% reduction in the number of convulsing

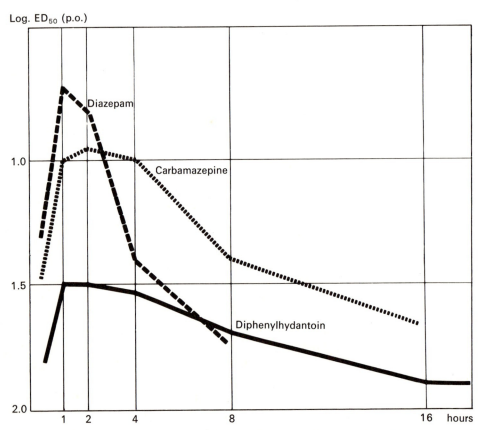

Fig. 2. Time course of the anticonvulsive effect of carbamazepine, diazepam, and diphenylhydantoin. The ED_{50} values are plotted against the time interval elapsing between drug administration and application of electroshock in rats. Note the short effect of diazepam as compared with that of carbamazepine and diphenylhydantoin.

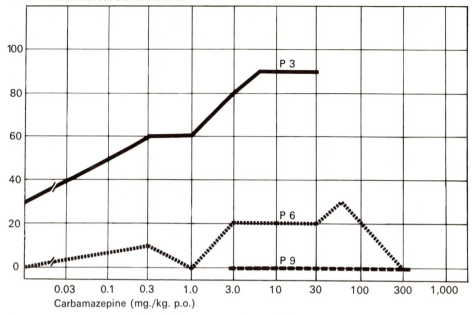

% of animals without clonic seizures

Fig. 3. Dose versus anticonvulsive effect curves (ED$_{50}$ values) of carbamazepine for various dosages of a convulsive drug (picrotoxin, 3, 6, and 9 mg./kg. i.p.)

animals; with higher doses this effect is reversed (Figure 3). Picrotoxin in a dose of 3 mg./kg. produces convulsions in only seven out of ten mice, and three of these animals are protected by 0.3 or 1.0 mg. carbamazepine per kg. Nevertheless, even in doses as high as 30 mg./kg., carbamazepine is unable to afford protection to all animals (Figure 3).

2.5. Against *strychnine*-induced convulsions and death in mice (2.5 mg./kg. strychnine i.p.) carbamazepine is less effective. In oral doses of 150 mg./kg. it protects 50% of the animals from death. In the same dose range it also reduces convulsions; but even oral doses of 300 mg./kg. are not sufficient to inhibit convulsions completely.

2.6. Following electrical stimulation of various structures belonging to the *limbic system* (e.g. the hippocampus), after-discharges can be recorded in the stimulated structure itself and in other areas interconnected with the challenged substrate[15]. According to AKERT and HUMMEL[1], the *hippocampal* after-discharge is possibly related to psychomotor epilepsy. This after-discharge has been shown to be sensitive to a number of anti-epileptic drugs and thus to be a good indicator of their anticonvulsive activity. In our laboratories we have investigated in cats the effect of carbamazepine and some of the other reference compounds on the hippocampal after-discharge induced by electrical stimulation of the hippocampus. Figure 4 illustrates a limbic epileptic seizure of this kind and its almost complete blockade by carbamazepine (3 mg./kg. i.v.). In Figure 5 the dose response/time relationships of carbamazepine are presented and compared with those of diazepam and diphenylhydantoin.

35

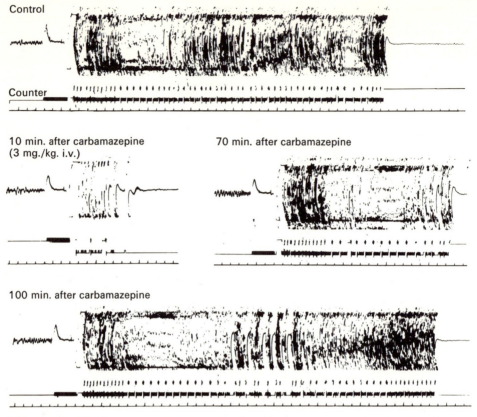

Control

Counter

10 min. after carbamazepine
(3 mg./kg. i.v.)

70 min. after carbamazepine

100 min. after carbamazepine

Fig. 4. After-discharge recorded from the dorsal hippocampus of a gallamine-immo-bilised cat following electrical stimulation of the same site (200 p.p.s., 10 volts, 0.1 msec. for 5 seconds).
Above: control. *Middle* and *below:* 10, 70, and 100 minutes after carbamazepine (3.0 mg./kg. i.v.).
"Counter" indicates number of spikes; each excursion = 10 spikes.

3. Profiles of some reference substances

For purposes of comparison, a number of other anticonvulsants, clinically proven to be effective in various forms of epilepsy, were subjected to our screening procedure under experimental conditions identical to those used for carbamazepine.

Table 1 presents the ED_{50} values and Figure 6 the dose-response curves for *phenobarbitone, sodium 2-propylvalerate* (®Depakine), *diazepam, clonazepam,* and *diphenylhydantoin,* compared with those for carbamazepine. The ED_{50} for diazepam in the *electroshock* test is about the same as that for carbamazepine. However, its anticonvulsive effect is of shorter duration (Figure 2). Diphenyl-hydantoin and phenobarbitone also show ED_{50} values against electroshock which are comparable with those of carbamazepine; clonazepam is effective in somewhat lower doses, whereas the ED_{50} of sodium 2-propylvalerate is very high.

36

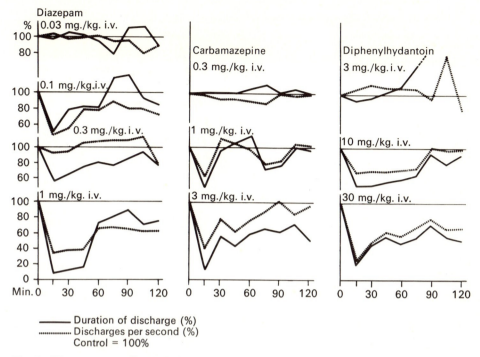

Duration of discharge (%)
.... Discharges per second (%)
Control = 100%

Fig. 5. Time-course effect of diazepam, carbamazepine, and diphenylhydantoin on hippocampal after-discharge. A hippocampal after-discharge was induced by electrical stimulation of the recording site at intervals of 15 minutes three times before and eight times after administration of the drugs. 100% = mean duration of discharge, or mean discharge rate, during the control period for the three animals in respect of each test substance and each dose level.

Table 1. ED$_{50}$ values (mg./kg.) of carbamazepine and some reference drugs in various screening procedures. The substances were invariably administered by mouth, except in the hippocampus test in which they were injected intravenously.

Test	Drug					
	Carbamaz-epine	Pheno-barbi-tone	Sodium 2-propyl-valerate	Diaz-epam	Clonaz-epam	Diphenyl-hydantoin
Electroshock (rat)	10	7	200	7	2	32
Electroshock (mouse)	12	13	350	5	1	20
Pentetrazole	30	2	200	0.5	0.05	⌀ 100
Strychnine (death)	150	75	650	7	5	300
Picrotoxin (12 mg./kg.)	⌀ 200	⌀ 100	⌀ 1,000	⌀ 100	30 (40%)	⌀ 100
Picrotoxin (9 mg./kg.)	⌀ 200	⌀ 30	500	10	0.08	⌀ 100
Picrotoxin (6 mg./kg.)	60 (30%)	10	≈ 100	1	0.015	0.5*
Picrotoxin (3 mg./kg.)	≈ 0.5	≈ 6	≈ 6	≈ 0.1	≈ 0.008	0.3*
Hippocampus	1.0		300	0.1 (max.)	0.03	10.0

⌀ No effect   * Biphasic effect

37

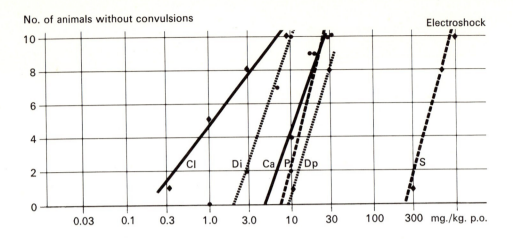

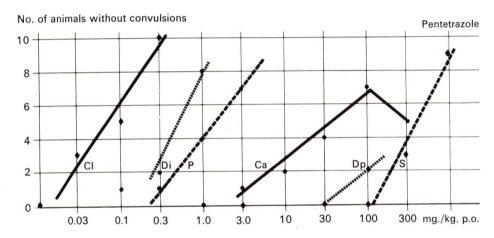

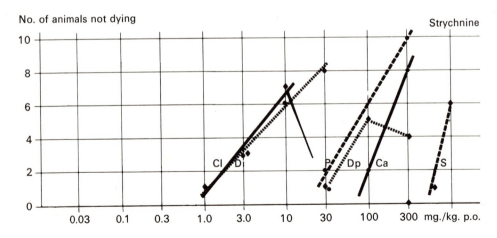

Fig. 6. Dose-response curves in the mouse for carbamazepine (Ca), phenobarbitone (P), sodium 2-propylvalerate (S), diazepam (Di), clonazepam (Cl), and diphenyl-hydantoin (Dp), all administered orally, in the electroshock test, the anti-pentetrazole test, and the anti-strychnine test.

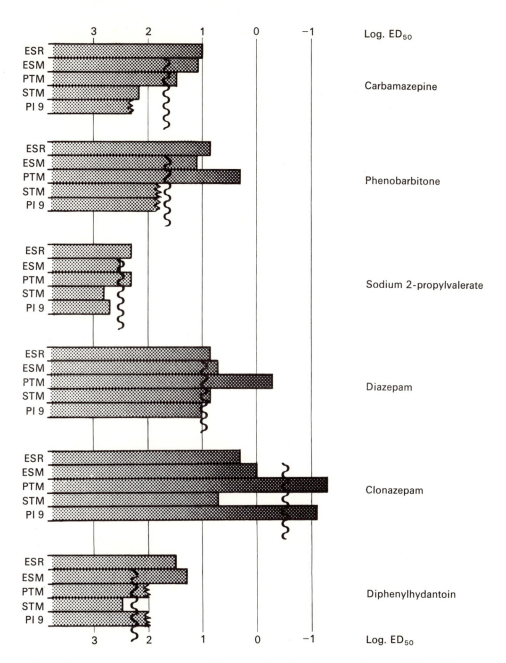

Fig. 7. Oral "potency" profiles (ED_{50} values) of carbamazepine and five reference drugs in various test situations. ESR = electroshock, rat; ESM = electroshock, mouse; PTM = anti-pentetrazole test, mouse; STM = anti-strychnine test, mouse; and PI 9 = anti-picrotoxin test, mouse (9 mg./kg. picrotoxin i.p.).

Abscissa: $-\log.\ ED_{50}$ values ($= \log.\ \dfrac{1}{ED_{50}}$) as a measure of potency.

The dose inducing sedation (in the mouse) is indicated in each instance by a vertical wavy line.

Note the low overall potency of sodium 2-propylvalerate and the high potency of clonazepam.

In the tests involving *chemically induced convulsions*, the two benzodiazepines are, milligramme for milligramme, the most powerful agents. The overall profile of phenobarbitone is somewhat akin to that of these two drugs, but the mean effective dose level is higher by a factor of about ten. Sodium 2-propylvalerate is effective only in very high doses; diphenylhydantoin is relatively weak in its action against strychnine and has hardly any effect worth mentioning on convulsions induced by pentetrazole or by picrotoxin.

The relative potency of these various drugs is indicated schematically in the form of profiles in Figure 7. In the *hippocampal after-discharge* procedure (cf. Figure 5) diphenylhydantoin in a dose of 30 mg./kg. i.v. reduces the duration of discharge and the number of single spikes as effectively as does carbamazepine in a dose of 3.0 mg./kg. Diazepam shows effects in doses as low as 0.1 mg./kg.; clonazepam is, milligramme for milligramme, even more potent than diazepam, whereas sodium 2-propylvalerate in this test is effective only in doses ranging from 30 to 300 mg./kg. i.v.

4. The effect of carbamazepine and of other anticonvulsants in additional epilepsy models

4.1. The phenomenon of *post-tetanic potentiation* (P.T.P.) was originally detected and put to experimental use in the realm of spinal reflexology. Typically, after short tetanic stimulation of a dorsal root, the reflex response to a single dorsal root stimulus recorded in the form of an action potential emanating from the homologous ventral root is temporarily enhanced, signalling facilitation of (monosynaptic) reflex transmission. This facilitatory effect is probably attributable to tetanisation-induced hyperpolarisation of the terminals of the afferent fibres. According to WOODBURY[25], it is probable that mechanisms related to P.T.P. are involved in the spread of the epileptic discharge at the supraspinal level.

THEOBALD et al.[22] reported in 1970 that carbamazepine depresses P.T.P., but recent experiments conducted in our laboratories suggest that the drug's pattern of activity in this model is more complex: intravenous doses of 3 or 10 mg./kg. at first reduce P.T.P. and then, after a delay of about 20–40 minutes, enhance it. Diphenylhydantoin[3, 4] and phenobarbitone[25] reduce P.T.P. quite effectively, whereas trimethadione is ineffective[26].

4.2. JULIEN[11] investigated the effect of carbamazepine on *penicillin-induced focal epileptic discharges* in the cat immobilised with D-tubocurarine. Local epileptic discharges were elicited by subpial injection of penicillin into the sensory motor cortex. Intraperitoneal injection of carbamazepine (5–15 mg./kg.) led to a gradual reduction in the spikes and in the cortical epileptiform bursts; 30–60 minutes after the application of carbamazepine the discharges were completely blocked. This relatively slow development of anticonvulsive activity is of interest in view of the fact that, following intraperitoneal injection, maximal blood levels of the drug (8–20 mcg./ml.) were attained within 15–30 minutes, whereas at the time of maximal anticonvulsive activity the blood levels had usually dropped to about 5–10 mcg./ml.

4.3. JULIEN[11] also investigated the influence of carbamazepine on the spontaneous discharge rate of *Purkinje cells in the cerebellar cortex*. Unlike diazepam and diphenylhydantoin, which increase Purkinje cell discharge[10], carbamazepine has no influence on this inhibitory cerebellofugal neuronal system. From these data, JULIEN[11] concludes that, while "the mode of carbamazepine's antiepileptic action has not been delineated, it appears to be different from that of diazepam or diphenylhydantoin".

4.4. KILLAM et al.[13] have described what they called a *"photomyoclonic epileptoid response"* in the Senegal baboon *(Papio papio)*. This seizure represents a model of epilepsy "which should provide an adequate stimulus for greater efforts at uncovering new molecules for the control of this disabling syndrome"[12]. In this model, seizures were induced by means of a flashing light. A series of electrodes were affixed to the experimental animals in order to record the E.E.G. Epileptic seizures consisted either of isolated E.E.G. changes (spikes-and-waves and spikes) or of E.E.G. changes together with muscular jerks or well-developed clonic seizures. These were either restricted to the face muscles or else involved parts or all of the body musculature.

Carbamazepine was effective in this model, although a clear-cut dose-response curve could not be established owing to the "wide variability in dose required to control seizures induced by flashing light"[12]. Still, from these authors' data (their Figure 2) it may be concluded that in a series of 19 animals the seizures could be blocked to varying degrees by carbamazepine in intramuscular doses ranging from 0.1 to 80 mg./kg. The authors did not observe any adverse side effects with doses as high as 40 mg./kg.

For phenobarbitone an ED_{50} (i.e. complete block of the seizures in 50% of the animals) of about 10 mg./kg. i.m. was found in this model. Diphenylhydantoin failed to block the seizure response in the baboon when administered in single doses of 50 mg./kg. i.m.; but in doses of 15 mg./kg. i.m. given three times, i.e. on three successive days, it completely blocked seizures in nine out of 12 animals and reduced the severity of the seizures in the remaining three.

Diazepam completely blocked these seizures in doses of 0.05–0.2 mg./kg. i.m. When low – yet initially effective – doses (e.g. 0.1 mg./kg. i.m.) were used, the animals began after several days to "escape", i.e. the drug became less effective. Doubling the dose usually re-established control of seizures.

4.5. According to MARCUS[16], *conjugated oestrogens* (®Premarin) induce seizures reminiscent of petit mal epilepsy, i.e. a 3/sec. spike-and-wave pattern in the cortical E.E.G. (as does also the injection of massive parenteral doses of penicillin[20]). While the Premarin-induced seizure responds to diphenylhydantoin, it is not influenced by carbamazepine[11].

4.6. Low-rate stimulation of the *non-specific thalamic* nuclei in cats induces the so-called *arrest reaction*, accompanied by a spike-and-wave pattern in the cortical E.E.G.[9]. In this epilepsy model, which is likewise somewhat reminiscent of petit mal, the effect of carbamazepine has not been clearly established[14]. Phenobarbitone diminishes the amplitude of the spikes-and-waves. However, trimethadione[14] and benzodiazepines[17] do not appreciably influence the discharge pattern in this model. Nor does diphenylhydantoin have any effect[21].

5. Effects of carbamazepine and of some other anticonvulsants that are not, or not directly, related to their anticonvulsive activities

5.1. Possible *sedative effects* of the drugs with which we are concerned here can be assessed to some extent on the basis of observations made in animals (mice, rats). These observations have shown that carbamazepine exerts a central depressant influence only when given in relatively high doses (Table 2). Similarly, high doses of carbamazepine are necessary to reduce spontaneous ambulatory activity as determined by the photocell technique (Table 3). The "therapeutic quotient", a semi-quantitative measure expressed by the ratio between anticonvulsive and sedative potency, is higher for carbamazepine than for most other compounds (Table 4). For phenobarbitone, whose initial excitatory effect is marked, it is difficult at the time of testing to assess "sedation" properly.

5.2. Carbamazepine is also "weak" in producing *muscular disturbances* and *motor incoordination*. Only doses well above those effective in anti-electroconvulsive tests induce signs of ataxia and of muscular hypotonia and eliminate the supporting function of the legs (Table 2). This has been corroborated by findings obtained in the *"test de la traction"*, in which mice are suspended by their forelegs and their ability to pull themselves up is measured (Table 3). In this test diphenylhydantoin is still weaker than carbamazepine. Diazepam and clonazepam already affect the pull-up reaction in doses which are about equal to, or smaller than, the anti-electroconvulsive ED_{50}.

Table 2. Minimal oral doses (mg./kg.) producing signs of sedation, ataxia, muscular hypotonia, prone position, lateral recumbency, paralysis, and convulsions in observation tests performed in the mouse (M) and rat (R).

	Carbamazepine M	R	Phenobarbitone M	R	Sodium 2-propylvalerate M	R
Light sedation	10–20	6–10	10–50	10	100–300	100–300
Clear-cut sedation	30–100	20	30	20	300	600
Ataxia	60–100	20–30	10	7	100–300	600
Muscular hypotonia	100–200	3	30		1,000	
Prone position		30	100–200	200	300	1,000
Lateral recumbency	200		100	200	1,000	
Paralysis	100					
Convulsions	600	1,000	300		1,000	

	Diazepam M	R	Clonazepam M	R	Diphenylhydantoin M	R
Light sedation	2–3	3	0.01–0.1	1	30	10–30
Clear-cut sedation	10	6–10	0.3	3	200	200
Ataxia	3	6	0.3–1	3	30–100	60–100
Muscular hypotonia	10–50	6	0.3	1–3	100	100
Prone position	30–100	30	1		100	
Lateral recumbency					400	
Paralysis						
Convulsions			30–100		200–600	2,000

Table 3. Some pharmacological effects not, or not directly, related to anticonvulsive activity.

Test	Carbam-azepine	Pheno-barbitone	Diazepam	Clonaz-epam	Diphenyl-hydantoin
Decrease in ambulatory activity (photocell), mouse	200		25		⌀ 1,000
Test de la traction, mouse	100	40	1.5	1	150
Reflex inhibition, cat					
Patellar tendon reflex	30 i.v.				
Flexor reflex	30 i.v.				
Linguomandibular reflex	0.1 i.v.		0.1		
Fighting reaction (foot shock), mouse	200*	30	4		
Fighting mice (isolation)	150	20	15		
Reserpine antagonism, ptosis, rat	⌀ 1,000				⌀ 1,000
Reserpine antagonism, ptosis, mouse	⌀ 300				750
Amphetamine antagonism, stereotypy, rat	⌀ 300				⌀ 300
Induction of catalepsy, rat	⌀ 300				⌀ 1,000
Tremorine antagonism, mouse	50		4		50

Doses: approximate ED_{50} (mg./kg.). Route: by mouth, except where otherwise stated
* Highest dose tested
⌀ No effect

Table 4. "Therapeutic quotient" $\dfrac{ED_{sed.}}{ED_{50} ES}$ in mouse (M) and rat (R). $ED_{sed.}$ = effective sedative dose, ES = electroshock.

	Carbam-azepine		Pheno-barbitone		Sodium 2-propyl-valerate		Diazepam		Clonaz-epam		Diphenyl-hydantoin	
	M	R	M	R	M	R	M	R	M	R	M	R
Therapeutic quotient	4	2	2	3	0.9	3	2	1	0.3	1.3	10	6

Only in doses of 30 mg./kg. or more (i.v.) does carbamazepine inhibit the patellar tendon reflex and the tibial flexor reflex in the cat anaesthetised with chloralose-urethan. Lower doses tend to facilitate both of these reflexes slightly. The linguomandibular reflex is depressed by carbamazepine in a dose-dependent manner, very low doses already being sufficient to produce a depression ($ED_{50} = 0.1$ mg./kg. i.v.). In this respect, the action of carbamazepine is similar to that of diazepam.

5.3. Two classic tests have been used to measure anti-aggressive or anxiolytic effects of the compounds under review. One is the fighting behaviour of mice kept in isolation. The other is the fighting behaviour of pairs of mice subjected to electric foot shocks. In both tests carbamazepine, in contrast to diazepam and phenobarbitone, is effective only in high doses. However, in as yet preliminary experiments in cats, in which a rage reaction was induced by electrical stimulation of the perifornical area[8], carbamazepine was found to raise the threshold voltage by 15% and 45% when given in oral doses of 30 mg./kg. and 60 mg./kg., respectively (Figures 8 and 9).

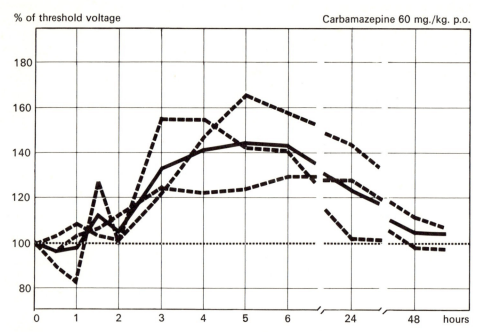

Fig. 8. Time course of threshold voltage required to elicit rage reaction in cats with an electrode chronically implanted in the hypothalamic perifornical area. 100% = control value. Note the increase in the threshold about 1–3 hours after oral administration of carbamazepine in a dose of 60 mg./kg. The threshold returned to the control level between 24 and 48 hours after administration. Uninterrupted line: mean value in three cats; interrupted lines: individual values recorded in each cat.

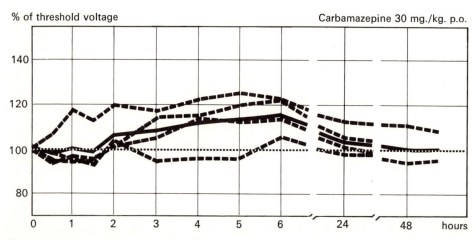

Fig. 9. Same experiment as in Figure 8, except that carbamazepine was administered in an oral dose of 30 mg./kg.

5.4. Carbamazepine is virtually ineffective in a number of test procedures commonly employed to detect antidepressive and/or neuroleptic properties of psychotropic compounds (Table 3). Also, tremorine-induced tremor, a model used to investigate antiparkinson and/or (central) anticholinergic properties, is affected by carbamazepine and by diphenylhydantoin only when these substances are administered in doses about five (carbamazepine) and two (diphenylhydantoin) times higher than the anti-electroconvulsive ED_{50}. Diazepam, by contrast, is quite effective in this test.

5.5. In cats anaesthetised with pentobarbitone sodium or chloralose, FROMM and KILLIAN[5] investigated with micro-electrodes the effect of carbamazepine on the *response to maxillary nerve stimulation of single cells in the spinal trigeminal nucleus*. In intravenous doses of 4–6 mg./kg., carbamazepine reduced the number of evoked spikes in these cells and increased the latency of the response. Diphenylhydantoin in doses of 3–5 mg./kg. had a considerably less pronounced, more erratic, and shorter effect. Phenobarbitone (0.75–1.0 mg./kg.) reduced the amplitude of the evoked neuronal spikes but did not change the latency of the response. Imipramine, in turn, tended to shorten the response latency, without affecting the number or height of the spikes.

Using gross recording techniques, HERNÁNDEZ-PEÓN[7] observed an effect of carbamazepine similar to that noted by FROMM and KILLIAN. The macro-potentials in the spinal nucleus of the trigeminal nerve evoked by electrical stimulation of the face area were reduced in amplitude by this compound.

6. *Discussion*

Carbamazepine shows remarkable anticonvulsive effects in a number of animal "epilepsy models". In small rodents, these anticonvulsive properties are most prominent against seizures induced by electroshock (oral ED_{50} about 10 mg. per kg.), whereas the drug's potency against chemically produced seizures (pentetrazole, strychnine, and picrotoxin) is less pronounced (Figure 7). The "after-discharge" in response to electrical stimulation of the hippocampus in unanaesthetised cats is well controlled by carbamazepine, the intravenous ED_{50} being about 1.0 mg./kg. Larger doses are able to inhibit such discharges almost completely.

Only in fairly large doses (about 50–100 mg./kg. p.o.) does carbamazepine produce sedation, muscular hypotonia, and faulty muscular coordination. In the mouse, there is evidently a good margin between the anticonvulsive (electroshock) dose, on the one hand, and clearly sedative and muscular hypotonic doses, on the other; in fact, compared with that of the other drugs studied, this margin is high.

In view of the clinically well-demonstrated "psychotropic" effects of carbamazepine – it has a proven ability to exert a beneficial influence on the personality changes typical of epileptics, such as aggressiveness, perseveration, and lability of affect – it is interesting to note that, in relatively low doses, the drug does not abolish aggressiveness in rodents. However, preliminary work in cats seems to indicate that hypothalamically induced rage is well checked by carbamazepine. This may suggest that the compound's "anti-aggressive" properties are selective, in the sense that they are directed only against particular (i.e. hypothalamic) types of aggression. More work is needed in this field in order to gain a better understanding of the drug's psychotropic effects by investigating the mechanisms involved.

The clear-cut effect of carbamazepine on the trigeminal sensory pathways may suggest an action which could have a bearing on its anticonvulsive potency and be related to the typical attenuating effect of anticonvulsants on post-tetanic potentiation. In view of the well-proven beneficial action of carbam-azepine in trigeminal neuralgia, this effect on synaptic transmission in the trigeminal nucleus may signal another fundamental aspect of the drug's action.

None of the "classic" anticonvulsive drugs used as reference compounds can be compared with carbamazepine in terms of their activity profile. Diphenyl-hydantoin, while almost as potent as carbamazepine in the electroshock tests, does not have an anti-pentetrazole effect. It is effective against hippocampal after-discharges only in doses ten times larger than those needed with car-bamazepine.

Sodium 2-propylvalerate reveals a rather uncharacteristic profile inasmuch as none of the tests used proves particularly sensitive; its overall potency is low (Figure 7).

The two benzodiazepines are characterised by an extremely prominent antag-onistic effect against pentetrazole – a characteristic which they share, on a relative basis, with phenobarbitone. Clonazepam, which in all tests – including sedation – was the most potent drug, also showed the absolutely and relatively strongest effect against picrotoxin.

Concerning the mechanism of action of carbamazepine or of any of the other anticonvulsive agents mentioned in this paper, the reader interested in this problem is referred to Woodbury's article[25], in which he mentions some pos-sible mechanisms of action of, in particular, diphenylhydantoin, trimetha-dione, bromide, and phenobarbitone.

Seizure discharge is certainly triggered off by faulty excitatory phenomena in single nerve cells, and these phenomena, in turn, may be due to faulty mem-brane properties and to an abnormal (i.e. probably subnormal) inhibitory input to these cells (cf. Creutzfeldt[2]; Prince[19]). Hence, the action of anti-convulsive drugs can be considered from a biophysical point of view.

However, biochemical factors – including, in particular, an imbalance of cen-tral nervous transmitter substances – seem to be of at least equal importance in the pathophysiology of seizure activity and, thus, possibly in the anticonvul-sive action of anti-epileptic drugs. To date, no conclusive evidence is available on the intimate mechanisms of action of any of the known anticonvulsive drugs, although the involvement of gamma-aminobutyric acid (GABA), a well-established central nervous inhibiting substance, has been considered. GABA levels have been shown to be lowered in some cases of experimental and clinical epilepsy (e.g. in epilepsy due to vitamin B_6 deficiency[23]). There is a significant correlation between the electroshock seizure threshold and the GABA concentration in the cerebral cortex[26]. Brain levels of GABA are elevated following administration of diphenylhydantoin, particularly in adrenalectomised animals[25]. Induced changes in the balance between glutamic acid decarboxylase and GABA transaminase activity have been suggested by WOOD and PEESKER[24] as being responsible for the anticonvulsive action of some compounds.

Although few detailed studies on the biophysical and biochemical mode of action of carbamazepine have yet been carried out, one excellent and careful investigation along these lines, performed at IVERSEN's laboratory (MINCHIN and IVERSEN, unpublished report), clearly indicates that carbamazepine does not influence GABA uptake into brain slices or into the satellite glial cells of dorsal root ganglia. Whole-brain GABA levels in mice were not changed by intraperitoneal injections of carbamazepine (15 mg./kg.). But carbamazepine did have a slight inhibitory effect on GABA transaminase activity in rat cerebral cortex. All in all, however, it would seem that the main anticonvulsive action of carbamazepine is related to the drug's influence on a system or systems different from GABA.

References

1 AKERT, K., HUMMEL, P.: Anatomie und Physiologie des limbischen Systems, 2nd Ed. (Hoffmann-La Roche, Basle 1968)
2 CREUTZFELDT, O.D.: Synaptic organization of the cerebral cortex and its role in epilepsy. In Brazier, M.A.B. (Editor): Epilepsy – its phenomena in man, p. 11 (Academic Press, New York/London 1973)
3 ESPLIN, D.W.: Effects of diphenylhydantoin on synaptic transmission in cat spinal cord and stellate ganglion. J. Pharmacol. exp. Ther. *120*, 301 (1957)
4 ESPLIN, D.W.: Criteria for assessing effects of depressant drugs on spinal cord synaptic transmission, with examples of drug selectivity. Arch. int. Pharmacodyn. *143*, 479 (1963)
5 FROMM, G.H., KILLIAN, J.M.: Effect of some anticonvulsant drugs on the spinal trigeminal nucleus. Neurology (Minneap.) *17*, 275 (1967)
6 GODDARD, G.V.: Development of epileptic seizures through brain stimulation at low intensity. Nature (Lond.) *214*, 1020 (1967)
7 HERNÁNDEZ-PEÓN, R.: Central action of G-32883 upon transmission of trigeminal pain impulses. Med. Pharmacol. exp. (Basle) *12*, 73 (1965)
8 HESS, W.R.: Das Zwischenhirn. Syndrome, Lokalisationen, Funktionen (Schwabe, Basle 1949)
9 HUNTER, J., JASPER, H.H.: Effects of thalamic stimulation in unanaesthetised animals. Electroenceph. clin. Neurophysiol. *1*, 305 (1949)
10 JULIEN, R.M.: Cerebellar involvement in the antiepileptic action of diazepam. Neuropharmacology *11*, 683 (1972)
11 JULIEN, R.M.: The effect of carbamazepine on experimental epilepsy in the cat. Proc. West. pharmacol. Soc. *16*, 126 (1973)
12 KILLAM, E.K., MATSUZAKI, M., KILLAM, K.F.: Studies of anticonvulsant compounds in the Papio papio model of epilepsy. In Sabelli, H.C. (Editor): Chemical modulation of brain function, p. 161 (Raven Press, New York 1973)
13 KILLAM, K.F., KILLAM, E.K., NAQUET, R.: Mise en évidence chez certains singes d'un syndrome photomyoclonique. C.R. Acad. Sci. (Paris) *262*, 1010 (1966)

14 Krupp, P., Monnier, M.: Action of anticonvulsants on cerebrospinal systems. In Mercier, J. (Editor): I.E.P.T. (International Encyclopedia of Pharmacology and Toxicology), Section 19, Vol. II, p. 371 (Pergamon Press, Oxford/New York 1973)

15 Liberson, W.T., Akert, K.: Hippocampal seizure states in guinea pig. Electroenceph. clin. Neurophysiol. 7, 211 (1955)

16 Marcus, E. M.: Experimental models of petit mal epilepsy. In Purpura, D., et al. (Editors): Experimental models of epilepsy – a manual for the laboratory worker, p. 113 (Raven Press, New York 1972)

17 Morillo, A.: Effects of benzodiazepines upon amygdala and hippocampus of the cat. Int. J. Neuropharmacol. 1, 353 (1962)

18 Morrell, F.: Secondary epileptogenic lesions. Epilepsia (Amst.) 1, 538 (1959/60)

19 Prince, D.A.: Neuronal correlates of epileptiform discharges and cortical DC potentials. In Rémond, A. (Editor-in-Chief): Handbook of encephalography and clinical neurophysiology, Vol. II, Part C, Creutzfeldt, O. (Editor): The neuronal generation of the EEG, p. 56 (Elsevier, Amsterdam 1974)

20 Prince, D.A., Farrell, D.: "Centrencephalic" spike-wave discharges following parenteral penicillin injection in the cat. Neurology (Minneap.) 19, 309 (1969); abstract of paper.

21 Stille, G.: Zur Frage der Wirkung von Diphenylhydantoin (DH) bei Schmerzzuständen. Eine neurophysiologische Analyse. Nervenarzt 31, 109 (1960)

22 Theobald, W., Krupp, P., Levin, P.: Neuropharmacologic aspects of the therapeutic action of carbamazepine in trigeminal neuralgia. In Hassler, R., Walker, A. E. (Editors): Trigeminal neuralgia. Pathogenesis and pathophysiology, p. 107 (Thieme, Stuttgart 1970)

23 Tower, D. B.: Neurochemical mechanisms. In Jasper, H. H., et al. (Editors): Basic mechanisms of the epilepsies, p. 611 (Little, Brown, Boston 1969)

24 Wood, J. D., Peesker, S. J.: The role of GABA metabolism in the convulsant and anticonvulsant actions of aminooxyacetic acid. J. Neurochem. 20, 379 (1973)

25 Woodbury, D. M.: Mechanisms of action of anticonvulsants, loc. cit.[23], p. 647

26 Woodbury, D. M., Esplin, D. W.: Neuropharmacology and neurochemistry of anticonvulsant drugs. Res. Publ. Ass. nerv. ment. Dis. 37, 24 (1959)

Discussion

M. Mumenthaler: I was impressed by your finding, Dr. Koella, that carbamazepine (®Tegretol), when given in certain doses, exerts a facilitatory effect on convulsions. How do you explain this in pharmacological terms?

W. P. Koella: Unfortunately I have no clear-cut explanation to offer as yet. It may be, though, that the drug has two effects – an inhibitory one and a facilitatory one. If so, this second effect would not appear until fairly high doses are administered, but it would exhibit a steeper dose-response curve. In other words, if sufficiently high doses are given, this facilitatory effect may break through, as it were. This, however, is pure speculation. What really happens with carbamazepine – and with a good many other drugs in similar test situations – we simply do not know. I might add that this facilitation is also encountered with the benzodiazepines in the picrotoxin test, and it is likewise observed with diphenylhydantoin if the doses used are large enough. Though this is a phenomenon that certainly exists, we don't yet know what to do about it. Incidentally, the facilitation of convulsions induced by low doses of picrotoxin is also a rather interesting additional effect of *antidepressive* drugs.

H. Petsche: I was somewhat puzzled by your finding, Dr. Koella, that the effect of clonazepam on strychnine-induced convulsions was reversed when higher doses were used. Have you any explanation for this strange phenomenon?

W. P. Koella: I'm sorry, but – as I said before – I'm afraid I can offer no explanation whatsoever.

S. Blom: Do you know anything about the effect of carbamazepine on ephaptic transmission in experimental models, Dr. Koella?

W. P. Koella: No, I don't, but perhaps Dr. Petsche does. If not, this may well be one of the more important questions to be studied in future research.

J. Kiffin Penry: In your paper, Dr. Koella, you mentioned that carbamazepine suppresses post-tetanic potentiation. Since suppression of post-tetanic potentiation is alleged to be one of the important mechanisms of action of diphenylhydantoin, it would be interesting to know whether you have any further data on carbamazepine in this connection.

W. P. Koella: Yes, we have. A few years ago, Theobald et al.* reported that carbamazepine has an inhibitory effect on post-tetanic potentiation. Recently, however, Hollister and Julien** published a paper indicating exactly the opposite, i.e. that carbamazepine enhances post-tetanic potentiation. Since we were interested in finding out who was right, we repeated the experiment in question over an extended period of time, and we discovered that both were correct. Initially carbamazepine inhibits post-tetanic potentiation, but, if one waits for about 20 minutes or so, the potentials return to control levels and then overshoot these levels by as much as 40–50% or even more, depending on the dose employed. In other words, carbamazepine exerts a biphasic effect in this test.

W. Grüter: I have two questions I should like to ask. The first concerns the inhibitory effect of carbamazepine and diphenylhydantoin on synaptic transmission in the trigeminal nucleus, an effect which might perhaps provide at least a hypothetical

---

* Theobald, W., Krupp, P., Levin, P.: Neuropharmacologic aspects of the therapeutic action of carbamazepine in trigeminal neuralgia. In Hassler, R., Walker, A. E. (Editors): Trigeminal neuralgia. Pathogenesis and pathophysiology, p. 107 (Thieme, Stuttgart 1970)
** Hollister, R. P., Julien, R. M.: Studies on the mode of the antiepileptic action of carbamazepine. Proc. West. pharmacol. Soc. *17*, 103 (1974)

49

explanation for the fact that substances of such differing chemical structure as the hydantoins and carbamazepine are effective not only as anticonvulsants but also in the treatment of trigeminal neuralgia. Have other cerebral nuclei or other afferent systems which might be of interest in this connection also been studied from this angle? And what is known about the behaviour of other anticonvulsants in this respect? My second question relates to the water balance, which is recognised as playing an important role in epilepsy. Since carbamazepine has also proved effective in diabetes insipidus, I should like to enquire whether any studies have been undertaken to determine what influence, if any, the anticonvulsants, including especially carbamazepine, exert on the water balance.

W. P. KOELLA: The answer to your first question, Dr. GRÜTER, as to whether other afferent sensory systems have also been investigated, is unfortunately "no", although a few preliminary studies are currently in progress. It is quite possible, however, that the various sensory modalities, such as the visual, auditory, or tactile afferent systems, may each react quite differently. As for your second question, I'm afraid I cannot yet supply any answer.

M. PARSONAGE: In animal experiments, Dr. KOELLA, you seem to have found positive evidence that carbamazepine has a tranquillising effect. Do you think this evidence supports the view that carbamazepine exerts a psychotropic effect in man? Many of us have felt that in clinical trials the "psychotropic" effect might have been due, at least in part, to the withdrawal of other medication.

W. P. KOELLA: I'm very glad, Dr. PARSONAGE, that you have raised this question. In my opinion, the effect that we find in animal experiments doesn't seem to have very much to do with sedation. We have used several experimental models in an attempt to find evidence that carbamazepine exerts an anti-aggressive effect. First of all, we studied the so-called fighting reaction in mice, which, when an electric shock is applied to the paw, start to attack their companions in the cage. In this model, carbamazepine has no effect: not even doses as high as 200 or 300 mg./kg. have any marked influence on this fighting reaction. On the other hand, sodium 2-propylvalerate, which – as indicated in the paper I presented – is a drug of very weak potency, does affect this fighting reaction, even in fairly low oral doses of 50–100 mg./kg.

We have also done some preliminary work using another model in which rats were given electroconvulsive treatment every day for as long as one month. In response to this treatment the rats became so aggressive that the laboratory technician was no longer able to touch them: as soon as she approached their cage, they would start to jump up and try to bite her. In this model, carbamazepine seemed to act very effectively. In oral doses of 10 and 30 mg./kg., it reduced or even eliminated the animals' aggressiveness, but did not sedate them.

Finally, there is the model in which rage is induced in the cat by means of hypothalamic stimulation; carbamazepine antagonises this rage – i.e. it raises the stimulus threshold – without producing any sedative effect.

The nosology of epilepsy in infancy and childhood

by B. Hagberg*

Convulsions are the commonest single symptom encountered in paediatric neurology. Epilepsy – whose prevalence works out at about 0.4% – is a symptom-complex which, once it has made its appearance in a child, often has far-reaching implications for the whole of the patient's future life. No less than 85–90% of all adult epileptics have a history of epilepsy dating back to their childhood or adolescence.

In children, the type of epilepsy from which the patient is suffering has a cardinal bearing on the developmental and social prognosis. Hence, it is all the more surprising to discover that very little information based on thoroughly investigated, non-selected series of cases is available from which to deduce the true incidence and prevalence of the various forms of epilepsy at different ages in a geographically well-defined region. Moreover, generally accepted classifications, definitions, and criteria for categorising fits of a minor nature in particular are still largely lacking.

Most series of cases presented in the literature are of the kind shown in Table 1, which indicates the distribution of various conventional types of epilepsy as recorded in 245 Finnish children seen in the paediatric department of a university hospital over a certain period of years. Such data, however, usually convey a false impression of the overall problem, because, among other things, they generally leave out of account many of the most serious epilepsy problems met with among mentally retarded institutionalised patients.

The manifestations of epileptic seizures assume varying forms at different ages, depending on the stage of functional development reached by the maturing brain. Those of us who are working in the paediatric field are therefore well

Table 1. Distribution of different types of epilepsy in 245 Finnish children ranging from neonates to patients aged 15 years. (From: SILLANPÄÄ[14])

Type of epilepsy	Number of patients	%
Partial cortical	11	4.5
Psychomotor	114	46.5
Secondarily generalised	36	14.7
Petit mal	12	4.9
Grand mal	131	53.5
Infantile spasms	11	4.5
Akinetic-myoclonic	11	4.5
Unclassified	12	4.9

* Department of Paediatrics, Östra Sjukhuset, University of Gothenburg, Sweden.

Table 2. Correlation between types of seizure occurring in children and the ages at which they are most common.

Type of seizure	Characteristic age
Amorphous fits in newborn infants	Neonatal period
Infantile spasms	3– 8 months
Myoclonic-astatic fits	1½– 4 years
Petit mal (3 c.p.s., spike-and-wave pattern)	3–20 years
Myoclonic petit mal	12–30 years
Partial motor seizures (Rolandic spike form)	5–10 years
Sensorial fits:	
Paroxysmal vomiting	1– 6 years
Paroxysmal abdominal pains	4–10 years
Paroxysmal headache	8–15 years
Paroxysmal vertigo	8–15 years

acquainted with the fact that seizures fall into distinct age-dependent categories, of which the main types are listed in Table 2. Unfortunately, however, we still lack reliable statistics on the incidence and prevalence of most of these types of seizure.

In the following paper I propose to consider certain forms of epilepsy which are characteristic of certain paediatric age groups and which are of particular relevance to the daily work of the neuropaediatrician.

Neonatal forms of epilepsy

Roughly 1% of all live newborn infants exhibit paroxysmal manifestations of one kind or another during the first four weeks of life. Since the incompletely developed neonatal brain reacts differently from a more mature brain, the forms of seizure encountered in newborn infants (Table 3) differ quite considerably from conventional fits.

With few exceptions, repeatedly occurring epileptic fits in neonates are of a symptomatic type, and their diagnosis therefore often calls for very thorough investigation. Perinatal brain damage due to asphyxia or to intracranial haemorrhages is a major causative factor, accounting for some two-thirds to three-quarters of all cases in which the aetiology either is known or can reasonably be inferred. Cases where the fits are attributable to hypoglycaemia, to inborn errors of metabolism, to early post-natal infections, or to C.N.S. malformations constitute small but clinically important groups. Cryptogenic epi-

Table 3. Types of seizure encountered in newborn infants.

Tonic extension fits	Episodes of limpness	Eye-rolling fits
Torsion fits	Apnoeic spells	Episodic colour changes

lepsy manifesting itself already in the newborn infant is extremely rare; if and when it does occur at this early stage of life, it often shows a remarkable tendency to familial clustering. BJERRE and CORELIUS[1], for example, have published a report on a family in which cryptogenic neonatal epilepsy appeared in no fewer than 14 members over five generations; the finding that in this family the boys and girls were equally susceptible would seem to suggest a simple, autosomal, dominant mode of inheritance. Characteristic features of cryptogenic neonatal epilepsy are the fact that, though unresponsive to anti-epileptic drugs, it is nevertheless benign, that it affects neither mental nor motor development, and that it never persists beyond the tenth year of age, but, on the contrary, already disappears within a matter of weeks in the majority of babies. This benign familial disorder should obviously be clearly differentiated from all other forms of epilepsy appearing in later stages of life.

Infantile spasms

The type of epilepsy which it is most important of all to recognise during the first year of the infant's life is that referred to in English as infantile spasms and in German as *Blitz-Nick-Salaam-Krämpfe*. Epilepsy of this kind should always be treated as an emergency, since adequate therapy instituted early on appears to be capable of preventing mental retardation in some cases, including those with a cryptogenic aetiology in particular.

For a long time, no statistics were available on the incidence of infantile spasms. On the basis of a series of cases recently reported from Denmark, however, MELCHIOR (personal communication, 1974) puts the incidence at 0.25 per 1,000 live births – which in Sweden would correspond to a figure of approximately 25 fresh cases per annum. In the absence of appropriate treatment, 22 or 23 of these children would be likely to be left with more or less pronounced mental retardation.

The mean age of onset of infantile spasms is five months. Since the clinical picture is so well known, I shall not describe it again here. I should, however, like to mention one particular observation emerging from an analysis of 44 cases which we have successfully treated with A.C.T.H. during recent years. In 28 of these infants (57%), consisting mainly of cryptogenic cases, irritability, autistic traits, and/or stagnation or even regression of psychomotor development had already been noted a couple of weeks before the onset of the fits (HAGBERG and RASMUSSEN, unpublished observations).

Factors indicative of, or conducive to, a favourable prognosis in cases treated with A.C.T.H. are believed to be the following:

a) Normal level of psychomotor development at the time of onset of the fits.
b) Unknown cause, i.e. cryptogenic infantile spasms.
c) Short duration of the spasms before diagnosis.
d) Absence of other types of seizure and/or of abnormal neurological signs.
e) Early and prompt institution of therapy.

In the above-mentioned series of 44 Swedish cases, what we considered as adequate therapy took the form of 120–180 units of ®Acton prolongatum daily. The mechanism of action of high doses of A.C.T.H. is still poorly understood. In the light of a thorough study of one case, ENEROTH et al.[7] recently advanced the interesting hypothesis that the anti-epileptic effect of A.C.T.H. in babies with infantile spasms and hypsarrhythmia may be mediated via the 3-beta-hydroxy-5-ene steroids, which are among the adrenocortical hormones secreted in increased amounts in response to the stimulus exerted by high doses of A.C.T.H.; some of these steroids had actually been undetectable in the patient's urine prior to treatment with A.C.T.H.

Myoclonic-astatic epilepsy in small children

Myoclonic-astatic epilepsy, which is perhaps the most problematic of all forms of epilepsy, constitutes in children aged 2–4 years a counterpart to infantile spasms in babies. In the Anglo-Saxon literature seizures of this type are variously designated as "akinetic seizures", "astatic epilepsy", or "myoclonic epilepsy", whereas German authors usually prefer the term *"myoklonisch-astatisches Petit mal"*.

In cases where these minor fits are associated with grossly abnormal E.E.G. activity, including slow spike-and-wave patterns, the condition is frequently referred to as "Lennox-Gastaut syndrome", of which mental retardation is often also a conspicuous feature. Some authors, however, such as DOOSE et al.[5], have objected that the criteria for this syndrome are not sufficiently precise, with the result that too many cases are being classified as belonging to this category.

Like infantile spasms, myoclonic-astatic epileptic fits have a polyaetiological background. Both the fits themselves and the accompanying E.E.G. changes seem to depend more upon the age of the child than on the nature of the brain damage it has sustained. KRUSE[10] succeeded in identifying obvious pre-natal, perinatal, or post-natal mechanisms in about two-thirds of the cases he had studied. Some two-thirds of the children already are, or later become, mentally retarded, and hyperkinetic behavioural problems also arise in roughly the same proportion of cases. No fewer than 50–70% of these children have major motor seizures in addition.

Whereas KRUSE[10] doubts whether centrencephalic myoclonic-astatic epilepsy can be accurately distinguished as such, DOOSE et al.[5] claim that, by reference to its combined clinical and electro-encephalographic characteristics, this form of epilepsy not only can, but most emphatically should, be differentiated. DOOSE et al. are in fact of the opinion that the centrencephalic type of epilepsy is a nosologically distinct disease in its own right; they also draw a parallel between this form of epilepsy and classic petit mal in older children. Finally, they believe that the susceptibility of these children to convulsions at various ages is of genetic origin and attributable, not to one simple cause, but to several heterogenetic factors.

So far as I am aware, the true incidence of myoclonic-astatic epilepsy is still unknown. As a neuropaediatrician working in a region of Sweden with a population of about one and a half million, it is my impression that this type of case is now being encountered more frequently at epilepsy clinics than it was ten years ago. Probably, however, this does not mean that there has been a genuine increase in the incidence of myoclonic-astatic epilepsy, but is simply a reflection of the fact that previously this form of epilepsy was often wrongly interpreted as some other entity, and also that, since these fits are more difficult to treat effectively than any others, the patients tend to return to hospital again and again.

Many patients of this type are to be found among the inmates of institutions for mentally retarded children. EEG-OLOFSSON[6], for example, recently reported that myoclonic-astatic seizures were present in 41% of all epileptic patients of all ages institutionalised on account of severe mental retardation; the percentage of patients subject to such seizures, the incidence of which was highest in those aged 5–20 years, was second only to that of grand mal (86%). In spite of its high incidence in this age group, myoclonic-astatic epilepsy may also occasionally be met with in an older patient – a fact which does not seem to me to be generally appreciated by neurologists who deal with adults. One thing is at all events quite clear: in Sweden at least, this type of epilepsy is by far the most frequently misinterpreted form of seizure occurring in mentally retarded patients.

The nature of the fits – consisting usually of more or less pronounced drop seizures with or without myoclonic components – may differ appreciably from patient to patient. To complicate matters, each child tends to have its own individual repertoire of various small and abortive or more dramatic fits, occurring in such a complex mixture that nurses working on the ward often find it difficult to describe them.

Petit mal during childhood

Not all epileptic seizures of brief duration are petit mal! Though every neuropaediatrician will regard this as a statement of the obvious, failure to appreciate its implications still frequently results in misinterpretations on the part of physicians to whose care children are entrusted. Defined on the basis of strict clinical and electro-encephalographic criteria, petit mal is in point of fact a relatively uncommon form of epilepsy occurring in only 2–5% of the patients belonging to series reported upon in recent years[2, 11]. The cases concerned represent a well-delineated and, in all probability, aetiologically homogeneous group in which simple, dominantly inherited, brain-reaction patterns are involved. The onset of petit mal usually occurs between the fourth and ninth year of age, and the fits persist for quite a number of years. Although the general prognosis may be considered good, it is estimated that not more than 25% of the patients become free from fits by the time they reach the age of 25 years.

Myoclonic petit mal

This rare condition, of which there are probably several subgroups, mainly affects teenage girls. Although it is believed to be closely related to pure petit mal, there is certain evidence in favour of the hypothesis that the two diseases are independent and separate types of cryptogenic epilepsy. The fits predominantly take the form of early-morning attacks characterised by sudden, symmetrical jerking confined mainly to the arms and neck.

Psychomotor epilepsy

Whereas petit mal was for many years grossly overdiagnosed, the opposite was the case with psychomotor epilepsy. Even as late as the mid-1950s it was still considered to be an unusual form of epilepsy in children. Today, by contrast, it is known to be one of the commonest epileptic disorders of childhood, accounting for 25–45% of the patients in case series investigated during more recent years[12].

Psychomotor fits may start at any age, and have even been observed in infants aged less than six months[12]. The clinical picture is so variable that any type of paroxysmal deviation from the normal should arouse at least the suspicion of psychomotor epilepsy. The commonest manifestations of psychomotor epilepsy are absence-like spells marked by more or less complete clouding of consciousness and often associated with various forms of stereotypy. These spells are frequently mistaken for pure petit mal attacks. Also characteristic of psychomotor epilepsy are such autonomic and sensorial signs as bouts of flushing, sudden onsets of pallor, attacks of sweating, vertigo, paroxysmal vomiting, paraesthesias, and colicky visceral pains. Aura and post-ictal symptoms are common and may provide important differential-diagnostic clues (cf. Table 4).

Table 4. Differential-diagnostic clues for the three main groups of minor seizures occurring in infancy and childhood. (From: HAGBERG and HANSSON[9])

	"Minor motor"	Petit mal	Psychomotor
Onset	0–3 years	3–15 years	All ages
Duration of fit	Seconds	Seconds	Minutes to hours
Aura	Never	Never	Common
Motor components	Prominent	Absent or minor	Stereotypy
Sensorial/affective signs	Never	Never	Common
Post-ictal stages	Never	Never	Common
E.E.G.	Characteristic	Pathognomonic	Variable
Effect of drugs:			
Ethosuximide	Occasionally good	Excellent	No effect
Phenytoin	No effect	No effect	Good
Carbamazepine	No effect	No effect	Good
Nitrazepam	Fair	No effect	Variable
Clonazepam	Fair	Variable	Variable

Partial motor seizures in children

Partial motor seizures probably constitute a separate benign form of childhood epilepsy with evidence in the E.E.G. of centrotemporal foci of the Rolandic type. There are several reasons why this form deserves to be differentiated from the broad heterogeneous group of grand mal seizures: not the least of these are the extremely good response it shows to ordinary anti-epileptic drugs and its decidedly good prognosis; what is more, despite the frequent presence of seizures of the focal type, this condition does not require neuroradiological investigation. Dr. BLOM and co-workers[3] have undertaken some very thorough studies on the clinical, electro-encephalographic, and genetic features of these partial motor seizures, and Dr. BLOM has promised to comment on their findings later in the discussion.

Grand mal epilepsy

Except in newborn infants, the symmetrical grand mal seizures of childhood do not differ from those occurring in adults. In many children, however, grand mal is accompanied by myoclonic-astatic fits, by petit mal or myoclonic petit mal, or by psychomotor seizures. Pure grand mal of the cryptogenic type can as a rule easily be brought under control with conventional anti-epileptic drugs, and many children suffering from this form of epilepsy tend to grow out of their paroxysmal brain-reaction patterns towards the end of their teens.

References

1 BJERRE, I., CORELIUS, E.: Benign familial neonatal convulsions. Acta paediat. scand. *57*, 557 (1968)

2 BLOM, S., BRORSON, L.O.: Barn med petit mal – en liten men avgränsbar grupp (Children with petit mal – a small but well-defined group). Opusc. med. (Stockh.) *11*, 138 (1966)

3 BLOM, S., HEIJBEL, J., BERGFORS, P.G.: Benign epilepsy of children with centro-temporal EEG foci. Prevalence and follow-up study of 40 patients. Epilepsia (Amst.) *13*, 609 (1972)

4 BRORSON, L.O.: Epilepsy in children and adolescents. A clinical, psychometric and social investigation in the county of Uppsala, Sweden (Stockholm 1970)

5 DOOSE, H., GERKEN, H., LEONHARDT, R., VÖLZKE, E., VÖLZ, C.: Centrencephalic myoclonic-astatic petit mal. Clinical and genetic investigations. Neuropädiatrie *2*, 59 (1970)

6 EEG-OLOFSSON, O.: Epilepsi hos utvecklingsstörda – frekvens, typer och behandlingsalternativ (Epilepsy in mentally retarded – prevalence, types and alternatives of treatment). In Lindström, B., et al. (Editors): Symp. psykiskt utvecklingsstörda (Symp. ment. retard.), Lidingö, Sweden, 1972, p. 119 (Lindgren, Mölndal 1973)

7 ENEROTH, P., GUSTAFSSON, J.-Å., FERNGREN, H., HELLSTRÖM, B.: Excretion and anticonvulsant activity of steroid hormones in an infant with infantile spasm and hypsarrhythmia treated with excessive doses of ACTH. J. Steroid Biochem. *3*, 877 (1972)

8 HAGBERG, B.: Kramper i barnaåren (2) [Seizures in infancy and childhood (2)]. Läkartidningen *65*, 2575 (1968)

9 HAGBERG, B., HANSSON, O.: Åldersberoende anfallsformer hos barn – diagnos och terapi (Age dependent seizures in infants and children – diagnosis and therapy). In Landström, B. (Editor): Epilepsy – medicinska och sociala aspekter, p. 168 (Sörmlands Grafiska, Katrineholm, Sweden 1974)

10 KRUSE, R.: Das myoklonisch-astatische Petit Mal (Springer, Heidelberg/New York 1968)

11 LIVINGSTON, S., TORRES, I., PAULI, L. L., RIDER, R. V.: Petit mal epilepsy. Results of a prolonged follow-up study of 117 patients. J. Amer. med. Ass. *194*, 227 (1965)

12 MATTHES, A.: Die psychomotorische Epilepsie im Kindesalter. Mitteilung I–III. Z. Kinderheilk. *85*, 455, 472, and 668 (1961)

13 MELCHIOR, J. C.: Infantile spasmer og tidlige vaccinationer i årene 1970–1972 (Infantile spasms and previous vaccination during the years 1970–1972). Ugeskr. Laeg. *135*, 1074 (1973)

14 SILLANPÄÄ, M.: Medico-social prognosis of children with epilepsy. Epidemiological study and analysis of 245 patients. Acta paediat. scand. Suppl. 237 (1973)

Discussion

W. BIRKMAYER: Thank you, Dr. HAGBERG, for the impressive review you have given us of the various clinical patterns of epilepsy encountered in children. The paediatricians among us in particular will no doubt wish to raise some points in connection with your paper.

S. BLOM: I should like to present some of the findings obtained by two paediatricians, Dr. J. HEIJBEL and Dr. P. G. BERGFORS, and myself in studies on benign epilepsy of childhood associated with centrotemporal (or Rolandic) discharges in the E.E.G., a form of epilepsy which has been extensively investigated by French authors in particular. The children concerned are usually aged between five and 15 years. Although they all display similar E.E.G. changes, the nature of their seizures may vary, inasmuch as some of them have partial motor attacks and others generalised attacks of the grand mal type. Our main interest, however, has centred not so much on the nature of the seizures, a question reviewed by LOISEAU and BEAUSSART* in 1973, as on the incidence, genetic aspects, and prognosis of this form of epilepsy.

The typical E.E.G. changes encountered in the children we studied, all of whom had seizures, are illustrated in Figure 1. The cortical distribution of these changes can be seen from Figure 2, which is reproduced from a paper published by LOMBROSO in 1967; they attain their maximal amplitude, not in the posterior frontal or anterior temporal regions as in psychomotor epilepsy, but in the centrotemporal area.

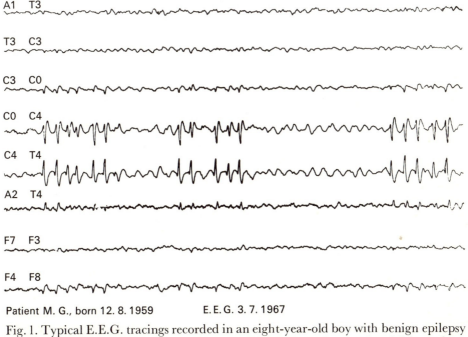

Patient M. G., born 12. 8. 1959   E. E. G. 3. 7. 1967

Fig. 1. Typical E.E.G. tracings recorded in an eight-year-old boy with benign epilepsy of childhood. [Reproduced, by kind permission of the authors and publishers, from BLOM, S., HEIJBEL, J., BERGFORS, P. G.: Benign epilepsy of children with centrotemporal EEG foci. Prevalence and follow-up study of 40 patients. Epilepsia (Amst.) *13*, 609 (1972)]

---

* LOISEAU, P., BEAUSSART, M.: The seizures of benign childhood epilepsy with Rolandic paroxysmal discharges. Epilepsia (Amst.) *14*, 381 (1973)

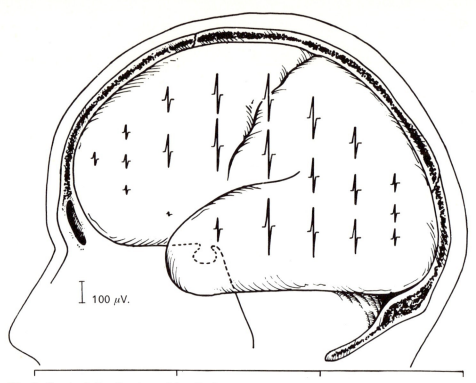

Fig. 2. Cortical distribution of the discharges encountered in benign epilepsy of child-hood. The discharges attain their maximal amplitude in the centrotemporal regions. [Reproduced, by kind permission of the author and publishers, from LOMBROSO, C.T.: Sylvian seizures and midtemporal spike foci in children. Arch. Neurol. (Chic.) *17*, 52 (1967). Copyright 1967, American Medical Association]

Early on in our studies we gained the impression that this form of epilepsy probably accounts for quite a large proportion of the total number of all cases of epilepsy oc-curring in childhood. From statistics on the prevalence of seizures in the Uppsala region of Sweden we calculated initially that it could be as much as seven times more common than "classic" petit mal. But, because we doubted whether this estimate was reliable, we decided to record over a period of one year all new cases of childhood seizures reported in the County of Västerbotten in the northern part of Sweden. The total population of this county was approximately 230,000, and the number of children aged up to 16 years came to just over 52,000. The incidence of febrile convulsions among these children was found to be 227 per 100,000 and that of true epilepsy 122 per 100,000. In order to establish how many of these cases of true epilepsy could be assigned to the category of benign epilepsy of childhood, we proceeded to classify the various types of seizure observed. Since our classification had to be based on a limited number of seizures in each child, it is of course open to criticism. However, our calculations showed that some 20% of the children with true epileptic seizures could be regarded as having benign epilepsy of childhood. This figure was more than four times higher than that for "classic" petit mal in the same population.

In view of the fact that in many children with this form of epilepsy the seizures occur only at night and may thus pass unnoticed by the parents, it is important in suspect cases to record E.E.G. activity both during sleep and while the child is awake.

As for the genetic aspect, we noticed at an early stage of our investigations that many of the children with Rolandic discharges had relatives with seizures. We therefore

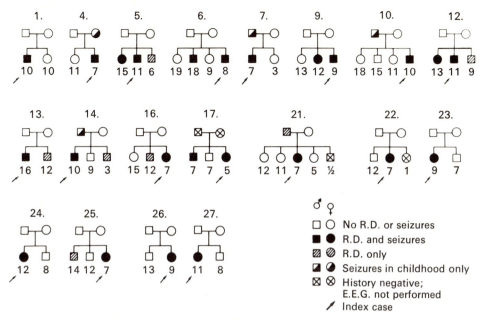

Fig. 3. Results of a genetic evaluation performed on the families of 19 children (index cases) displaying Rolandic discharges (R.D.). The numerals below each set of symbols indicate the ages of the children. [Reproduced, by kind permission of the authors and publishers, from HEIJBEL, J., BLOM, S., RASMUSON, M.: Benign epilepsy of childhood with centrotemporal EEG foci; a genetic study. Epilepsia *16*, 285 (1975)]

carried out a genetic study on a relatively small number of families whose members included one child with Rolandic discharges and seizures. One difficulty met with in this part of our investigation was that the E.E.G. changes associated with benign epilepsy of childhood can, by definition, only be detected in children and not, for example, in their parents. Hence, our evaluation, the results of which are shown in Figure 3, was restricted to siblings of the children with Rolandic discharges. When we calculated the mode of inheritance of the E.E.G. pattern by applying the so-called *"a priori"* method, we came to the conclusion, after consultation with Professor MARIANNE RASMUSON of the Department of Genetics, University of Umeå, that the E.E.G. trait is most probably inherited in an autosomal dominant manner. The possibility of a recessive mode of inheritance, or of a multifactorial heredity, was also examined but was found to be considerably less likely.

In addition, we studied the question of prognosis in a limited number of children whom we had been able to follow up until their late teens or even longer. The results of this study, from which Figure 1 has been taken, showed that, though the prognosis was good, many of the children subsequently encountered social difficulties; some of them, for example, were unable to obtain a driver's licence, or even to find a job, although they had been free of seizures for years.

To sum up, we believe that benign epilepsy of childhood associated with centro-temporal E.E.G. foci is characterised by the following features:

1. The E.E.G. trait in question is inherited in an autosomal dominant manner, with an age-dependent penetrance which reaches its maximum between the ages of five and 15 years.
2. The E.E.G. discharges show an increase during sleep, and may in fact in some cases appear only during sleep.

61

3. The prognosis is good, most of the children becoming free from seizures after puberty.
4. Benign epilepsy of childhood accounts for a large proportion (approximately 20% in our studies) of all children subject to true epileptic seizures.
5. This form of epilepsy is readily amenable to treatment. The seizures are of the partial motor, secondarily generalised, or sometimes even primarily generalised type.

D. JANZ: I'd like to comment briefly on what Dr. HAGBERG has referred to as "myoclonic petit mal", a condition which SCHORSCH* once called "myoclonic petit mal of adolescence". HERPIN, who was the first to publish an account of this syndrome, described the manifestations as "impulsions" – which in turn led us** to coin the expression "impulsive petit mal". You stated in your paper, Dr. HAGBERG, that this is a rare condition which mainly affects teenage girls. But, in our experience, this syndrome is not all that infrequent. It merely appears to be so uncommon because, of all the epileptic syndromes, it is the one most likely to be passed over – the reason being the age of the patients concerned, which is such that they tend to fall between the two stools of paediatrics and neurology. Hardly ever are they still referred to a paediatrician, whereas they are relatively seldom seen by a neurologist. Among our own patients, however, this form of epilepsy is just as frequent as myoclonic-astatic petit mal, i.e. its incidence works out at about 3.5% of cases. I was also surprised, Dr. HAGBERG, at your statement that it chiefly affects girls. It has been our finding that boys and girls are equally susceptible. TSUBOI and CHRISTIAN*** recently published a report on a genetic study involving over 300 cases, in which they too found an equal distribution between the sexes.

B. HAGBERG: These comments of yours, Dr. JANZ, are very interesting. However, I can only repeat that, as far as the children followed in Scandinavia are concerned, myoclonic petit mal has been rare. In the Finnish series, its incidence was – if I remember rightly – less than 1%; and during the last ten years I myself have seen in the paediatric age group only about half a dozen girls and only one boy with this form of epilepsy.

M. BONDUELLE: May I at this point revert to a question already touched upon by Dr. HAGBERG in his paper, namely, the extent to which petit mal is liable to persist into adulthood. This is always a difficult problem, one of the reasons being that the doctors who see the patients as adults are not the same as those who saw them as children. Almost all epileptic children are dealt with by paediatricians, who lose sight of them when they grow up. Dr. HAGBERG implied that petit mal frequently persists in the adult. It is my impression, on the contrary, that petit mal persisting into adulthood is exceptional – but that those cases in which this does happen pose very difficult therapeutic problems. I believe, on the other hand, that persistence of *myoclonic* petit mal in the adult is a more frequent occurrence, although I can't quote any precise figures in support of this belief.

---

* SCHORSCH, G.: Epilepsie: Klinik und Forschung. In Gruhle, H.W., et al. (Editors): Psychiatrie der Gegenwart. Forschung und Praxis, Vol. II: Klinische Psychiatrie, p. 646 (Springer, Berlin/Göttingen/Heidelberg 1960)
** JANZ, D.: Die Epilepsien. Spezielle Pathologie und Therapie (Thieme, Stuttgart 1969)
   JANZ, D.: The natural history of primary generalized epilepsies with sporadic myoclonias of the impulsive petit mal type. In Lugaresi, E., et al. (Editors): Evolution and prognosis of epilepsies (Gaggi, Bologna 1973)
   JANZ, D., CHRISTIAN, W.: Impulsiv-Petit mal. Dtsch. Z. Nervenheilk. *176*, 346 (1957)
*** TSUBOI, T., CHRISTIAN, W.: On the genetics of the primary generalized epilepsy with sporadic myoclonias of impulsive petit mal type. Hum. Genet. *19*, 155 (1973)

Just another brief remark on a point of terminology: the word "aura" strikes me as involving some risk of confusion. Its original meaning in Latin was "breath", but it does not appear to be applicable to the context of psychomotor epilepsy. In the classic descriptions it was applied to that fleeting impression which the patient experiences immediately before losing consciousness in an attack of grand mal, i.e. in an attack assuming a generalised form *from the very outset*. When Dr. HAGBERG referred to "aura" in his description of psychomotor epilepsy, however, it seemed to me that he was applying the term to the first manifestation – whether sensorial or otherwise – of the psychomotor seizure, which becomes generalised only *secondarily*, i.e. as it develops further. I suggest at all events that "aura" is an ambiguous expression and, as such, difficult to accept.

I. GAMSTORP: May I first of all say something about seizures in the newborn. I certainly agree with Dr. HAGBERG that the commonest cause of these seizures is perinatal asphyxia or intracranial bleeding, but I would add a word of warning against assuming that the cause is always asphyxia. The asphyxia may often be complicated by a metabolic disorder which should be diagnosed and treated. Moreover, a vitamin B_6 deficiency syndrome may also present in the form of neonatal asphyxia – in which case, if you don't do a test with pyridoxine, you will fail to make the correct diagnosis. It is also important to bear in mind that children showing signs of asphyxia in the first few minutes of life may have some other underlying disorder which can be treated by taking appropriate measures.
In addition, I should like to point out that the possibility of tuberous sclerosis should be considered in all cases of infantile spasms and neonatal convulsions, particularly in cases where such seizures are found to have occurred in several members of the same family. With reference to Dr. JANZ's comments on myoclonic petit mal, I too think that this condition is a little more common than Dr. HAGBERG suggested. In my experience, about one-third of the patients are boys.

B. HAGBERG: I quite agree that in newborn infants with convulsions it is very important to carry out thorough neurometabolic examinations. In unselected series of such patients, however, the proportion found to be suffering from genuine neurometabolic disorders amounts to no more than 2–4%.

G. NISSEN: As a child psychiatrist, I am particularly grateful to Dr. HAGBERG for having emphasised in his paper how difficult it is in some forms of epilepsy to arrive at a satisfactory differential diagnosis and differential typology. In this connection, I should like to mention that we have had some six or eight children under observation who, over the course of several years, have exhibited – sometimes even simultaneously – various forms of attack comprising infantile spasms, absences, and twilight attacks, as well as twilight states and grand mal seizures. Although, when discussing epilepsy, we have to make use of classifications based on differential typology if we are to understand one another, the examples I have just referred to illustrate the artificial nature of such classifications.
Incidentally, it is my impression too that psychomotor attacks are much commoner in children than was previously assumed, and I would remind you that French epileptologists have always put the incidence of psychomotor attacks in epileptic children at some 40–50%. I have also encountered cases of "masked" psychomotor epilepsy which, though few in number, were very impressive and associated with more or less typical E.E.G. patterns. A case in point was that of a 14-year-old boy who, every 6–8 weeks or so, would get out of bed at four o'clock in the morning, pull up the blinds in the bathroom, and proceed to wash himself and clean his teeth. His E.E.G. recordings showed clear evidence of psychomotor epilepsy. Treatment with carbamazepine, in the form of one tablet of ®Tegretol taken every evening, eliminated the symptoms. In children in particular, behavioural anomalies of indeterminate origin may well be accompanied by borderline or frankly pathological E.E.G. findings which should not be overlooked when considering the problem of diagnosis and treatment.

L. Oller-Daurella: I'd like to ask Dr. Hagberg a question concerning the various types of seizure mentioned in his paper. He made no reference to tonic seizures, which are very frequent in children, especially between the ages of two and five years. Did you perhaps include these seizures in the category of grand mal, Dr. Hagberg? If so, I'm not sure whether that would be justified. This type of seizure, by the way, is more likely to be detected if electro-encephalographic recordings are made during sleep.

With regard to myoclonic-atonic or myoclonic-astatic seizures, I believe that in our country their incidence among children is far higher than the figure of 3.5% quoted by Dr. Janz. For atypical petit mal (Lennox-Gastaut syndrome) we, at all events, have recorded higher percentages in Spain, where the incidence amounts to some 10–15%.

In his contribution to this discussion, my friend Dr. Bonduelle raised the question as to the evolution of petit mal. It is our impression that the condition which we in our statistical data classify as *typical* petit mal does indeed sometimes disappear with age – probably after puberty. But it does not always disappear completely, and minor absences lasting only a few seconds may persist; to obtain proof that these so-called micro-absences are in fact occurring, however, one has to perform recordings or even carry out tests to determine the patient's level of consciousness. I cannot entirely agree with what either Dr. Hagberg or Dr. Bonduelle have said about the way in which petit mal evolves with age, because in our experience at least 50% of cases exhibiting typical absences eventually develop into grand mal – as Dr. Janz* has also shown in a paper published 20 years ago.

B. Hagberg: I did not make any special mention of tonic seizures, but included them instead under the other main headings. Regarding the question of petit mal and its evolution with age, I followed up a series of patients some years ago in whom 50% still had their petit mal absences at the age of 25 years. Despite this, and although such absences are very common between the ages of 15 and 20 years, I think that probably in most, if not all, of the cases they disappear completely by the age of 30 years.

A. Rett: In his paper, Dr. Hagberg drew attention to the fact that in a very high percentage of children with myoclonic-astatic epilepsy the condition is associated with mental retardation. This is something that I can fully confirm. I should like to point out, however, that the cause of the retardation plays no role in this connection and that myoclonic-astatic attacks are always apt to occur in the presence of mental retardation, regardless of its aetiology. It is for this reason that, whenever we examine a mentally retarded child for the first time, i.e. already when making our initial interpretation of the disorder, we invariably warn the parents that epileptic attacks – though they may not yet have occurred – are liable to set in sooner or later. Unfortunately, these warnings of ours all too often prove well founded.

* Janz, D.: Die klinische Stellung der Pyknolepsie. Dtsch. med. Wschr. *80*, 1392 (1955)

Problems encountered in the treatment of epilepsy

by D. JANZ

Introduction

Only a few years ago it seemed that such a sound body of knowledge and experience had been acquired in the treatment of epilepsy that the only problem remaining was to put it into practice. A note of proud self-assurance can in fact be detected in a number of my own papers dating from the 1950s and 1960s. In these papers the various anti-epileptic drugs are listed in the chronological order of their development, the various types of epilepsy are described by reference to their clinical and electro-encephalographic characteristics, the specific indications for drugs in the different forms of epilepsy are outlined, attention is drawn to certain of their side effects, and, finally, the important bearing which psychological factors have on the success or failure of treatment is duly stressed. It is my impression that this approach is no longer appropriate to the situation confronting us today, and this impression is reflected in a certain change of emphasis: whereas I was wont to dwell upon what I referred to as "specific treatment for epilepsy"[11,12], I should now prefer to concentrate more on the "problems of treatment for epilepsy".

It is true that certain of the principles underlying the concept of "specific anti-epileptic therapy" still retain their validity. Here, I am thinking primarily of the establishment of special indications on the basis of which a particular drug is selected for use in a particular form of epilepsy. It is a well-known fact, for example, that ethosuximide proves effective in absences – especially pyknoleptic absences, which occur frequently and are associated with regular 3/sec. spikes-and-waves. On the other hand, both in infantile absences, characterised by slow spike-and-wave patterns, as well as in juvenile absences, which are marked by fast spike-and-wave patterns, ethosuximide yields less satisfactory results. It is completely ineffective against focal attacks and against major, generalised tonic-clonic seizures. For use in major seizures the drugs chiefly employed are, of course, the hydantoins or the barbiturates, the most popular compounds in these two groups being diphenylhydantoin and primidone. The decision as to which of these latter two drugs to prescribe when initiating treatment will depend on whether the major seizures occur chiefly during sleep or chiefly after waking: at least in our experience[15], diphenylhydantoin elicits better responses in so-called sleep epilepsy, whereas primidone is likely to prove more effective in epilepsy occurring upon awakening. Both drugs

---

* Abteilung für Neurologie im Klinikum Charlottenburg der Freien Universität, Berlin.

are also of approximately equal efficacy in focal attacks[15, 17]. Nowadays, however, it is carbamazepine (®Tegretol) that is mainly used in focal epilepsy, since it is probably just as effective as diphenylhydantoin or primidone but less likely to provoke unpleasant side effects. Carbamazepine is undoubtedly every bit as good as diphenylhydantoin in the treatment of psychomotor seizures. This has recently been confirmed by a controlled comparative study of the two drugs[29], and it must therefore be concluded that, thanks to its lower incidence of side effects, carbamazepine is the drug of first choice in the type of focal epilepsy which is accompanied by psychomotor seizures. In this indication, carbamazepine is nevertheless still by no means ideal – as evidenced by the fact that, whereas complete freedom from attacks can be achieved with ethosuximide in 78% of cases of pyknoleptic absences, with diphenylhydantoin in 72% of cases of sleep epilepsy, and with primidone in 65%[15] of cases of epilepsy on awakening, the corresponding percentage for carbamazepine in psychomotor epilepsy is only 40%[41].

As for those specifically childhood forms of epilepsy which, as such, constitute special indications, here there have been no new developments in recent years: in West's syndrome (otherwise known as infantile spasms or propulsive petit mal) A.C.T.H., dexamethasone, or nitrazepam are still the drugs of preference, and in children subject to febrile convulsions phenobarbitone is still awarded pride of place as a prophylactic agent[8].

There are several reasons, however, why I prefer to discuss problems met with in the treatment of epilepsy rather than simply to repeat what are already accepted as dogmatic tenets:

1. Quite a few of the failures we encounter in this field should serve as a reminder that the success of treatment depends not only on the knowledge and skill of the treating physician but also on the patient's motivation. It certainly cannot be taken for granted that a patient suffering from epilepsy will always have a *positive motivation with regard to treatment*.

2. Bound up with this problem is that of deciding *under what circumstances treatment should in fact be initiated* at all, and

3. of ensuring *compliance* once it has been initiated.

4. If the drugs employed are to be properly handled, it is also essential that the patient concerned be given all the necessary *information on the treatment*.

5. In the conduct of drug therapy a role of major importance is played by *questions relating to dosage schedules*, e.g. how the medication should be built up, changed, reduced, or discontinued, what dosage level should be selected, how the dosage should be divided over the day, and whether treatment should take the form of monotherapy or combined therapy.

6. The correct handling of drugs also implies *choice of the most appropriate dosage form* for the needs of a given case, e.g. parenteral administration with a view to achieving a therapeutically effective blood concentration as quickly as possible in a patient with status epilepticus, or prescription of suppositories in order to maintain a steady state in a patient who is temporarily unable to take drugs by mouth.

7. Neither drugs themselves nor, for that matter, the patient who is required to use them can be satisfactorily handled unless the treating physician has a certain basic understanding of the *pharmacokinetics of anti-epileptic agents*, i.e. of their distribution and fate in the organism. Of practical significance in this connection is a knowledge, firstly, of those factors which determine the concentrations attained by an anti-epileptic drug in the serum and, secondly, of the way in which the preparation interacts with other drugs. Since these, however, are questions which will be discussed later on in this symposium, I shall not dwell upon them here.

8. Finally, problems also arise from the possible *side effects of anti-epileptic agents*, two of which have claimed particular attention in recent years – the first being the occurrence of osteoporosis, chiefly in children and adolescents receiving diphenylhydantoin, and the second the possible teratogenic risk of anti-epileptic drugs. But, as I believe the toxicological aspects of anti-epileptic medication are to be dealt with in Dr. DREYER's paper, I need not go into this question of side effects either.

Motivation to seek treatment

Although epilepsy is by no means uncommon, few patients subject to epileptic attacks visit a doctor regularly. It is estimated that 30% of all persons suffering from repeated epileptic seizures, i.e. from chronic epilepsy, never consult a doctor at all[19] and that, of the remainder, quite a few are never seen by a specialist[5].

An epidemiological study carried out in Iceland revealed that, of all epileptics living on the island at a given date, 32% had never undergone any treatment and only 42% were in receipt of regular therapy[9]. A field survey recently undertaken in Warsaw actually disclosed that 37% of all patients who had had more than two epileptic attacks had never taken an anti-epileptic drug and that, at the time of the survey, only 35% were being given drug treatment[43]. The finding that almost two-thirds of all epileptic patients are receiving no medical attention whatsoever provides food for thought. Admittedly, of the patients in the Warsaw study who had never been treated, most were suffering from mild forms of epilepsy; only one-quarter of them had consulted a doctor, and one-third had been free of seizures for more than five years. Among these untreated patients were many subject to focal attacks or absences which they did not regard as requiring treatment, even though major seizures occasionally occurred. There were also other patients, including those with major seizures in particular, who simply did not want to be treated, who thought that epilepsy was untreatable, or who refrained from consulting a doctor because they were afraid of being admitted to hospital and subjected to various diagnostic procedures. Among those who had in fact been treated at some time or other, several had discontinued the medication because of side effects; most of them, however, had ceased taking their drugs either because they considered them ineffective or because they had become free from attacks[43].

In our experience, reluctance to seek or pursue treatment may be attributable to a wide variety of causes: for example, the attacks may occur so infrequently or in such a mild form that the patient does not feel handicapped by them; he may be worried at the thought of having to undergo examinations or at the idea of his illness being discovered and becoming known to others; on the other hand, in the past he may perhaps have run up against an impatient doctor or have suffered unduly from the side effects of sedative drugs. Another, though admittedly rare, possibility to be borne in mind is that the patient may have become addicted, as it were, to his epileptic attacks, i.e. that he may actually derive pleasure from the aura or from the manoeuvres of precipitation[14].

Less uncommon are cases in which the patient – especially if he has suffered from epilepsy for many years, if the results of treatment have proved disappointing, and if he has been habitually pampered and molly-coddled – derives a secondary gain from his illness which robs him of all incentive to seek treatment[26]. It is a well-known fact that patients in receipt of a pension for reasons of ill-health tend to be no longer interested in submitting to systematically conducted treatment[1].

If, despite all the possible reasons I have just outlined, it may still seem curious that so many epileptics either do not consult a doctor at all or fail to pursue their treatment conscientiously, allow me also to point out that epilepsy differs from most other illnesses insofar as it is not so much the epileptic attacks as such which entail suffering for the patient, but rather their repercussions vis-à-vis society. The manifestations of epilepsy which make the strongest impression upon the onlooker – the epileptic's sudden cry, his falling to the ground, and the muscle contractions typical of a generalised tonic-clonic seizure – are, it is true, suffered by the patient, but not really experienced by him. What actually impinges upon the patient's consciousness during an attack is at all events in no way comparable with the shock sustained by the onlooker, particularly since epileptics – who, incidentally, cannot be regarded as "patients" in the strict sense of the term – experience the attacks the less, the more violent they are.

With the exception of auras, Jacksonian attacks, and the brief myoclonic jerks occurring in cases of impulsive petit mal, epileptic attacks are for the most part experienced by the patient indirectly, so to speak, inasmuch as he is only able to draw inferences about them from the expressions he sees on the faces of bystanders when he regains consciousness after an attack. By and large, and at the risk of oversimplification, it may therefore be stated that epileptic patients experience their illness chiefly as mirrored in the reactions of their fellow-men[13].

Indications for the initiation of treatment

The question of the patient's motivation is one that must be given due consideration when deciding whether or not to institute therapy, because it will prove impossible to carry out treatment properly if he himself is not convinced that it is both beneficial and necessary. By the same token, a patient's non-compliance can generally be taken as a sign that he expects to derive no profit from the treatment. Consequently, before initiating therapy, one should carefully ascertain to what extent the patient really feels the need for treatment, and, if he obviously lacks the requisite motivation, one should also have the courage to refrain from treating him.

Now that more has become known about the risks of long-term medication with anti-epileptics and about the complex pharmacokinetics of these drugs, there is a general tendency to apply stricter criteria in deciding whether or not treatment is indicated[7, 16]. No treatment should be initiated, for example, in a case of so-called latent epilepsy characterised by purely subclinical epileptic activity in the E.E.G. In such cases there is no rational justification for *prophylactic therapy*. In the first place, we simply do not know what risk there is that this subclinical activity might later lead to overt attacks – quite apart from the fact that such "patients" would not be inclined to accept regular treatment. Secondly, the danger of seizures occurring as a reaction to withdrawal of the medication far outweighs such benefit as might be derived from performing what amounts to a "cosmetic operation" on the patient's E.E.G.

Prophylactic treatment to offset the threat of epilepsy can, on the other hand, be considered in cases of complicated febrile convulsions. Here, the relevant criteria are as follows: positive heredity, pre-existing cerebral damage, signs of focal seizures, onset either during early infancy or after the fourth year of life, three previous relapses, occurrence of several attacks during an infection or of attacks lasting longer than 30 minutes, pathological interseizure E.E.G. records[7]. Furthermore, prophylactic treatment can be considered after all acute cerebral lesions due, in particular, to trauma or to surgery.

Prophylactic medication should invariably be given in cases involving penetrating injuries of the centroparietal region, as well as following surgery for cerebral abscesses, because it is in these two types of brain damage that the incidence of post-traumatic epilepsy is greatest (50–60%)[2, 4, 27, 30].

Preventive treatment is, in fact, advisable in all patients who have sustained any type of penetrating injury to the brain, since in such cases the likelihood of epilepsy ensuing averages 37%[28]. In Czechoslovakia it is the routine practice to administer prophylactic therapy to all patients with closed cerebral contusions. SERVÍT[37, 38] quotes both experimental[34-36] and clinical findings[3, 10, 24, 25] in support of this practice; but the validity of these findings has been disputed on methodological grounds[27]. The Czechoslovak authors in question, however, have also reported that even in the group of untreated control cases it was still possible to prevent the recurrence of attacks, and thus to guard against the development of chronic epilepsy, by instituting treatment after the first attack had already occurred. In view of this, I wonder whether – at least until such time as KIFFIN PENRY is in a position to report on the results of the collaborative study in which he is acting as coordinator – it might not be preferable simply to carry out routine follow-up examinations in patients who have sustained cerebral injuries, rather than to give them prophylactic therapy as a matter of course.

I would in any case not consider it justifiable to institute drug treatment if there had been only one previous attack or series of attacks or even if status epilepticus had occurred on one single occasion -- unless, of course, the patient himself insisted upon being treated. From a medical standpoint, I can see no necessity for treatment in such cases, not even if the patient's E.E.G. is abnormal or possibly specific, if he has a history of epilepsy in his family, if there is residual evidence of previous damage, or if he is suffering from a progressive disease of the brain. I say this because there are no grounds for supposing that an attack will recur in the absence of medication; nor can I conceive of any social handicap that might be guarded against by giving the patient drugs. Patients working in dangerous occupations, for example, are in any case obliged to find alternative employment, even after they have had only one seizure; and others, even if they were receiving treatment, would have to refrain from driving a vehicle for a certain time.

At all events, a physician who already treats patients after they have had only a single seizure will certainly achieve good results as far as *statistics* are concerned. This seems to be borne out by the fact that, according to the results of a general-practice study which was undertaken in Great Britain, only one out of every eight patients presenting with so-called first fits is likely to suffer any subsequent attacks[5].

On the other hand, a follow-up survey of patients admitted to our clinic as "first-fit" cases revealed that, over a period of 4–8 years, one out of two had experienced further attacks[18]. Since the general practitioners who participated in the British study also included febrile convulsions among the cases they recorded, and since patients referred to a neurological clinic probably represent a negative selection as regards prognosis, it is perhaps safe to assume that the truth lies somewhere in the middle, i.e. that three out of every four adults with first fits suffer no further attacks, even in the absence of medication.

The only absolute indication for drug therapy is thus chronic epilepsy, irrespective of its origin; and by chronic epilepsy I mean the repeated occurrence of attacks at fairly frequent intervals. Also to be included in this category are cases of epilepsy due to cerebral tumours; here, even following excision of the tumour, epilepsy – in the form of post-traumatic epilepsy – is liable to recur after a seizure-free period if the pre-operative treatment has not been continued for at least 6–12 months after the operation.

The problem of compliance

That medication is likely to be successful only if patients take their drugs conscientiously and systematically in adequate doses over sufficiently prolonged periods of time, and only if they report for regular check-ups, may appear to be a statement of the obvious; but, though an absolute *sine qua non* in the management of epilepsy, it often proves difficult to achieve. Any failure to fulfil this requirement may be fraught with baneful consequences, particularly since the occurrence of relapses in the course of half-heartedly conducted treatment is liable to result in disappointment and lack of cooperation on the patient's part. If only the physician who actually institutes anti-epileptic medication also had as a rule to supervise the conduct of treatment in the years to follow, patients would be spared many a disappointment and the doctors responsible for maintenance therapy would, for their part, also be spared a great deal of drudgery. There are nevertheless certain aids which have given proof of their worth as a means of improving compliance, i.e. of helping to ensure that the patient takes his medication regularly. By monitoring the concentrations of diphenylhydantoin in the serum, LUND[21], for example, has demonstrated that the following measures are conducive to better compliance: providing the patient with information designed to underline the necessity for the regular ingestion of a drug, shortening the periods between check-ups, and issuing the patient with a small container for his daily dose. Further measures which probably help to foster compliance include: making fixed appointments for check-ups, and simplifying the regimen by prescribing, if possible, only two fractional doses daily, by aiming wherever feasible at monotherapy, and by refraining – as far as possible – from employing any additional drugs.

Information on the treatment

Even an investigation which simply reveals that a self-evident truth can also be confirmed scientifically may be considered to have served a useful purpose – as, for example, when proof is furnished that a negative motivation with regard to treatment correlates with poor compliance, this poor compliance resulting not only in underdosage but sometimes also in overdosage. Among such self-evident truths which have recently been rediscovered, as it were, is the finding that if one takes the trouble to inform the patient about the medication – i.e. if, when starting treatment, one explains to him the principles underlying it and the way in which the drug in question works – even this simple effort will pay dividends in the form of higher and steadier serum concentrations[21]. When giving the patient his initial briefing, one should, I think, also endeavour to strike an optimistic note, but at the same time explain to him what conditions he will have to fulfil if his hopes are to be realised; what is more, besides telling him how the drug is believed to act, one should inform him of its possible side effects as well. Finally, the whole object of the exercise should be to describe and justify the plan of treatment to the patient in such a way that he willingly accepts his own share of responsibility; in this connection, one can likewise help to create a positive motivation in a variety of seemingly minor ways – for instance, by not only discussing the electro-encephalographic recordings with the patient, but by also actually inspecting them together with him.

Building up to an adequate dosage level poses few if any problems, provided one makes it a practice to begin with small, gradually increasing doses. In the case of diphenylhydantoin, this means that – except in hospitalised patients – one should never exceed weekly dosage increments of 100 mg. The dosage of succinimides, primidone, carbamazepine, and dipropylacetate (®Ergenyl), on the other hand, can be raised by one unit every 3–4 days; where primidone is prescribed, however, the very first dose (given, if possible, in the evening) should be half a tablet at the most, and preferably only one-quarter of a tablet.

If the need arises *to transfer a patient to another drug*, this should never be done by replacing one type of tablet by another. Instead, one should begin by adding the new drug to the old regimen, wait and see what effect this combined medication produces, and only then – if necessary – withdraw the old drug step by step while making no change in the dosage of the new drug. Only in this way can one accurately assess the effects of the previous medication alone, of the combined treatment, and of monotherapy with the new drug.

The *daily dosage* should be decided upon solely by reference to the ratio of therapeutic effects to side effects. If attacks are still occurring, but no side effects have been encountered, the dosage should be increased – either until the patient can no longer tolerate the drug or until the attacks cease. In many cases, freedom from attacks can be purchased only at the price of side effects during the initial stages of treatment; and failures are often attributable to the fact that, precisely during this critical phase of adjustment, there has not been sufficiently close contact between doctor and patient. Monitoring of the serum concentrations will probably in future prove of value in helping the treating physician to arrive at the optimum individual dosage.

Although the therapeutically effective serum concentrations exhibit such a broad scatter that it is impossible to lay down any hard-and-fast rules, it may be helpful at this juncture to point out that, in the case of diphenylhydantoin, values of less than 10 mcg./ml. are too low for an optimum therapeutic effect and that at values exceeding 30 mcg./ml. one is almost certainly overshooting the limits of tolerability.

With regard to *fractionation of the daily dosage*, one should not adopt a schematic approach, but should base the dosage schedule on the drug's half-life. The time taken for one-half of a given dose to be eliminated from the body is 20–25 hours in the case of diphenylhydantoin, 2–3 days for ethosuximide, and as much as 3–6 days for phenobarbitone[20]. This means that the entire daily dosage of diphenylhydantoin, phenobarbitone, primidone, or ethosuximide could quite well be taken in a single dose without incurring the risk of the serum concentration diminishing to any appreciable extent over a 24-hour period. Studies in which the serum concentrations of diphenylhydantoin following a single dose were compared with those following fractionated doses have shown that the fluctuations recorded remain within clinically acceptable limits[39]. Since there may be some cases, however, in which the enzyme responsible for catabolising the drug displays exceptionally high activity, one certainly cannot go wrong by adhering to the principle of prescribing diphenylhydantoin and the other aforementioned drugs twice daily. This procedure is particularly to be recommended in children, because they break down anti-epileptic drugs more rapidly than adults and therefore require, and are also able to tolerate, relatively larger doses. In view of what has just been said about the half-lives of these anti-epileptic agents, it should be noted that there is no point in trying to adapt the daily dosage schedule to the time of day at which attacks are wont to occur, e.g. by arranging for the bulk of the daily dosage to be taken before rising if the patient happens to be subject to epilepsy on awakening, or before going to bed in the evening if he suffers from sleep epilepsy.

Similarly, the pharmacokinetic properties of these drugs are such that it is also pointless to vary the dosage in an attempt to cope with changing circumstances – e.g. to raise the doses around the time of menstruation in a woman who is allegedly more susceptible to attacks during her periods – because, at least in the case of oral medication, it always takes a few days for the serum concentration to rise in response to an increase in the dosage.

Fractionation of the daily dosage poses certain special problems in patients receiving carbamazepine. Although in healthy subjects carbamazepine has the same half-life as diphenylhydantoin[23, 40], in patients with epilepsy its serum concentrations, even where a divided dosage is employed, fluctuate markedly during the day and show a decrease at night[31]; the daily dosage of carbamazepine should therefore be prescribed in at least two, but preferably three, fractional doses.

Choice of dosage forms

In circumstances where oral medication with anti-epileptic drugs is impossible, the choice of an alternative dosage form sometimes gives rise to problems. I am thinking here of patients who are unable to swallow drugs or to absorb them properly through the gastro-intestinal tract, as may be the case, for example, after tonsillectomy, in the presence of vomiting, or where – as in status epilepticus or following a cerebral contusion or an operation on the brain – the patient is unconscious. In such instances, diphenylhydantoin and phenobarbitone can be administered intravenously, whereas the other drugs will have to be given in the form of suppositories.

Parenteral administration of diphenylhydantoin or phenobarbitone is practicable only via the intravenous route. Therapeutically effective serum concentrations cannot be achieved by means of intramuscular injections[6, 32], because these lead, at or around the site of the injection, to haemorrhages, necrosis, and crystal formation which appreciably delay absorption of the drug[33, 42]. This, at all events, has been demonstrated both clinically and experimentally in the case of diphenylhydantoin.

The use of suppositories, which any dispensing chemist can produce and which should contain the equivalent of one and a half times the oral dose, has yielded good clinical results in our experience. So far, however, only in the case of carbamazepine – and only in one patient at that – has it actually been demonstrated that adequate serum levels can be attained by the rectal route[22].

Here, once again, it is apparent that determination of the serum concentrations has a major role to play in connection with drug treatment for epilepsy[20]. It sheds valuable light on questions ranging from the patient's psychological motivation to selection of the most suitable form of administration. The importance of monitoring the serum concentrations serves in fact to emphasise that nowadays informed discussion of the treatment of epilepsy is no longer possible without some basic knowledge of the pharmacokinetics of anti-epileptic drugs.

References

1 ARNOLD, O. H.: Epilepsie. Eine statistische Studie am Material einer Epileptikerambulanz. Wien. Z. Nervenheilk. *9*, 359 (1954)

2 ASCROFT, P. B.: Traumatic epilepsy after gunshot wounds of the head. Brit. med. J. *1941/I*, 739

3 BIRKMAYER, W.: Die Behandlung der traumatischen Epilepsie. Wien. klin. Wschr. *63*, 606 (1951)

4 CREDNER, L.: Klinische und soziale Auswirkungen von Hirnschädigungen. Z. ges. Neurol. Psychiat. *126*, 721 (1930)

5 CROMBIE, D. L., CROSS, K. W., FRY, J., PINSENT, R. J. F. H., WATTS, C. A. H.: A survey of the epilepsies in general practice. Brit. med. J. *1960/II*, 416

6 DAM, M., OLESEN, V.: Intramuscular administration of phenytoin. Neurology (Minneap.) *16*, 288 (1966)

7 DOOSE, H.: Indikationen zur Einleitung und Beendigung einer antiepileptischen Therapie im Kindesalter. In Kruse, R. (Editor): Epilepsie. Therapie-Indikation – Neue Antiepileptika – Therapie-Resistenz, p. 9 (Thieme, Stuttgart 1971)

8 FAERØ, O., KASTRUP, K. W., LYKKEGAARD NIELSEN, E., MELCHIOR, J. C., THORN, I.: Successful prophylaxis of febrile convulsions with phenobarbital. Epilepsia (Amst.) *13*, 279 (1972)

9 GUÐMUNDSSON, G.: Epilepsy in Iceland. Acta neurol. scand. *43*, Suppl. 25 (1966)

10 HOFF, H., HOFF, H.: Fortschritte in der Behandlung der Epilepsie. Mschr. Psychiat. Neurol. *114*, 105 (1947)

11 JANZ, D.: Gezielte Therapie der Epilepsien. Dtsch. med. Wschr. *82*, 1158 (1957)

12 JANZ, D.: Gezielte Therapie der Epilepsien. Med. Welt (Stuttg.) *1962*, 629

13 JANZ, D.: Soziale Aspekte der Epilepsie. Psychiat. Neurol. Neurochir. (Amst.) *66*, 240 (1963)

14 JANZ, D.: Über das Suchtmoment in der Epilepsie. Nervenarzt *39*, 350 (1968)

15 JANZ, D.: Die Epilepsien. Spezielle Pathologie und Therapie (Thieme, Stuttgart 1969)

16 JANZ, D.: Indikationen zur Einleitung und Beendigung einer antiepileptischen Therapie bei Jugendlichen und Erwachsenen, loc. cit. [7], p. 15

17 JANZ, D.: Wegweisung zu einer differenzierten medikamentösen Behandlung der Epilepsien, 6th Ed. (Dtsch. Sekt. Int. Liga Epilepsie, Kork/Kehl 1972)

18 JANZ, D.: Results of long term treatment in epilepsy. Riv. Pat. nerv. ment., p. 72 (1972)

19 JANZ, D., COPER, H., CREUTZFELDT, O., DOOSE, H., DREYER, R., LATSCH, G., PENIN, H., VEITH, G.: Denkschrift Epilepsie (Boldt, Boppard 1973)

20 KUTT, H., PENRY, J. K.: Usefulness of blood levels of antiepileptic drugs. Arch. Neurol. (Chic.) *31*, 283 (1974)

21 LUND, M.: Failure to observe dosage instructions in patients with epilepsy. The short term effect of a daily dispenser. Acta neurol. scand. *49*, 295 (1973)

22 MEIJER, J.W.A., KALFF, R.: Less usual ways of administering anti-epileptic drugs. In Schneider, H., et al. (Editors): Clinical pharmacology of anti-epileptic drugs, Proc. Workshop on the determination of anti-epileptic drugs in body fluids – II, Bethel 1974 (Springer, Berlin/Heidelberg/New York 1975; printing)

23 MORSELLI, P.L., GERNA, M., MAIO, D. DE, ZANDA, G., VIANI, F., GARATTINI, S.: Pharmacokinetic studies on carbamazepine in volunteers and in epileptic patients, loc. cit. [22]

24 POPEK, K., HOLUB, V.: Klinický pokus o prevenci posttraumatické epilepsie po těžkých zraněních mozku u dětí (Clinical trial to prevent posttraumatic epilepsy after severe brain injuries in children). Čas. Lék. čes. 108, 148 (1969)

25 POPEK, K., MUSIL, F.: Klinický pokus o prevenci posttraumatické epilepsie po těžkých zraněních mozku u dospělých (Clinical trial to prevent posttraumatic epilepsy after severe brain injuries in adults). Čas. Lék. čes. 108, 133 (1969)

26 RABE, F.: Die Kombination hysterischer und epileptischer Anfälle (Springer, Berlin/Heidelberg/New York 1970)

27 RAPPORT II, R.L., PENRY, J.K.: Pharmacologic prophylaxis of posttraumatic epilepsy. A review. Epilepsia (Amst.) 13, 295 (1972)

28 RODIN, E.A.: The prognosis of patients with epilepsy (Thomas, Springfield, Ill. 1968)

29 RODIN, E.A., RIM, C.S., RENNICK, P.: The anticonvulsant effects of carbamazepine in patients with psychomotor epilepsy: results of a double-blind study. Epilepsia (Amst.) 15, 275 (1974)

30 RUSSELL, W.R., WHITTY, C.W.M.: Studies in traumatic epilepsy. I. Factors influencing the incidence of epilepsy after brain wounds. J. Neurol. Neurosurg. Psychiat. 15, 93 (1952)

31 SCHNEIDER, H., STENZEL, E.: Carbamazepin: Tageszeitlicher Verlauf des Serumspiegels unter Langzeitmedikation. Paper presented at XVIth Ann. Meet. Dtsch. Sekt. Int. Liga Epilepsie, Berlin 1974

32 SERRANO, E.E., ROYE, D.B., HAMMER, R.H., WILDER, B.J.: Plasma diphenylhydantoin values after oral and intramuscular administration of diphenylhydantoin. Neurology (Minneap.) 23, 311 (1973)

33 SERRANO, E.E., WILDER, B.J.: Intramuscular administration of diphenylhydantoin. Arch. Neurol. (Chic.) 31, 276 (1974)

34 SERVÍT, Z.: Prophylactic treatment of post-traumatic audiogenic epilepsy. Nature (Lond.) 188, 669 (1960)

35 SERVÍT, Z.: The role of subcortical acoustic centres (colliculi inferiores laminae quadr.) in seizure susceptibility to an acoustic stimulus and in symptomatology of audiogenic seizures in the rat. Physiol. bohemoslov. 9, 42 (1960)

36 SERVÍT, Z.: Preventive treatment of posttraumatic epilepsy in rats. Physiol. bohemoslov. 9, 408 (1960)

37 SERVÍT, Z.: Patofyziologické základy prevence posttraumatické epilepsie (Pathophysiological basis of the prevention of post-traumatic epilepsy). Čas. Lék. čes. 108, 129 (1969)

38 SERVÍT, Z.: Preventive treatment of posttraumatic epilepsy. Clinical effects and physiopathological interpretations. In Fusek, I., Kunc, Z. (Editors): Present limits of neurosurgery, Proc. Europ. Congr. Neurosurg., Prague 1971 (Avicenum, Prague 1972)

39 STRANDJORD, R.E., JOHANNESSEN, S.I.: One daily dose of diphenylhydantoin for patients with epilepsy. Epilepsia (Amst.) 15, 317 (1974)

40 STRANDJORD, R.E., JOHANNESSEN, S.I.: A preliminary study of serum carbamazepine levels in healthy subjects and in patients with epilepsy, loc. cit. [22]

41 VASCONCELOS, D.: Die Behandlung der Epilepsie mit Tegretal. Nervenarzt 38, 506 (1967)

42 WILENSKY, A.J., LOWDEN, J.A.: Inadequate serum levels after intramuscular administration of diphenylhydantoin. Neurology (Minneap.) 23, 318 (1973)

43 ZIELIŃSKY, J.J.: Epileptics not in treatment. Epilepsia (Amst.) 15, 203 (1974)

The long-term administration of anti-epileptic agents, with particular reference to pharmacotoxicological aspects

by R. DREYER*

Current approaches to the treatment of epilepsy

The treatment of epilepsy calls, as it always has done, for a psychosomatic approach. Any physician who in the course of his efforts at treatment forgets or neglects the implications of this statement – and, for example, places his trust solely in the use of one of the numerous anti-epileptic drugs available – cannot hope to achieve successful results in severe forms of epilepsy. My reason for emphasising this self-evident truth is that the risk of its being disregarded is particularly great at the present time when drug therapy for epilepsy is going through a period of reappraisal. We are now witnessing a phase in which purely empirical methods of treatment are being replaced to an increasing extent by an approach to therapy that is based on pharmacokinetic data, including especially the findings yielded by blood-level determinations. The epileptologist, too, has to familiarise himself with the information obtained from studying the concentration patterns of drugs or their metabolites within the various compartments of the organism as a whole. Monitoring of the blood levels should be undertaken in severe forms of epilepsy, i.e. in the forms which are usually refractory to treatment, and also in the event of complications arising – that is, if attacks recur following a fairly long seizure-free period, or if they show a marked, unaccountable increase in frequency or severity. Blood levels should likewise be determined in patients who display overt signs and symptoms of overdosage or who suddenly develop side effects in response to drugs or dosages which they have hitherto tolerated satisfactorily for some considerable time.

Monotherapy versus combined therapy

Since, in cases where combined treatment with several anti-epileptic drugs is being administered, blood-level determinations are still very difficult to perform and their results have to be assessed with extreme caution, a categorical demand has recently again been voiced that monotherapy should be employed in all forms of epilepsy. It is also argued – certainly with some degree of justification – that the interactions occurring between different drugs make it impossible to evaluate their efficacy, duration of action, or properties and give rise to serious toxicological problems.

* Nervenfacharzt, Bielefeld-Bethel, German Federal Republic.

As far back as 1952 TOMAN and TAYLOR[18] expressed the view that it was unlikely for both theoretical and practical reasons that any one single anti-epileptic drug could be developed which would exert an equally good and equally potent effect in all forms of seizures. These authors went on to say that certain types of stimuli will continue to elicit attacks unless cortical activity is suppressed to the point where only very primitive subcortical reflexes are still present. Moreover, we know today that epilepsy is not one uniform entity but a symptom-complex due to various causes and assuming various forms. Experienced epileptologists agree that epilepsy is not an hereditary disease; they know that, as in the case of diabetes, only a predisposition – which varies very considerably from one individual to another – can be inherited. The predisposition to seizures is transmitted by a multifactorial system involving several genes, additive gene effects, and threshold effects. Little is known about how these various constitutional factors become manifest or about which structures they affect in order to produce the functional disorder of epilepsy. Also to be borne in mind is the fact that the causes capable of acting as so-called irritative noxae and thus of provoking an epileptic seizure are many and varied. Hence, it can only be concluded that the pathways by which the various irritative noxae and manifold genetic factors lead to epileptic reactions must be equally multifarious.

In the light of these considerations, it seems improbable that epilepsy in all its many forms can ever be controlled by *monotherapy* with any one of the four or five recognised basic anti-epileptic agents, even where these drugs are administered in the maximum tolerated doses.

The plurality of factors which underlie epileptic reactions and which cannot be influenced by monotherapy also include genetically determined individual peculiarities in the enzyme system responsible for breaking down anti-epileptic drugs and in the epileptic's metabolism as a whole. Patients with refractory epilepsy are as a rule subject to several types of seizure and often display at the same time behavioural disorders which are to some extent a consequence of the epileptic process or of secondary neurotic developments. Furthermore, it is highly likely that the disturbance in normal brain excitability and in the balance between excitation and inhibition in nerve-cell aggregates is not due to one simple basic neuronal disorder. Complicated and refractory cases of epilepsy therefore call for treatment with several substances, especially as some drugs influence the development of excitation and some its propagation, while others probably increase membrane stability and thus affect the exchange of electrolytes.

In the course of many years' experience in the management of severe cases of epilepsy I have repeatedly had to revert to the practice of administering combined treatment with several drugs after an initial attempt at monotherapy had failed. In many cases, for example, I followed suggestions from others to give a single drug a trial in certain patients; but it almost invariably became clear after a few weeks that this approach could not bring about any decisive improvement in the patient's condition. To employ combined therapy properly, however, a physician must have wide clinical experience, he must adhere to strict guidelines, and he must give due consideration to the possibility that anti-epileptic drugs may interact in such a way as to upset each other's binding to proteins or to interfere with each other's degradation. In practice, it is impossible to predict in every case exactly what the long-term consequences of these metabolic interactions will be, especially as such interactions may be subject to considerable modification by exogenous and endogenous factors.

Prophylactic administration of additional drugs

In recent years, it has become increasingly common to administer additional drugs for prophylactic purposes. Calcium and vitamin D preparations, for instance, are prescribed in order to counter the risk of bone diseases, and also in the hope that they will at the same time raise the convulsion threshold; according to some reports (cf. CHRISTIANSEN et al.[2]), this hope has indeed been fulfilled. However, bone diseases occurring as a result of anti-epileptic medication are relatively rare; KRUSE[14] estimates the incidence to be 5% in children, and in adults it is most probably even lower. An incipient rachitogenic bone disease can be recognised in good time by performing serum determinations of alkaline phosphatase activity, as well as X-ray check-ups, twice a year; its treatment does not pose any problems, because hitherto all cases have proved responsive to vitamin D.

The possibility that primidone, for example, may give rise to the formation of megalocytes has led some therapists – in my view mistakenly – to administer vitamin B_{12} prophylactically, while the presence of low serum folic acid levels has prompted others to use drugs containing folic acid, particularly as such preparations have also been reported to improve disturbances in behaviour and performance and to reduce seizure frequency[16]. But, as long as the cause and significance of the low folic acid levels have not been completely elucidated, folic acid preparations should not be prescribed as additional medication, because folic acid can also have the effect of provoking seizures.

I have considerable doubts about the wisdom of giving epileptic patients vitamin K to prevent bleeding, vitamin E to step up their performance, and vitamin B complex to guard against possible polyneuropathy – to say nothing of the habit of prescribing vitamin B_6 to offset the psychic side effects of oral contraceptives in women subject to epilepsy. Provided patients are kept under close supervision, such polypragmatic prophylaxis is not indicated, and in many cases it is definitely harmful. The fact that we still know far too little about the metabolic interactions of specific anti-epileptic agents must not be allowed to undermine our confidence in using them for severe cases of epilepsy.

Long-term anti-epileptic medication very often arouses the fear of irreversible liver-cell damage. Recently, the finding that gamma-glutamyl transpeptidase activity may increase during long-term treatment with anticonvulsants has persuaded many physicians to resort to intensive measures designed to protect the liver. Determination of gamma-glutamyl transpeptidase – a serum enzyme which, if its values are excessive, indicates the presence of cholestasis – is an extremely sensitive test. Elevated values are in fact found in numerous disorders and diseases, including, for example, mild infections. Anti-epileptic agents very rarely cause toxic liver damage[3, 8, 20].

An increase in serum gamma-glutamyl transpeptidase activity on an isolated occasion during long-term treatment with anti-epileptic drugs is not a sign of damage to the hepatobiliary system[1], but merely reflects the presence of a microsomal enzyme-induction process and is thus of no pathological significance. Only regularly demonstrable and appreciable increases in gamma-glutamyl transpeptidase, coupled with increased serum activities of cytoplasmic and mitochondrial liver enzymes, constitute serious signs of a change in liver-cell metabolism. Such findings call for further intensive diagnostic measures and also require that careful consideration be given to the question of differential diagnosis, because they may not necessarily be attributable either solely or even primarily to the anti-epileptic medication. At all events, it is essential to carry out additional studies in an attempt to classify such enzyme findings nosologically. It should also be remembered that even substances regarded as exerting a protective effect on the liver cells may themselves impose an added strain on the liver.

The effect of intercurrent infections on medication with anti-epileptic drugs

Some 15 years ago, HUNTER[11] mentioned "internal withdrawal" of anticonvulsive agents – occurring, for example, during an infection marked by high fever – as a cause of status epilepticus. In my experience, complications of this kind in the course of long-term medication with anti-epileptics are rare. What I much more frequently encounter in patients with intercurrent infections are life-threatening toxic states in which the seizures cease altogether. The patient's relatives – as well as the treating physician and nursing staff, if they are not familiar with this type of situation – anxiously continue to administer anti-epileptic drugs even though the patient is eating hardly anything and drinking only a little fluid. Under such circumstances, metabolic conditions are completely changed, and the ability of the liver to break down drugs and of the kidneys to excrete them is impaired. Difficulty in swallowing, due to secondary toxic effects of the drugs ingested, is often marked in these patients and, coupled with a decrease in the cough reflex, may well simulate pneumonia. Parenteral administration of ample fluids and adjustment of the medication to the changed metabolic conditions usually bring about a dramatic improvement in the patient's status. It is my experience that, in the overwhelming majority of cases, infections do not give rise to any internal drug withdrawal, but lead as a rule to a considerable accumulation of non-metabolised anticonvulsive substances. It should also be remembered that an infection may cause a change in the blood-brain barrier, thus allowing increased quantities of anti-epileptic drugs to enter the central nervous system.

Once a patient has completely recovered from an intercurrent infection characterised by the type of complication I have described, either the previous medication should be resumed in good time, or else it should be readjusted on the basis of the patient's convulsive threshold as ascertained by clinical or electro-encephalographic examination; such readjustments should also take account of any new advances that have been made in the treatment of epilepsy.

West's syndrome and myoclonic-astatic epilepsy

The management of infantile spasms (West's syndrome) and of myoclonic-astatic epilepsy in small children (also referred to as "akinetic seizures" or "Lennox-Gastaut syndrome") still poses considerable difficulties despite the progress that has been achieved in this field. The use of the benzodiazepine derivatives nitrazepam, clonazepam, and diazepam often yields good results, but the percentage of relapses is high and the side effects are by no means negligible. In patients who show massive clinical signs of a convulsive tendency and marked E.E.G. changes, and who have amorphous grand mal seizures at the same time, basic drugs such as carbamazepine (®Tegretol) and primidone must be prescribed in addition. In cases where carbamazepine and primidone are combined with benzodiazepine derivatives, the administration of fairly high doses leads to impairment of the sensorium and of motor activity; this can be so pronounced that some children, who had previously been able to run about without tiring, now become quickly exhausted. The adverse effect of the treatment on alertness reduces the child's ability to concentrate and to absorb new knowledge. Moreover, even the benzodiazepine derivatives very often fail in the long run to provide the more severe cases with effective help. Nevertheless, what can be achieved in a relatively high proportion of these children is a clear-cut reduction in the frequency and severity of the seizures. In some instances the seizures occurring during the day can be successfully eliminated, but in return the nocturnal attacks often prove resistant to treatment. The children, however, surmount these nocturnal attacks much better and are as a rule surprisingly fresh on the following morning.

If the attacks associated with West's syndrome or with Lennox-Gastaut syndrome fail to show any appreciable improvement in response to the combined therapy already referred to, an attempt must be made to achieve freedom from attacks, or at least a therapeutic breakthrough, by resorting to dexamethasone or A.C.T.H. It is customary to start with dexamethasone (0.3–0.7 mg./kg. daily). The exact dosage level to be selected will depend on the tolerability of the drug and on the child's general condition, as well as on the degree to which Cushing's syndrome proves a problem. If it is impossible to elicit a decisive response with dexamethasone, A.C.T.H. should be given a trial. Some very experienced epileptologists carry out a brief course of combined treatment with both A.C.T.H. and dexamethasone. Certain children – provided they can be completely relieved of their seizures in this way for a matter of weeks or months – will make a sudden leap forward in their development, even though seizures may recur later.

80

In cases where the basic drugs, carbamazepine or primidone, singly or in combination, fail to exert an adequate effect on grand mal seizures associated with West's syndrome or Lennox-Gastaut syndrome, recourse should be had to phenobarbitone or barbexaclone. And, if none of the measures described succeeds in producing a substantial and lasting response, an attempt should be made to combat the infantile spasms or myoclonic-astatic attacks with succinimides. As a rule, it is advisable to begin with ethosuximide and to give this drug a thorough test before abandoning it. The aim should be to interrupt the automatic repetition of seizures by using high doses, even at the risk of provoking toxic symptoms for a while. If no progress can be achieved with ethosuximide, mesuximide should be used. Medication with mesuximide must be particularly carefully supervised, and a clear-cut improvement in the patient's condition is the only justification for continuing treatment with this drug for any length of time.

Recently, 2-propylvalerate (dipropylacetate) has come to be employed in the treatment of West's syndrome and Lennox-Gastaut syndrome, despite reports[15] that this drug yields poor results in such cases. MATTHES and SCHMUT-TERER[15] believe that it is virtually only in cases of primarily generalised epilepsy that 2-propylvalerate displays a therapeutic effect, and that this effect is due to an increase in the transmitter substance gamma-aminobutyric acid (GABA). It was thought that 2-propylvalerate would make it possible for the first time to provide causal treatment for the tendency to epileptic reactions. However, definite confirmation that 2-propylvalerate increases brain levels of GABA has not been obtained, and it has been found that the drug may also elicit a response in seizure patterns which are not assignable to the category of the primarily generalised epilepsies. In some cases of Lennox-Gastaut syndrome, for example, 2-propylvalerate brings about a considerable improvement in the convulsive tendency and may even relieve the patient of his attacks for fairly long periods. But it is important to bear in mind that this drug may markedly potentiate other anti-epileptic agents, particularly in children. Hence, the use of 2-propylvalerate can give rise to massive signs of overdosage in cases where the doses of the other drugs employed have not been reduced in good time.

Petit mal epilepsy

The so-called petit mal drugs continue to be indicated in cases of primarily generalised epilepsy, including in particular pyknoleptic petit mal accompanied by a generalised 3/sec. spike-and-wave activity which is most pronounced in the frontal region. Here, however, the succinimides and the oxazolidines are increasingly being thrust into the background by 2-propylvalerate. This preparation is at present to be regarded as the drug of first choice for the treatment of primarily generalised epilepsy associated with petit mal attacks. In cases where it achieves a substantial improvement or even freedom from attacks, 2-propylvalerate is far less likely to impair intellectual performance. 81

This drug is the first anti-epileptic displaying a structural formula that lacks a nitrogen atom and a ring formation. It is not only indicated in pyknoleptic petit mal attacks, but also achieves good results in pure grand mal epilepsy and in mixed epilepsies featuring grand mal and petit mal seizures. Unlike the oxazolidines and the succinimides, 2-propylvalerate shows little, if any, tendency to provoke grand mal seizures. In some cases it improves mental impairment caused by succinimides or oxazolidines, and it may also sometimes exert a beneficial influence on behavioural or psychotic disorders. As far as the drug's side effects are concerned, bleeding anomalies due to a decrease in the platelet count have been described, and the possibility that 2-propylvalerate may impair platelet formation requires further scientific investigation in a large series of patients. The risk of its giving rise to a haemorrhagic complication must at all events be borne in mind. If, for example, a patient receiving 2-propylvalerate reports a marked tendency to bruising, or if a woman complains that her periods have become considerably longer and heavier, blood coagulation tests should be carried out immediately. Another possible side effect of 2-propylvalerate is pronounced alopecia, which either stops later of its own accord or else regresses completely following withdrawal of the drug. In adults, too, the administration of 2-propylvalerate in combination with other anti-epileptics such as phenobarbitone, primidone, carbamazepine, and diphenylhydantoin may lead to potentiation effects and to severe signs of overdosage, which cannot always be avoided by readjusting the doses of these other drugs when instituting treatment with 2-propylvalerate. Reports that 2-propylvalerate may impair thyroid function and cause abnormalities to appear in the electrocardiogram call for further investigation in a representative series of patients selected as being particularly suitable for such studies.

Grand mal epilepsy

Primarily and secondarily generalised grand mal epilepsy, in cases where the attacks occur chiefly at night, is treated for the most part with diphenylhydantoin, to which small doses of phenobarbitone or primidone are added where necessary. One beneficial effect which may be expected of diphenylhydantoin is normalisation of sleep periodicity and diminution in depth of sleep[12]. When using diphenylhydantoin in fairly high doses – either alone or, in particular, in combination with other anti-epileptic agents – one should invariably keep a careful look-out for signs of cerebellar or peripherally induced ataxia. If these signs are not heeded in good time, permanent damage may result[3,4,9,10,19].

Grand mal epilepsy marked by attacks occurring after the patient gets up in the morning responds well to primidone and barbexaclone. Cases in which seizures occur both during the day and at night show a beneficial response to optimally combined therapy with diphenylhydantoin, phenobarbitone, primidone, and carbamazepine.

The guidelines I have just given for the treatment of the various forms of grand mal epilepsy are, of course, mere suggestions and should not be regarded as in any way binding. In particular, they must not be allowed to discourage the treating physician from using the entire range of basic drugs available. My own experience has led me to believe that sultiame, for example, possesses intrinsic anti-epileptic properties, i.e. that it improves a convulsive tendency not simply by perhaps delaying or diminishing the metabolism of diphenyl-hydantoin or phenobarbitone. If one uses carbamazepine, one should note that, according to the investigations of SCHNEIDER[17], this drug is metabolised relatively quickly and should therefore be administered several times daily.

Psychomotor epilepsy

Epilepsies associated with both grand mal and psychomotor seizures, as well as pure psychomotor epilepsies, are difficult to treat. Where the patient displays only psychomotor attacks, carbamazepine should be given alone to begin with, in an attempt to achieve a decisive response. If no such response is elicited, carbamazepine can then be combined with diphenylhydantoin. If this combination proves insufficient, primidone should be included in the regimen, assuming that each of the three substances – carbamazepine, diphenylhydantoin, and primidone – exerts at least a detectable effect when added to the previous drug or drugs.

Clonazepam and diazepam produce good responses in some cases of psychomotor epilepsy, especially those marked by anxiety states, abnormal sensations, and fairly pronounced autonomic nervous symptoms. Clonazepam, diazepam, and chlordiazepoxide in daily doses of 5–30 mg. are quite suitable for use in patients exhibiting these sensations and symptoms, which can be extremely tormenting. The pharmacological explanation for the success of such substances in cases of this kind is that they exert a depressant effect on the limbic system, which plays a major role in imparting to these symptoms their emotional overtones. The therapist, however, must always bear in mind that substances belonging to the benzodiazepine group have introduced for the first time into the treatment of epilepsy an addiction factor which has to be taken seriously. Patients with pronounced neurotic symptoms and psychomotor seizures should only be given benzodiazepine derivatives after the risk/benefit ratio has been carefully weighed up; what is more, strict supervision of the patient is essential during such medication.

Status epilepticus

In cases where long-term treatment for epilepsy is carried out by physicians familiar with all the advances that have been made in this field, status epilepticus occurs far less often nowadays than it used to. I have not seen any severe cases of grand mal status for a long time now. Status epilepticus lasting

83

days or weeks and proving very refractory to treatment is encountered most frequently in small children suffering from Lennox-Gastaut syndrome (myoclonic-astatic epilepsy). In such children, whose immature brain shows a remarkable degree of excitability, there is always a risk of status epilepticus developing for no detectable external or internal reason, even where nitrazepam or clonazepam in combination with carbamazepine and primidone have yielded relatively good results. The parenteral administration of diazepam in these cases is not without risk, since it may give rise to so-called tonic seizures which are extremely difficult to control. It is for this reason that most authors have gone over to using clonazepam as treatment for status epilepticus in patients with Lennox-Gastaut syndrome. If clonazepam in an intravenous dose of 1–6 mg. fails to elicit a response, paraldehyde should be given. In small children, paraldehyde is best administered via a nasal tube, for which purpose the contents of a 5 or 10 ml. ampoule for intramuscular injection can be used. Even small children are able to tolerate a dose of 5–10 g. paraldehyde.

When faced with a patient displaying grand mal status for the first time, I begin by injecting diphenylhydantoin intravenously in a dose of 250–500 mg. If this fails to produce an immediate effect, I increase the intravenous dose to 750–1,000 mg., the exact amount depending on the patient's physical condition and on the severity of the grand mal status. As every experienced epileptologist knows, the first appearance of a grand mal status is invariably to be regarded as a serious cerebral complication. Hence, the patient should be hospitalised at once in order to elucidate the cause. Since diphenylhydantoin does not exert any depressant effect on the respiratory system and does not affect the patient's state of consciousness, it is the first drug that a practising physician should use in a case of grand mal status; with other drugs there is a risk of their radically modifying the primary cerebral syndrome. In my experience, diphenylhydantoin administered by the intravenous route usually produces the rapid therapeutic effect desired. In severe cerebral complications of this kind the blood-brain barrier is probably more permeable, and at the same time high protein levels in the C.S.F. increase the uptake of diphenylhydantoin in the brain. If diphenylhydantoin nevertheless fails to interrupt the status epilepticus, diazepam should be used and then, if necessary, paraldehyde or diethylamine barbiturates (®Somnifene). Paraldehyde can be given in high doses of 10–40 g. daily.

Patients with severe grand mal status should be placed in an intensive care unit where there are facilities for recording a continuous E.E.G., monitoring the cardiovascular system, and regulating respiratory function. Proper parenteral feeding and electrolyte replacement can only be carried out in such a unit. Given these optimal conditions, it is almost invariably possible gradually to reduce the massive increase in brain excitability and to arrest the status epilepticus.

Status psychomotoricus is more common than might have been assumed on the basis of the first description of this form[5]. Among institutionalised patients suffering from very severe epilepsy, it is in fact no rarity and occurs as a rule in refractory cases with a poor prognosis. Its course should be carefully watched; if the occasion warrants it, this type of status can be interrupted by resorting to treatment with diazepam or clonazepam.

Petit mal status no longer poses any therapeutic problems today and can almost always be dramatically arrested by administering diazepam.

Conclusion

In conclusion, I should like to stress that it is the clinician himself who continues to play the decisive role in the long-term treatment of epilepsy, even though he must of course take due account of all laboratory and clinical findings, as well as of the overall situation of the individual patient. While it is extremely useful to determine the blood levels of drugs, the importance of such determinations should not be overestimated, particularly since the blood levels do not supply any direct information on the nature and extent of the effect exerted by an anti-epileptic substance on the excitable membrane. As I pointed out at the beginning of my paper, we should not allow the availability of techniques for the manipulation of the patient to blind us to his mental and emotional problems and needs.

References

1 BARTELS, H., PETERSEN, C., SCHULZE, W.: Der Einfluss von antikonvulsiver Langzeitbehandlung auf die Aktivitäten einiger in der Diagnostik hepatobiliärer Erkrankung gebräuchlicher Serumenzyme. Mschr. Kinderheilk. *112*, 674 (1974)

2 CHRISTIANSEN, C., RØDBRO, P., LUND, M.: Incidence of anticonvulsant osteomalacia and effect of vitamin D: controlled therapeutic trial. Brit. med. J. *1973/IV*, 695

3 DREYER, R.: Therapieschäden durch antiepileptische Mittel unter besonderer Berücksichtigung schwerer Nebenwirkungen an Hand der Literatur und eigener Fälle. Fortschr. Neurol. Psychiat. *27*, 401 (1959)

4 DREYER, R.: Die Behandlung der Epilepsien. In Gruhle, H.W., et al. (Editors): Psychiatrie der Gegenwart, Vol. II, p. 778 (Springer, Berlin/Göttingen/Heidelberg 1960)

5 DREYER, R.: Zur Frage des Status epilepticus mit psychomotorischen Anfällen. Ein Beitrag zum temporalen Status epilepticus und zu atypischen Dämmerzuständen und Verstimmungen. Nervenarzt *36*, 221 (1965)

6 DREYER, R.: Erfahrungen mit Tegretal. Nervenarzt *36*, 442 (1965)

7 DREYER, R.: Kleinhirndauerschädigung infolge Diphenylhydantoinintoxikation. Fortschr. Neurol. Psychiat. *34*, 224 (1966)

8 DREYER, R.: Pharmakotoxikologie der antiepileptischen Arzneimittel (Hansisches Druck- und Verlagshaus, Hamburg 1972)

9 DREYER, R.: Die Pharmakotherapie der Epilepsien. In Kisker, K.P., et al. (Editors): Psychiatrie der Gegenwart, Vol. II/Part 2, 2nd Ed., p. 713 (Springer, Berlin/Heidelberg/New York 1972)

10 DREYER, R.: Überlegungen und Beobachtungen zur Pharmakotoxikologie der antiepileptischen Arzneimittel. Nervenarzt *45*, 115 (1974)

11 HUNTER, R.A.: Status epilepticus. History, incidence and problems. Epilepsia (Amst.) *1*, 162 (1959/60)

12 Jovanović, U.J.: Die sich aus dem natürlichen Schlaf der Epileptiker ergebenden therapeutischen Konsequenzen. Nervenarzt *39*, 199 (1968)

13 Kruse, R.: Osteopathien bei antiepileptischer Langzeittherapie (Vorläufige Mitteilung). Mschr. Kinderheilk. *116*, 378 (1968)

14 Kruse, R.: Osteopathien unter antiepileptischer Langzeittherapie. Paper presented at XVIth Ann. Meet. Dtsch. Sekt. Int. Liga Epilepsie, Berlin 1974

15 Matthes, A., Schmutterer, J.: Klinische Erfahrungen mit einem neuen Antiepileptikum: Dipropylessigsäure. Dtsch. med. Wschr. *96*, 63 (1971)

16 Neubauer, C.: Mental deterioration in epilepsy due to folate deficiency. Brit. med. J. *1970/II*, 759

17 Schneider, H.: Serum levels of carbamazepine in in-patients under various drug regimes. In Schneider, H., et al. (Editors): Clinical pharmacology of anti-epileptic drugs, Proc. Workshop on the determination of anti-epileptic drugs in body fluids – II, Bethel 1974 (Springer, Berlin/Heidelberg/New York 1975; printing)

18 Toman, J.E.P., Taylor, J.D.: Mechanism of action and metabolism of anticonvulsants. Epilepsia (Boston) *1*, 31 (1952)

19 Utterback, R.A.: Parenchymatous cerebellar degeneration complicating diphenylhydantoin (Dilantin) therapy. Arch. Neurol. Psychiat. (Chic.) *80*, 180 (1958); abstract of paper

20 Ziegler, H.-K., Sinazadeh, M.: Antiepileptika und Leberschaden. J. Neurol. (Berlin) *208*, 207 (1975)

Discussion

P. KIELHOLZ: I should like to thank Dr. JANZ most warmly for the extremely clear paper he has presented and especially for having given us some important practical tips on how to cope with the problems of treatment for epilepsy. There is one major therapeutic problem, however, to which he made no reference, namely, that of epileptic mood disorders. Not only do these disorders impose a tremendous burden on the patient himself, as well as on his family and on others with whom he comes in contact, but they are also the factor most often necessitating the admission of epileptic patients to a psychiatric hospital. In a large number of cases, they chiefly take the form of disturbances which are marked by dysphoria and irritability or by depression, and which may occur not only before and after paroxysms but also during the intervals between attacks. Our own experience in the treatment of such cases suggests that one should first prescribe ®Tegretol (carbamazepine), and that – if this fails to eliminate the disorders – one should resort to an antidepressant in addition. But I'd be interested to hear from Dr. JANZ how he treats these epileptic mood disorders, which, since they also prove so tormenting for those who have to put up with the patient, constitute a very serious practical problem.

M. PARSONAGE: I, too, was greatly interested in Dr. JANZ's remarks, and I would agree that the confidence we used to have in the treatment of epilepsy may have become a little undermined as a result of the new knowledge that has been acquired, especially in the field of pharmacokinetics, and as a result of our increasing awareness of short-term and long-term side effects. On the other hand, I would also agree that some of our principles still retain their validity, such as, for example, the use of ethosuximide in the treatment of absences. Of course, since the introduction of sodium dipropylacetate we may have to revise our thinking in this respect, because this agent seems to have a much broader spectrum of action. It is, as far as I can recall, the first drug that has proved to be effective both against various types of absence and against generalised tonic-clonic attacks. It also seems to act well in some cases where there is evidence of associated brain damage.

While I largely share Dr. JANZ's opinion about the use of hydantoins and barbiturates, I think that, owing to the increasing interest which is being taken in the adverse effects of these agents, some of us now have doubts about employing them in the same carefree way that we used to do. For example, clinical psychologists are always telling us nowadays about the dulling effects of barbiturates on intellectual function, and the paediatricians draw attention to the adverse effects of phenobarbitone in children. Diphenylhydantoin, too, has been widely studied in relation to its adverse effects, perhaps more so than any other drug – in fact, so much so that some of us have begun to wonder if we should use the drug at all. Recently I have seen reports indicating that the long-term administration of diphenylhydantoin – and possibly also of other anti-epileptic drugs – may lead to a gradual coarsening of facial features due to an effect on connective tissue.

I also agree entirely with what Dr. JANZ had to say about the value of Tegretol. I have long taken the view that this is the drug of first choice in the treatment of complex partial seizures. It seems to me to be better than any other drug we have in this context, even though it may not be ideal; and I should like to add that, so far, I have not been impressed by the results of treatment with sodium dipropylacetate in seizures of this kind. I was also interested in Dr. JANZ's remarks about the practical problems that one encounters in treating epilepsy. I personally believe that the most important single variable is the individual patient's personality and attitude to treatment. It has been my experience that, if the patients are unwilling to cooperate, there is really not a great deal that we can do for them. This may sound a little pessimistic, but it underlines the necessity for securing the cooperation of our patients. It takes time, of course, to achieve this cooperation, but it is time well spent. I sometimes find

87

this difficult to get across to those we are trying to train in the field of epilepsy, and I wonder what the experience of others has been in this connection.

Another point of interest raised by Dr. JANZ in his paper was the use of blood-level determinations of anti-epileptic drugs. These determinations have made it possible for us to revise our dosage schedules and to minimise the harmful effects of drug interactions. The realisation that many patients can be effectively treated with a twice-daily dosage regimen has marked a very useful step forward which has been greatly welcomed by many sufferers from epilepsy. As regards the avoidance of drug inter-actions, it has become my practice now to make every endeavour to secure control of seizures with a single drug or with two drugs at the most. In my opinion there has been an all too common tendency not only to resort to multi-drug therapy but also to add psychotropic drugs as well with the aim of curing so-called psychological symp-toms. It should, however, be borne in mind that these psychological symptoms may in fact be due to the effects of the anti-epileptic therapy itself.

Concerning the question of patients not seeking treatment, my impression is that, in England at all events, more patients are nowadays being referred for treatment than ever before. A more commonly encountered difficulty, in my experience, is the insti-tution of inadequate treatment, i.e. treatment either with the wrong drug or with the right drug in the wrong dosage.

The problem of when treatment should be started was referred to. This should not usually be a matter of great difficulty, although it may be so in certain cases, and I would fully agree with Dr. JANZ that we are treating patients with epilepsy and not those with E.E.G. abnormalities. Prophylactic treatment is obviously something to be considered very seriously in high-risk cases such as seizures associated with fever, although it seems that paediatricians, in England at least, still disagree as to what form this prophylaxis should take. My own feeling is that Dr. JANZ was perfectly right to say that the only real indication for the institution of anti-epileptic therapy is the existence of chronic epilepsy. This is sometimes forgotten. Once treatment has been instituted, it is of paramount importance that it be continued under properly con-trolled conditions. Our problem in England is that, while patients are being referred to us at quite an early stage of their illness, we unfortunately lack sufficient staff to give them the kind of expert and continued care they certainly ought to be having.

With regard to the parenteral administration of anti-epileptic drugs, it has been well established that there are difficulties in using diphenylhydantoin in this way. How-ever, in England diazepam by the parenteral route is now being widely used for the treatment of generalised convulsive status, both in hospital and in general practice. On the other hand, I have no personal experience in the administration of anti-epileptic drugs in the form of suppositories.

In conclusion, I think we would all agree that the introduction of methods for de-termining the serum levels of anti-epileptic drugs has undoubtedly been a major ad-vance. Nevertheless, it is essential that we use these techniques with great care and discrimination, and that we regard them as an aid, but not as a short-cut, to effective treatment. Indeed, they can only be regarded as a part of the comprehensive approach which is so necessary in the management of all cases of epilepsy.

M. BONDUELLE: I have a few remarks to add which merely endorse and supplement those that Dr. PARSONAGE has just made. But, before I go any further, may I say how deeply impressed I was by the quality of the paper Dr. JANZ presented. What he ex-pounded in this paper was not only good therapeutics but also good medicine. Now for the few points I wanted to raise:

I must say that I was astonished – as Dr. PARSONAGE seems to have been too – at the percentages Dr. JANZ quoted for epileptic subjects receiving no treatment at all. I don't think the figures can be as high as that in France. Many of the epileptics we see are cases referred to us by general practitioners as being in need of more suitable therapy, and in such cases we do indeed often find that the treatment they have been receiving was either inappropriate or badly conducted. I have also been struck by the fact that epileptics tend to be dutiful and faithful patients; in this respect they contrast with many of the patients suffering from other types of neurological disorder – as a study which I am currently engaged upon in cases of narcolepsy serves to prove. Generally speaking, it is possible to keep a very close check-up on one's epileptic patients, because they return regularly for their consultations. Though they may frequently also be subject to behavioural disturbances, they nevertheless carry out their treatment most conscientiously; and those who might be inclined not to do so are watched over, often very attentively, by members of their family.

I don't think one should necessarily be discouraged if such a patient has a seizure. If and when a patient returns to me before the date of his next appointment because he has had an intervening attack, I always ask him whether he had forgotten or been careless about his treatment, and I find that this is almost invariably the explanation. He tells me that he had mislaid his prescription, that he had been travelling and forgotten to take his tablets with him, or simply that he hadn't been taking them regularly as instructed. I now seize the opportunity to give him a little lecture on the necessity for taking his medicine with unfailing regularity. The fact that he has had a seizure is then not a reason for disappointment but, on the contrary, an encouragement for the patient to stick to his treatment.

Now just a couple of points of detail concerning the conduct of treatment. Firstly, it has long – if not always – been my practice to make every attempt to reduce the number of doses to a minimum, as advocated by Dr. JANZ; if possible, I prescribe only one dose per day, and at the most two. If only for psychological reasons, it is important that the patient should not have to take several doses in the course of the day. Secondly, with regard to treatment with carbamazepine, it is certain that – as has already been stated and reiterated at this symposium, and as I, too, pointed out in my earliest reports on this drug – carbamazepine occupies a privileged place in the management of psychomotor seizures. But its use should not be confined to this indication, because it is, for example, also eminently suitable for the treatment of grand mal and partial motor seizures.

Finally, a word or two on the subject of "prophylactic" treatment in patients convalescing from neurosurgical operations. In France, and no doubt in most other countries as well, the patient leaves the neurosurgical department armed with a standard prescription for 200 mg. phenobarbitone daily, which is obviously an excessive dose. In this connection, I should like to raise the question whether it is in fact necessary to prescribe prophylactic medication in each and every one of these patients recovering from neurosurgery.

L. MARQUES-ASSIS: May I take this opportunity of reporting briefly on my experience with Tegretol in the treatment of epilepsy in Brazil. The Epilepsy Department at the São Paulo Clinical Hospital is responsible for the care of epileptic patients living not only in São Paulo itself, but also in a wide area around the town. The total population of this region is over ten million. The number of epileptic patients registered in the department amounts to approximately 10,000. Each month we see about 70 new cases and 450 old ones. Some of our patients have been in our care for more than ten years. Epileptics displaying chiefly mental disorders are not treated by us but are referred to the psychiatric clinic.

As in other parts of the world, in São Paulo, too, wide use is made of phenobarbitone and diphenylhydantoin in cases of epilepsy. In our department recourse is often had to combined therapy. In fact, monotherapy with anti-epileptic drugs is employed in only 6% of our patients; in 49% of cases barbiturates are given in association with diphenylhydantoin.

Following its introduction in Brazil, Tegretol rapidly acquired for itself an important place in the management of epilepsy. It is now being used in 20% of our patients (as monotherapy in 10% of them and in combination with other drugs in 90%).

In one series of 40 patients treated with Tegretol, 29% had primarily generalised convulsions and 42% secondarily generalised convulsions developing from focal discharges. In 58% of cases, focal manifestations were present alone or in association with convulsions. Headache was a major feature in 13% of cases. The duration of illness ranged from three months to 29 years, and the time of observation was 1–14 years. Examination of the C.S.F. yielded normal findings in all cases. The E.E.G. tracings were normal in 20% of the patients; focal abnormalities were found in 70% and diffuse abnormalities in 10%. It is interesting to note that 83% of the focal abnormalities were in the temporal-lobe region.

As regards the results obtained with Tegretol, the response was classified as good (reduction of 50% or more in the frequency of seizures) in 62% of the patients, and a total remission of symptoms was obtained in 30%. In only 8% of cases did the patients' condition deteriorate under treatment with the drug. No side effects of any importance were observed.

Increasing use is now being made of Tegretol in our department. In the medical treatment of adult epileptics, Tegretol ranks at present as our drug of third choice, after barbiturates and hydantoins. In the management of temporal-lobe epilepsies, however, in which its anticonvulsive efficacy has been corroborated by a number of authors, Tegretol plays an even bigger role.

In conclusion, may I draw attention to one indication for Tegretol that is becoming increasingly common in our department – namely, headache presenting as the principal symptom in epileptics. We have found that Tegretol yields good results in these cases of paroxysmal or continuous headache associated with epilepsy.

G. NISSEN: With reference to the various problems arising in the management of epilepsy, Dr. JANZ stressed among other things the necessity for providing the patient with adequate information on the treatment he is receiving. I would like to add that not only adult patients but also children as well can and should be given the benefit of such information and advice. In this way, even children who are not yet old enough to attend school can be successfully motivated to take their drugs regularly and, indeed, to carry out one's instructions more reliably than do certain parents. We must not forget that unfortunately there are still some kindergarten and school teachers – and even a few doctors – who persuade parents either to reduce the doses of drugs that have been prescribed for their children or to discontinue the treatment altogether.

Regarding the medication itself, we now have such a variety of anticonvulsive agents at our disposal that we can pick and choose our drugs to suit the basic mood of the epileptic child we are treating. In children lacking in drive, for example, we obtain good results with Tegretol, whereas in those exhibiting excessive drive we give preference to anticonvulsants exerting a mild sedative action.

In connection with drug treatment for children, I should like to conclude with an appeal to the pharmaceutical industry. I suggest that, when dosage forms are being developed for new preparations, as many different forms as possible should be produced for children, including young children in particular, and that drugs already on the market should be suitably modified for paediatric use. Tablets, for instance, should be scored so that they can more easily be halved or quartered. The aroma of liquid dosage forms should be tested to ensure that their taste appeals to children. I know of a succinimide preparation, for example, which many children refused to take because it had an excessively strong aroma of the type favoured in America. Sometimes it is a good idea to give the child, while it is actually in the surgery, a sample of the medicine to taste, or to show the parents how to break the tablets into equal fractions. Quite a number of subsequent telephone enquiries from parents can thus be avoided.

H. REISNER: I have two questions for you, Dr. JANZ, but before asking them I should like to endorse most strongly what you said in the introduction to your paper. You were absolutely correct in pointing out that until a few years ago we thought we knew well nigh all there was to know about the treatment of epilepsy. You have now drawn our attention to the many problems that still confront us in this field, and rightly so. During the last 20 years I have been successively responsible for three large neurological clinics; when I was younger, I used to seize upon new findings obtained in the treatment of epilepsy and try to put them immediately into practice in the clinic, but these attempts were seldom rewarded with success. I have since become much more cautious. It's not enough simply to believe in the therapeutic efficacy of a given drug; one also has to have a thorough knowledge of it. There's a certain similarity here with the use of antiparkinsonian agents and probably of psychopharmaceuticals too, inasmuch as one doesn't really get to know drugs of this type until and unless one has been employing them for some considerable time.

Now I come to the two questions I wanted to ask. Firstly, I am aware of the fact that the use of carbamazepine is particularly justified in psychomotor attacks; and, from what you have said, Dr. Janz, it would seem that the same also applies to Jacksonian epilepsy. Dr. Rett will, I expect, recall the discussion we had a few years ago in which I expressed doubts as to the therapeutic effect of carbamazepine in grand mal. I should now like to hear your views on this point, Dr. Janz; and I should perhaps add that I for my part have meanwhile somewhat revised my opinion in this connection. Secondly, Dr. Janz, you stated – quite rightly as I see it – that not every patient who has once had a grand mal attack, or even status epilepticus, should immediately be placed on long-term anti-epileptic medication. This is something that I don't do either. I gather that the only form of epilepsy which you would regard as an absolute indication for drug therapy is chronic epilepsy, irrespective of its origin. You defined chronic epilepsy as "the repeated occurrence of attacks at fairly frequent intervals". May I ask precisely what you understand by "fairly frequent intervals"?

I also have a query for Dr. Dreyer. His plea in favour of combined therapy does, I think, certainly deserve to be upheld. Personally, however, I only believe in free combinations, i.e. in the use of single substances that I prescribe in combinations of my own choosing, as opposed to combined preparations marketed by the pharmaceutical companies. On the other hand, I feel that there are certain types of case in which one can manage satisfactorily with only one drug and that such monotherapy is in fact the ideal solution. As regards combined therapy, Dr. Dreyer, would you agree with me that preference should invariably be given to free combinations?

I should also like to comment on the question of fever and epilepsy which Dr. Dreyer touched upon in his paper. As most of us will recall, there was a time when induced pyrexia used to be employed as a form of treatment for epilepsy. When general paralysis of the insane was still quite a common disease (curiously enough, we are now once again seeing more cases of this kind), it was the practice at our clinic in Vienna to make use of chronic epileptics as hosts for strains of malarial parasites, and in such patients an improvement in the epileptic attacks was sometimes observed. I think that in epileptics one should therefore beware of combating fever too vigorously, particularly with high doses of penicillin. Every now and again I come across cases in which an epileptic patient suffering from a relatively mild intercurrent infection has been given penicillin in a dosage of ten million units twice daily; I consider this utterly nonsensical. In my experience, such treatment is liable to result in status epilepticus – which explains why, in contrast to you, Dr. Dreyer, I do in fact even sometimes encounter grand mal status in the presence of infections.

One last question, Dr. Dreyer: don't you ever use clomethiazole in the treatment of status epilepticus?

J. Kiffin Penry: I would like to disagree slightly with Dr. Janz on the question of treating milder forms of epilepsy. He advocates that only patients with recurrent epilepsy should be treated. But every chronic epileptic patient had at one time only one seizure. Rodin* has shown that the longer the duration of the illness, the poorer the

---

* Rodin, E. A.: The prognosis of patients with epilepsy (Thomas, Springfield, Ill. 1968)

prognosis. There is a lot of other information, both experimental and clinical, to support this. For example, the very nice epidemiological surveys of KURLAND* and, later, of HAUSER and KURLAND** show that the average lapse of time between the first manifestation of epilepsy – that is, the first seizure – and definitive diagnosis and treatment is about three years. We have had the same experience with absence seizures in the State of Virginia. These seizures are not treated, because it is believed that only severe and chronic cases require therapy. It is, of course, true that a great deal of harm can be done if you treat every patient who has had a seizure, because there are certainly many who don't require treatment. But we need to find some way of detecting at an early stage those patients who are going to have recurrent seizures. In a study of 100 adults who had had a single seizure, JOHNSON et al.*** carried out complete neurological evaluations, including E.E.G., spinal taps, skull X-rays, etc., and found no abnormalities. These patients were then followed for one year, and 40% of them had a second seizure. If only we could detect and predict this 40%, we would be able to institute preventive treatment in good time. A recent study by WASTERLAIN and PLUM**** at Cornell University has shown that in animals D.N.A. levels are reduced by recurrent seizures. MCINTYRE and GODDARD***** at Dalhousie University in Nova Scotia have demonstrated in studies on kindling phenomena that the greater the number of seizures, the lower the convulsive threshold. I was reminded of this point today when Dr. KOELLA described his experiments showing that after-discharge was increased later on. As physicians, therefore, we must pay careful attention to the preventive aspect, and at the same time look for better predictors. Admittedly, the fact that 40% of patients have a second seizure doesn't give us the right to make the other 60% sick on anticonvulsants, but we must find ways of detecting the patients who are going to have recurrent seizures.

With regard to the treatment of subclinical seizures, I think we should consider carefully what is meant by "subclinical". DOOSE and GERKEN****** have advocated treating the relatives of children with absences who have generalised spike-and-wave discharges, and we have published a series of papers******* showing that these generalised spike-and-wave discharges are really not subclinical. If you measure simple reaction time in these cases, you will find that it is impaired. We have also shown

---

* KURLAND, L.T.: The incidence and prevalence of convulsive disorders in a small urban community. Epilepsia (Amst.) 1, 143 (1959)

** HAUSER, W.A., KURLAND, L.T.: The epidemiology of epilepsy in Rochester, Minnesota, 1935 through 1967. Epilepsia 16, 1 (1975)

*** JOHNSON, L.C., DeBOLT, W.L., LONG, M.T., Ross, J.J., SASSIN, J.F., ARTHUR, R.J., WALTER, R.D.: Diagnostic factors in adult males following initial seizures. A three-year follow-up. Arch. Neurol. (Chic.) 27, 193 (1972)

**** WASTERLAIN, C.G., PLUM, F.: Vulnerability of developing rat brain to electroconvulsive seizures. Arch. Neurol. (Chic.) 29, 38 (1973)

***** MCINTYRE, D.C., GODDARD, G.V.: Transfer, interference and spontaneous recovery of convulsions kindled from the rat amygdala. Electroenceph. clin. Neurophysiol. 35, 533 (1973)

****** DOOSE, H., GERKEN, H.: Possibilities and limitations of epilepsy prevention in siblings of epileptic children. In Parsonage, M.J. (Editor): Prevention of epilepsy and its consequences, Proc. Vth Europ. Symp. Epilepsy, London 1972, p. 32 (International Bureau for Epilepsy, London 1973)

******* GOODE, D.J., PENRY, J.K., DREIFUSS, F.E.: Effects of paroxysmal spike-wave on continuous visual-motor performance. Epilepsia (Amst.) 11, 241 (1970)

PORTER, R.J., PENRY, J.K., DREIFUSS, F.E.: Responsiveness at the onset of spike-wave bursts. Electroenceph. clin. Neurophysiol. 34, 239 (1973)

BROWNE, T.R., PENRY, J.K., PORTER, R.J., DREIFUSS, F.E.: Responsiveness before, during, and after spike-wave paroxysms. Neurology (Minneap.) 24, 659 (1974)

that, if you eliminate the very brief bursts of E.E.G. activity in these children, you can improve their performance at school. Hence, I think it's wrong to call these cases of epilepsy "subclinical", because measurable effects of the illness can in fact be found. If we can document these effects in specific types of seizure, we shall be in a position to institute treatment at an earlier stage and thus to improve the prognosis.

W. GRÜTER: You stated in your paper, Dr. JANZ, that drug treatment was not indicated in cases where specific electro-encephalographic changes are unaccompanied by any epileptic manifestations. In this connection you were thinking simply of prophylactic medication designed to prevent attacks, and I am sure we would all agree with you on this point. From various accounts that have been published, however, and from my own experience too, it would seem to be precisely in cases of this kind that one encounters a particularly high incidence of behavioural abnormalities and psychic changes, including mood disorders, of the type to which Dr. KIELHOLZ referred at the beginning of this discussion. Often, in fact, it is these psychic changes which prompt the patient to consult a doctor in the first place. Would you agree with me, Dr. JANZ, that these patients certainly do require anticonvulsive medication – preferably with a drug like Tegretol – and that the need for medication is all the greater the more closely the psychic disturbances resemble those which epileptics are known to exhibit?

C. GROH: Among the problems referred to by Dr. JANZ in his paper was that of motivation to seek treatment, and this question of motivation undoubtedly has an important bearing on the success or failure of therapy. In the case of children the situation is somewhat different, inasmuch as here it is the parents who as onlookers experience the full impact of the seizures and who are therefore as a rule strongly motivated to seek treatment for their child. But, where the child has had only one attack, the doctor will often be well advised to try and reassure the parents and to explain to them that he does not regard this one attack as justification for instituting long-term therapy.

Dr. DREYER, may I ask whether 2-propylvalerate can, as you claimed in your paper, really be considered the drug of first choice in pyknoleptic petit mal? Although I have only limited experience of this compound, it is my impression that in patients with pyknoleptic petit mal the succinimides produce freedom from attacks in a higher percentage of cases.

Finally, I have a brief remark to make on the subject of prophylactic treatment designed to prevent grand mal seizures in myoclonic-astatic petit mal and myoclonic petit mal in adolescents. I should like to question the wisdom of employing carbamazepine in this indication, because – although I cannot quote any statistics – I have quite often found that, when prescribed for the prevention of grand mal seizures, carbamazepine caused either an aggravation or a recurrence of petit mal attacks.

H. REMSCHMIDT: In his paper, Dr. JANZ mentioned that anti-epileptic medication, as a routine form of prophylaxis, could be considered following severe cerebral trauma. In this connection, one problem which has lately been preoccupying us is that of the precise criteria on which one should base one's decision to *discontinue* such prophylactic medication in patients with cerebral trauma, including penetrating injuries.

Like others who have already contributed to this discussion, I too attach great importance to the question of motivation. But it is extremely difficult to lay down any simple guidelines as to how patients can best be motivated. We have made a special study of this problem with reference to epileptic children, for which purpose we have carried out detailed investigations that also took account of the family situation and of the personality structure of the parents. One finding to emerge from this study was that the parents' attitude and personality structure have a very decisive influence on motivation. We also actually discovered a correlation between, on the one hand, certain psychic peculiarities of the children as reported by the parents and, on the other hand, corresponding personality traits in the parents themselves. I am afraid that in the realm of child-parent relationships we have hitherto achieved far less progress than in the pharmacological field. If one were to do a sort of time-and-motion study on the treatment of epilepsy, I am sure one would find that two-thirds to three-quarters of our time is devoted to problems of psychological guidance in the broadest sense of the term, despite the fact that we may have succeeded in establishing quite a good or even an optimum drug regimen for the patient.

A. RETT: I'd like to ask Dr. JANZ whether his statement that chronic epilepsy is the only absolute indication for drug therapy also applies to children. I believe that in children in particular a so-called "first fit" is often like the tip of an iceberg. When one proceeds to take down the case history after a "first fit", it is by no means unusual to discover that in fact attacks have already occurred on previous occasions. What approach should we therefore adopt when confronted with a child who has had one of these "first fits"? The answer, I suggest, is that we should pay due attention to the attitude of the family (parents vary greatly in their reactions, some either ignoring or making light of the attack, and others lapsing into what almost amounts to an anxiety neurosis), and that we should also examine the child's overall situation, i.e. its behaviour, its psychology, its general performance, and especially its E.E.G. recordings. If this procedure is followed, it will be found that there are some cases in which one can certainly afford to postpone treatment, others in which one should preferably not delay treatment, and, finally, some in which it would be absolutely wrong to wait a moment longer.

Another question arising in this connection is the frequency with which attacks are apt to occur in the future. Dr. JANZ has quoted findings from the British study reported by CROMBIE et al. which showed that only one out of every eight patients with so-called first fits is likely to suffer any subsequent attacks. Among his own patients with first fits, Dr. JANZ found that some 50% experienced further attacks over a period of 4–8 years. It is my opinion, however, that – at least in the case of children – one has to reckon with the possibility of an even longer period between the first fit and subsequent recurrences. We, for example, have seen many children who had their first fit at the age of one or two years, but whose second fit did not occur until they were 11 or perhaps even 15 years of age; some of them, moreover, then developed manifest epilepsy. Even in cases where the epilepsy did not assume a chronic form, quite a few of these children who had had fits at an early age – often on only one or two occasions – later became problem patients who frequently required treatment for behavioural disorders.

Dr. DREYER referred in his paper to the fact that some therapists are in the habit of administering folic acid preparations in addition to anti-epileptic medication. Among our own patients, we have found that folic acid neither provokes seizures nor has the effect of improving them. Could you perhaps tell us, Dr. DREYER, in what dosage these folic acid drugs are usually given?

Dr. DREYER also mentioned the repercussions produced by intercurrent infections. In this connection, I should like to say that we have seldom encountered toxic states as an accompaniment to acutely febrile infections in patients receiving anticonvulsive therapy. I think it is simpler for the paediatrician if he can treat both the epilepsy and the infection simultaneously. Whereas less experienced general practitioners quite often abruptly withdraw anti-epileptic medication if and when an infection occurs, we find that – at any rate in some cases – the problem of whether or not to interrupt anti-epileptic medication tends to arise, not when the infection is at its height, but during the subsequent phase of post-infective exhaustion – i.e. after subsidence of the fever, which often occurs very rapidly. Assuming that the anti-epileptic treatment has in fact been withdrawn, the question as to when it should be resumed is certainly a difficult one to answer.

D. JANZ: Since I'm afraid there isn't time enough for me to deal with all the comments arising from my paper, and, since the remarks made by Dr. PARSONAGE, Dr. BONDUELLE, and Dr. REISNER largely confirmed what I had already said, I propose now to confine myself chiefly to answering the concrete questions that have been asked.

One of the questions you put to me, Dr. REISNER, was whether, in the light of my own experience, I think that carbamazepine is effective against grand mal attacks. In 1967 VASCONCELOS from our clinic published a report* on the effect of carbamazepine in 125 of our own cases; in response to this drug, 47% of the patients with grand mal became free from attacks. I therefore believe that the effectiveness of carbamazepine against grand mal seizures can be taken as proven. Whether it is more effective or less effective than other drugs indicated in grand mal, however, is a question I cannot answer, because I haven't carried out any comparative studies.

Another question which not only you, Dr. REISNER, but also Dr. RETT raised was that of deciding, by reference to the time elapsing between a first fit and subsequent fits, whether or not treatment should be instituted in cases of what is sometimes referred to as "oligo-epilepsy", i.e. cases in which the attacks are separated by seizure-free intervals lasting several years. You will, I am sure, appreciate that I neither wish to, nor am able to, quote any absolute figures in this context; any attempt to do this might easily be misinterpreted as suggesting that a sort of rule of thumb exists based on the number of years intervening between one fit and the next. All I can say is that whether or not treatment is in fact indicated has to be decided from patient to patient in the light of the overall circumstances of the case.

Also to some extent related with this whole problem was the question posed by Dr. REMSCHMIDT as to when and under what conditions one should discontinue anti-epileptic medication. This, unfortunately, is a question about which nothing more is known than was reported by JUUL-JENSEN** several years ago. Dr. REMSCHMIDT, however, was referring specifically to the withdrawal of anti-epileptic drugs administered prophylactically following cerebral trauma. The Czechoslovak authors whose studies I briefly mentioned in my paper discontinue such medication after two years and – so far as one can gather from their reports – they have encountered no relapses after this two-year period. In my paper, however, I added that RAPPORT and PENRY had expressed doubts about the methodology employed in these Czechoslovak studies, and I must admit that I share their misgivings on this score.

Now I come to what was probably the most interesting question of all. This question, raised by Dr. KIELHOLZ and also touched upon by Dr. NISSEN and Dr. GRÜTER, concerns treatment for epileptic mood disorders or, as I would prefer to term them, mood disorders associated with epilepsy. I may not perhaps be quite competent to discuss this problem, because, as you know, I am a neurologist and, as such, I do not often see epileptic patients suffering from mood disorders that are so pronounced as to require psychiatric treatment. What I feel we are lacking in this connection is first and foremost a phenomenological classification of the mood disorders encountered in cases of epilepsy. So far as I know, no investigations have yet been carried out to determine the frequency of mood disorders in the various forms of epilepsy or to establish under precisely what circumstances they are apt to arise. These are therefore questions to which no general answers can be given; instead, one can only make statements about certain individual, specifically defined, mood disorders. I myself, for example, have found that mood disorders are definitely liable to occur in connection with anti-epileptic medication, e.g. in the presence of very high phenobarbitone levels or in patients receiving diphenylhydantoin as treatment for generalised epilepsy. It is also known that ethosuximide may give rise to mood disorders and that these ethosuximide-induced disorders are probably just about the most difficult of all

---

* VASCONCELOS, D.: Die Behandlung der Epilepsie mit Tegretal. Nervenarzt *38*, 506 (1967)

** JUUL-JENSEN, P.: Frequency of recurrence after discontinuance of anticonvulsant therapy in patients with epileptic seizures. A new follow-up study after 5 years. Epilepsia (Amst.) *9*, 11 (1968)

to treat. If you were to ask me, Dr. KIELHOLZ, to what I ascribe the favourable response to carbamazepine that you yourself have observed in mood disorders associated with epilepsy, I would suggest as one possible explanation the results of pharmacokinetic studies which have shown that the addition of carbamazepine to anti-epileptic treatment with phenobarbitone or diphenylhydantoin has the effect of lowering the serum concentrations of these drugs. The beneficial influence which sodium dipropylacetate (®Ergenyl) or carbamazepine have been observed to exert on behavioural disturbances or even on psychotic symptoms might, as Dr. PARSONAGE has already implied, also have been due simply to the fact that, when treatment with one of these two preparations was instituted, the other anti-epileptic drugs – which had actually been responsible for the psychic changes – were withdrawn. In view of the two possible interpretations I have just mentioned, we must realise that the psychotropic effect of a drug such as carbamazepine may conceivably be an indirect one, i.e. it may perhaps merely be due to a reduction in the activity of other drugs or to their elimination from the regimen.

R. DREYER: To answer the first of the three questions you asked me, Dr. REISNER, I would say that it is of course up to the treating physician, and to him alone, to decide what form of combined therapy may be required and how it can best be adapted to the patient's individual needs. Like you, I consider it wrong to employ combined preparations in rigid dosage schedules.

Regarding the question of intercurrent febrile infections in epileptic patients, I know that general practitioners tend to withdraw all anti-epileptic drugs at once in the event of any complications. I make it a rule to warn parents and, of course, all patients against this practice. The cases to which I was referring in my paper involved severe forms of epilepsy. In an institute responsible for the care of 2,000 epileptics, circumstances repeatedly arise in which a doctor, faced with the problem of a feverish patient, decides – albeit with some trepidation – to continue the anti-epileptic medication, because he knows what a serious form status epilepticus is liable to take in a case of this kind. This continuation of the medication then leads to severe intoxication. Dr. REISNER has uttered a warning against resorting overhastily to large doses of penicillin in patients with febrile infections. I know that the use of penicillin involves a considerable risk of provoking epilepsy. But, as a rule, this hazard arises only when the penicillin comes into direct contact with the meninges or with the surface of the brain; there is seldom any danger when it is given orally or intravenously.

Your third question, Dr. REISNER, was whether we also use clomethiazole. Though the answer is "yes", I must add that – bearing in mind its possible effects on respiration and the circulation – I personally do not consider this drug to be as harmless as other therapists apparently do.

With reference to your query regarding 2-propylvalerate, Dr. GROH, I can only repeat that, in the light of my extensive experience with this compound over a period of some five years, I regard it as the drug of first choice in pyknoleptic petit mal, i.e. in classic forms of epilepsy characterised by 3/sec. spike-and-wave activity.

So far as prophylactic treatment for grand mal in cases of myoclonic-astatic epilepsy is concerned, it is of course once again experience that counts. I'm sure you will agree that in a thirty-minute paper it is impossible to tackle all the relevant problems in detail. I should therefore like to add at this point that in patients showing a marked susceptibility to grand mal, as also reflected to some extent in their E.E.G. tracings, 2-propylvalerate or primidone deserves preference. But in my experience carbamazepine, too, affords effective protection against grand mal seizures. In cases of pure grand mal epilepsy – provided they are not severe ones – I prescribe carbamazepine alone, so as not to make the treatment unnecessarily complicated, and I find that in such cases it yields good results.

Dr. RETT raised a question concerning the practice which some doctors adopt of administering prophylactic doses of folic acid preparations. Unfortunately I do not know how frequently, how regularly, or under what conditions the folic acid levels are monitored in patients receiving such treatment. As regards the efficacy of this form of prophylaxis, my own personal view is that folic acid shows, if anything, a slight tendency to provoke seizures and that it certainly does not serve to diminish them. Moreover, although some authors have suggested that treatment with folic acid helps to improve impaired mental performance, I don't believe that this has been convincingly demonstrated.

Just a final word about mood disorders: it is of course true that mood disorders may be induced, aggravated, or prolonged by drugs such as ethosuximide, but it should not be forgotten that mood disorders were also a problem before the advent of drug therapy for epilepsy and that they tended then to be much more severe and deep-rooted than the mood disorders we encounter in epileptic patients today.

Carbamazepine in the treatment of epileptic disorders in infancy and childhood

by I. GAMSTORP *

Carbamazepine (®Tegretol) became available for clinical use in the late 1950s. Initial results obtained with the drug in Swedish children with epilepsy were published first by HAGBERG[6] and then by GAMSTORP[2], whose reports also summarised previous papers on the subject. From these findings it was apparent that carbamazepine could be an effective form of treatment for epilepsy in childhood, particularly for focal attacks of all kinds, including psychomotor fits.

Brief review of the relevant literature

Although numerous other reports dealing with the effect of carbamazepine on epilepsy in childhood have since been published, only a few will be discussed here. HANEKE[7] tried carbamazepine in 92 children, 38 of whom had psychomotor attacks alone and 16 psychomotor attacks combined with grand mal. Of these 54 children, 24 became entirely seizure-free, and only eight failed to respond at all. The response was poorer in other types of epilepsy. The dose used is not stated in relation to body weight, but seems to have been about 10–15 mg./kg. Side effects consisted of fatigue, apathy, ataxia, abdominal pains, and decreased appetite during the initial phase of therapy, particularly if the drug was introduced rapidly.

FICHSEL and HEYER[1] gave carbamazepine to 106 children, 83 of whom had grand mal, focal attacks, or psychomotor fits. Twelve out of 40 children with grand mal became seizure-free, as did also 18 out of 43 with focal attacks, including psychomotor fits. Poorer results were obtained in other types of epilepsy. The dose used by these authors was 15–20 mg./kg. body weight. The side effects reported consisted of ataxia (three cases) and skin rash (17 cases). The skin rash was interpreted as an allergic reaction, but in only two patients was it considered necessary to withdraw carbamazepine permanently.

SCHEFFNER and SCHIEFER[12] tried carbamazepine in 74 children, 69 of whom had grand mal seizures, focal seizures (including psychomotor fits), or both. Twenty-six out of 30 patients with grand mal, 25 out of 26 with focal attacks, and 11 out of 13 patients with a combination of both became seizure-free. The results obtained in the remaining five children were not indicated. The dose employed was, on the average, 20 mg./kg. in children weighing 10–20 kg. and 11 mg./kg. in children weighing 50–60 kg. The authors state that no side effects at all were noted.

---

* Department of Paediatrics, University Hospital, Uppsala, Sweden.

GRANT[5] gave carbamazepine to 25 schoolchildren with multiple handicaps. He found no overall reduction in the number of seizures. In 14 out of the 17 who did show some degree of reduction, the frequency of fits decreased by at least half; six of these 14 patients had grand mal and eight psychomotor attacks. The dose used ranged from 7.3 to 30.5 mg./kg. No side effects were observed in this series of patients.

RETT[11] has treated several hundred epileptic children with carbamazepine and carried out psychological tests on 300 of them. According to his findings, carbamazepine is the only anti-epileptic drug without a sedative effect. Thus, when other drugs are replaced by carbamazepine, their sedative effect disappears and the children seem more alert, but when carbamazepine is given as the first drug, no improvement in mood is seen. In RETT's experience, carbamazepine is more effective in older children than in young ones.

O'DONOHOE[9] reported his results with carbamazepine therapy in 36 children. Complete or adequate control was achieved in four out of seven children with grand mal, in nine out of 11 with psychomotor attacks, in three out of ten with mixed grand mal and psychomotor fits, in two out of three with myoclonic epilepsy, in two out of two with reflex epilepsy, and in one out of two with petit mal; in one case of infantile spasms the drug proved ineffective. Various other drugs were also used, and the dose of carbamazepine is not stated in relation to body weight. One boy developed a psychotic syndrome characterised by withdrawal and almost schizophrenic behaviour; no other side effects were noted.

Results of the author's own studies

Carbamazepine became available to me in 1963, and my first patient was started on the drug in February of that year. At the time my first report was published[2], the longest follow-up period was two and a half years. The patients were kept under observation subsequently, and a further report on them was published in 1970[3], by which time the longest follow-up period had amounted to seven years.

The original group consisted of 58 children, 55 of whom were included because their epilepsy had not responded to other drugs available, and two because they had proved allergic to other drugs; in one patient carbamazepine was used as the first drug. In 30 of these children the initial response was good, 22 of them (Group A) becoming entirely seizure-free and eight (Group B) experiencing a reduction of at least 75% in the incidence of their seizures. Of these 30 children, 12 had grand mal, five short focal motor seizures, seven grand mal plus psychomotor seizures, five psychomotor fits, and one petit mal. The drug was tried in three children with grand mal plus mixed short seizures, as well as in nine with infantile spasms, and proved ineffective in all of them (Table 1).

Of the 22 children who initially became seizure-free, one had a severe relapse within the first six months, two after one year, and one after one and a half

99

Table 1. Initial results in 58 patients treated with carbamazepine.

Group	Grand mal	Short focal motor seizures	Grand mal plus mixed short seizures	Grand mal plus psycho-motor seizures	Psycho-motor seizures	Petit mal	Infantile spasms	Totals
A	8	4	0	5	4	1	0	22
B	4	1	0	2	1	0	0	8
C	5	3	3	2	4	2	9	28
Totals	17	8	3	9	9	3	9	58

Group A: No attacks. This group also includes four children who became seizure-free on a combination of carbamazepine and acetazolamide after monotherapy with each of the two drugs had proved of no avail, as well as two patients who had had a single attack, one when he was acutely ill with viral meningitis and the other when he had by mistake been given no carbamazepine for three days.
Group B: Attacks reduced by at least 75%
Group C: Poor or no response

Table 2. Results of follow-up in the 22 patients of Group A (cf. Table 1).

Follow-up period	No. of patients still in Group A	No. of patients transferred to Group B because of mild relapse	No. of patients with severe relapse
6 months			1
1 year		3 (transferred back to Group A or still in Group B 3½–6 years later)	2
1½ years	1		1
3½ years	1	2 (still in Group B 2–3 years later)	
4 years	1		
5 years	1		
6–7 years	9		
Totals	13	5	4

Table 3. Results of follow-up in the eight patients of Group B (cf. Table 1).

Follow-up period	No. of patients still in Group B	No. of patients seizure-free and transferred to Group A	No. of patients with severe relapse
6 months			1
1 year		1 (still in Group A 5 years later)	2
2 years	1		
2½ years			1
5½ years	1		
6 years	1		
Totals	3	1	4

years. Three had a mild relapse after one year and two after three and a half years; these five children either remained in Group B or became seizure-free again during a follow-up period lasting 2–6 years (Table 2). In three cases the treatment was stopped after the children had been seizure-free for at least five years; none of them has relapsed. Of the eight children originally belonging to Group B, one had a severe relapse after six months, two after one year, and one after two and a half years; by 1970 one had been seizure-free for five years, while the remaining three still belonged to Group B (Table 3).

Hence, out of 30 children who initially showed an excellent or good response, eight relapsed during the first three and a half years, whereas 22, of whom 20 were followed for three and a half to seven years, remained well[3].

During the first few months of treatment some side effects were noted, including an allergic skin rash in one patient and severe ataxia in another. Drowsiness and ataxia, not severe enough to necessitate interruption of the treatment, were also observed initially in several patients, particularly before we had learned to introduce the drug slowly. No side effects were recorded after the first couple of months.

Since then carbamazepine has become a routine method of treatment, and patients are no longer followed up so intensively. I do not know the exact number of patients I have treated with carbamazepine, but it must amount to some 300–500. About two-thirds of those with focal seizures, including psychomotor fits, have shown a good response to carbamazepine, irrespective of whether or not the focal seizures were combined with generalised grand mal. Furthermore, a substantial number of patients with grand mal seizures alone have responded to the drug. I have given carbamazepine a trial in a few more cases of petit mal, but have seen no new patient responding to it. In patients with grand mal seizures alone, phenytoin remains my drug of first choice; if the patient is allergic to phenytoin or fails to respond to it, I try carbamazepine as the second drug. In focal seizures, including psychomotor fits, the order tends to be reversed. However, phenytoin is much cheaper than carbamazepine and, since several patients with psychomotor fits respond to it, I try it first in many cases. In common with RETT[11], I have found that older children seem to respond better to carbamazepine than younger ones, and consequently it is particularly in young children with psychomotor fits that I tend to use phenytoin first. In a child with petit mal it may be worthwhile to give carbamazepine a trial if the child does not respond to anything else. I consider it pointless to resort to carbamazepine in cases of infantile spasms.

Dosage and tolerability

The dosage of carbamazepine, regardless of the type of fits, is 20 mg./kg. body weight daily, administered in two divided doses, if the child weighs less than 50–60 kg.; I seldom exceed a daily dosage of 1.2 g. If one starts immediately with the full dose, many children will develop unpleasant side effects, and one may have trouble in making the parents or the patient continue the medication. Carbamazepine should therefore be introduced slowly. I commence treatment with one-quarter to one-third of the calculated final dosage and give this as a single dose every evening for one week. A morning dose is then introduced and the daily amount increased once a week until the final dosage is reached, which takes 2–4 weeks. Most children tolerate this regime well; some become drowsy and dizzy for a day or two after each increase in dosage, and in a few cases the increments have to be made at longer intervals, with the result that it takes 6–8 weeks to reach the final dosage. Exceptionally, a child may fail to tolerate a daily dose of 20 mg./kg., and in such cases one may have to stop at a lower level.

In my personal experience, the only side effects noted have been an allergic skin rash and initial drowsiness, fatigue, dizziness, and ataxia. If the child develops a skin rash, I withdraw the medication. If the child has the common initial side effects described, I continue the drug, usually in the same dose, but occasionally at a lower dosage; these problems usually disappear even if the dose is not changed, and they invariably do so when the dose is reduced or the drug withdrawn. I have so far seen no new side effects appear after a child has been on the drug for two months.

As far as I can discover in the literature, serious side effects have been reported only once in a child. These occurred in an 11-year-old girl, who, three weeks after the commencement of treatment with carbamazepine, developed a skin rash, fever, and agranulocytosis, and also displayed jaundice and other evidence of hepatic involvement. Symptoms and signs disappeared without the medication being changed, but returned three weeks later; the drug was then withdrawn, and the girl made a complete recovery (Prieur et al.[10]).

Livingston et al.[8] reported a case in which a patient who had ingested 15 g. carbamazepine made an uneventful recovery in response to symptomatic therapy alone. Irreversible side effects in children seem not to have been reported in the literature, nor have they so far occurred in any of my own cases. Hence, neither in the literature nor in my own experience can I find any support for the statement by Gold[4] that carbamazepine is a toxic drug calling for the performance of blood counts and liver function tests at regular intervals. Ten years ago I carried out these checks in every case, but, as they always yielded normal results, I have long since stopped doing them. Incidentally, Gold does not say why he considers carbamazepine to be toxic.

Summary

Carbamazepine is effective in childhood epilepsy, particularly in focal attacks, including psychomotor fits. Roughly two-thirds of children with focal fits, several of whom fail to respond to other drugs, become seizure-free or greatly improved on carbamazepine. Carbamazepine may also be effective in generalised grand mal, but in this type of epilepsy phenytoin remains the drug of first choice. Since a child with petit mal may exceptionally respond to carbamazepine, this drug can also be given a trial in such cases if other preparations have proved ineffective. A trial of carbamazepine in children with infantile spasms seems pointless, as a positive effect of the drug has never been reported in this condition. It is possible that older children respond better than young ones to carbamazepine.

Regardless of the type of seizures, the dosage is about 20 mg./kg. body weight daily, administered in two divided doses; a daily dosage of 1.2 g. is, however, seldom exceeded. The drug should be introduced stepwise – the full dose being attained after 2–4 weeks (occasionally 6–8 weeks) – in order to avoid initial unpleasant side effects consisting of drowsiness, fatigue, dizziness, and ataxia. These side effects usually disappear even if the dosage is not changed, and they invariably do so when the dose is reduced or the drug withdrawn. An allergic skin rash may develop and necessitate the discontinuation of treatment. One case of reversible psychotic behaviour and one of reversible bone-marrow depression and hepatic involvement have been described in the literature; other serious side effects have to my knowledge not been reported in childhood.

References

1 FICHSEL, H., HEYER, R.: Carbamazepin in der Behandlung kindlicher Epilepsien. Dtsch. med. Wschr. *95*, 2367 (1970)
2 GAMSTORP, I.: A clinical trial of Tegretol in children with severe epilepsy. Develop. Med. Child Neurol. *8*, 296 (1966)
3 GAMSTORP, I.: Long-term follow-up of children with severe epilepsy treated with carbamazepine (Tegretol, Geigy). Acta paediat. scand. *59*, Suppl. 206: 96 (1970); abstract of paper
4 GOLD, A.P.: Psychomotor epilepsy in childhood. Pediatrics *53*, 540 (1974)
5 GRANT, R.H.E.: The use of carbamazepine (Tegretol) in patients with epilepsy and multiple handicaps. In Wink, C.A.S. (Editor): Tegretol in epilepsy, Rep. int. clin. Symp., London 1972, p. 16 (Nicholls, Manchester 1972)
6 HAGBERG, B.: Psykomotorisk epilepsi hos barn, kombinationsbehandling med Tegretol (Psychomotor epilepsy in children, combination treatment with Tegretol). Opusc. med. (Stockh.) *10*, 288 (1965)
7 HANEKE, K.: Tegretal bei kindlichen Anfallsleiden. Med. Klin. *61*, 804 (1966)
8 LIVINGSTON, S., PAULI, L.L., NEIMS, A.H.: Use of carbamazepine (Tegretol) in epilepsy. In Abstr. Vth World Congr. Psychiat., Ciudad de México 1971, p. 398 (Prensa Médica Mexicana, Mexico 1971)
9 O'DONOHOE, N.V.: A series of epileptic children treated with Tegretol, loc. cit. [5], p. 25
10 PRIEUR, A.-M., LE BOUAR, Y., GRISCELLI, C., MOZZICONACCI, P.: Agranulocytose à la carbamazépine. Ann. Pédiat. *20*, 909 (1973)
11 RETT, A.: Tegretol therapy of epileptic children, loc. cit. [5], p. 12
12 SCHEFFNER, D., SCHIEFER, I.: The treatment of epileptic children with carbamazepine. Follow-up studies of clinical course and EEG. Epilepsia (Amst.) *13*, 819 (1972)

Carbamazepine in the treatment of severe epilepsy

by R. H. E. Grant*

Introduction

Before I present the results obtained in a small clinical trial of carbamazepine
(®Tegretol) in severely handicapped people with epilepsy, let me give you an
outline of the general clinical situation in which these patients were studied.
The David Lewis Centre for Epilepsy is an independent organisation for the
treatment of the very small proportion of people with severe epilepsy who are
unable, for variable periods of time, to function in the community. "Severe"
in this context refers to the global condition of the patient, including emotional
and personality difficulties, intellectual handicap, and behavioural disturbances; many have severe and frequent seizures, but this is not always so and
may not be the primary reason for admission to the Centre.

At the present time there are just under 300 adults and 74 children in residence,
the children attending the special residential school. The sex distribution in the
adults is approximately equal, but in the school about 70% of the pupils are
boys. Some 15% of the patients are physically handicapped owing to brain
damage, and the average intelligence is in the low normal/educationally subnormal range. The population is thus highly selected, and this must be borne in
mind when considering the results of any form of anti-epileptic treatment.

In a previous study of carbamazepine[4], I presented the results obtained in
42 patients, 25 of whom were schoolchildren. Although the overall effect on
seizure control was not statistically significant, it was clear that, in those
patients who did experience a reduction in seizure frequency, this was clinically
highly significant to the individual. One of the purposes of this study was to
assess the effect of carbamazepine in controlling disturbed behaviour. No
attempt was made to assess this in the 17 adults because of the wide range
of individual circumstances. However, in the case of the schoolchildren it was
possible to make a reasonably objective assessment by careful observation in
a structured environment. In 20 of the 25 children treated with carbamazepine,
behaviour was sufficiently disturbed for us to consider trying the drug irrespective of seizure frequency. The results are shown in Table 1 and are statistically
significant ($P < 0.01$). The improvement consisted mainly of a smoothing-out
of abnormal behaviour patterns, reduction in the frequency of temper outbursts, and improvement of interpersonal relationships.

This trial was conducted during my first three years at The David Lewis Centre,
in the course of which many changes were made in the approach to medical

 * The David Lewis Centre for Epilepsy, near Alderley Edge, Cheshire, England.

Table 1. Effect of carbamazepine on behaviour in children.

Effect	No. of children
Worse	1
No change	5
Improved	14
Total	20

P < 0.01

Table 2. Additional anti-epileptic drugs used in 27 patients.

Drug	No. of patients
Primidone	17
Phenytoin (D.P.H.)	15
Phenobarbitone	6
Pheneturide	4
Ethosuximide	4
Nitrazepam	2
Sultiame	1

treatment, social work, and administration. Control of epilepsy was much less effective then than it has been over the last five years (in spite of an increasingly difficult population), and biochemical control of anti-epileptic treatment was not available.

It was therefore decided to carry out a further clinical trial to study the effect of carbamazepine specifically on grand mal and psychomotor seizures only, and furthermore to restrict this study to adults, because it is impossible to be certain of seizure frequency in children during school holidays.

Clinical material and methods

A total of 27 patients with mixed grand mal and psychomotor epilepsy were treated. There were 15 females ranging in age from 21 to 65 years (mean 36.8) and 12 males aged 19 to 54 years (mean 26.7). All the patients were on stable anti-epileptic treatment which had not been altered for six months prior to commencing carbamazepine in 23 patients, and for three months in the remaining four patients; moreover, this anti-epileptic treatment was continued unchanged for a similar length of time after medication with carbamazepine had been started. All the patients had previously been treated with various drug combinations in varying doses with no further improvement, and it was thus considered unnecessary to use a double-blind crossover trial. The other anti-epileptic drugs employed and the frequency distribution are shown in Table 2.

As in the first trial, treatment with carbamazepine was always introduced gradually. The usual initial dosage of 300 mg. daily in three divided doses was

Table 3. Final dosages of carbamazepine.

Range	400–1,200 mg./day 7.6–21.1 mg./kg.				
Mean	13.2 mg./kg.				
Distribution	Daily dose (mg.)	400	600	800	1,000	1,200
	No. of patients	1	11	9	2	4

Table 4. Total number of seizures recorded over a six-month period (A) or a three-month period (B) before and after treatment with carbamazepine.

	Patient	Sex	Age	Body weight (kg.)	Dose of carbamazepine		Grand mal seizures			Psychomotor seizures		
					mg./day	mg./kg.	Before	After	% change	Before	After	% change
A	1. F.C.	F	29	45.0	800	17.8	41	2	− 95.12	115	96	−16.52
	2. B.M.	F	35	63.6	600	9.4	54	16	− 70.37	29	30	+ 3.45
	3. J.W.	F	31	55.0	800	14.6	2	0	−100.00	61	35	−42.62
	4. G.R.	F	26	50.9	1,000	19.7	32	5	− 84.38	67	49	−26.87
	5. M.W.	F	47	41.8	600	14.4	0	0	–	21	16	−23.80
	6. M.R.	F	61	58.5	600	10.3	5	2	− 60.00	0	0	–
	7. P.B.	F	26	60.0	600	10.0	5	5	–	16	15	− 6.25
	8. H.P.	F	21	58.2	1,000	17.2	0	0	–	23	18	−21.74
	9. A.S.	F	65	63.6	600	9.4	0	0	–	60	20	−66.67
	10. E.T.	F	26	54.5	800	14.7	8	14	+ 75.00	121	106	−12.40
	11. J.B.	F	52	55.0	800	14.6	8	0	−100.00	3	2	−33.33
	12. H.W.	F	30	63.6	1,200	18.9	115	124	+ 7.84	Data unreliable		
	13. J.C.	F	28	54.6	600	11.0	1	0	−100.00	10	11	+10.00
	14. T.D.	F	32	62.7	800	12.8	0	0	–	65	27	−58.46
	15. S.W.	M	20	69.8	800	11.5	3	4	+ 33.33	59	49	−16.95
	16. W.H.	M	24	72.7	600	8.3	101	43	− 57.43	29	16	−44.83
	17. D.B.	M	27	57.0	1,200	21.1	66	10	− 84.85	11	3	−72.73
	18. P.C.	M	21	53.5	800	15.0	33	21	− 36.36	1	1	–
	19. P.C.	M	28	52.0	600	11.5	0	0	–	33	28	−15.15
	20. A.G.	M	19	61.0	600	9.8	0	0	–	17	2	−88.23
	21. K.P.	M	22	72.0	800	11.1	21	23	+ 9.52	1	1	–
	22. H.M.	M	28	60.0	800	13.3	0	0	–	74	37	−50.00
	23. D.G.	M	30	67.7	600	8.9	42	24	− 42.85	7	6	−14.29
B	24. G.S.	F	43	50.0	600	12.0	0	0	–	9	5	−44.44
	25. E.H.	M	54	53.0	400	7.6	13	2	− 84.61	0	0	–
	26. N.W.	M	19	70.9	1,200	16.9	17	18	+ 5.88	124	15	−87.90
	27. S.S.	M	28	83.8	1,200	14.3	9	7	− 22.22	12	4	−66.66

administered for at least seven days and sometimes longer, after which it was raised to 600 mg. daily or more, depending on the clinical situation. The final doses of carbamazepine are shown in Table 3, and it can be seen that 56% of the patients were given more than 600 mg. daily.

Results

Details of the patients, the frequency of grand mal and psychomotor seizures before and after treatment, and the percentage change in seizure rate are shown in Table 4. Seizure frequency was reduced in 13 (68.4%) of the 19 patients with grand mal and in 20 (83.3%) of the 24 with psychomotor seizures. The mean reduction in grand mal was 44.4%, with a slightly lower reduction of 38.8% in the psychomotor seizures (Table 5 and Figures 1 and 2). The reason for the higher significance of the figure for psychomotor seizures is that these seizures were more consistently reduced than the grand mal attacks. Some of the patients were very substantially improved not only in respect of seizure control but also in respect of general temperament and behaviour.

Table 5. Total and mean number of seizures before and after treatment.

	Grand mal		Psychomotor	
	Before	After	Before	After
Total	576	320	968	592
Mean	30.3	16.8	40.3	24.7
Reduction	44.4%		38.8%	
	$P < 0.02$		$P = 0.0001$	

Side effects

Carbamazepine has been reported to cause a wide variety of side effects, including drowsiness, ataxia, nausea and vomiting, skin rashes, depression and confusion, and various haematological abnormalities. For example, in a review of the use of carbamazepine in the treatment of trigeminal neuralgia, GAYFORD and REDPATH[3] found that 309 out of 510 patients (60.6%) had been reported as suffering from side effects due to the drug. One-third of these side effects were referable to the nervous system, with ataxia, vertigo, and drowsiness accounting for 20.4% of the total. These symptoms were usually transient, but in elderly patients they could be quite disabling. Aplastic anaemia occurred in four (0.8%) of the 510 patients and was fatal in three of them. The authors recommended that regular haemoglobin and white cell counts be carried out during treatment. On the other hand, BOWER[1] found remarkably few side effects in his patients.

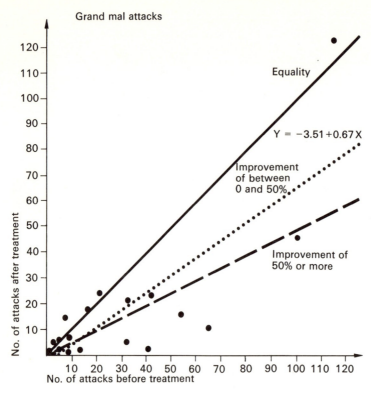

Fig. 1. Comparison of number of grand mal attacks before and after treatment.

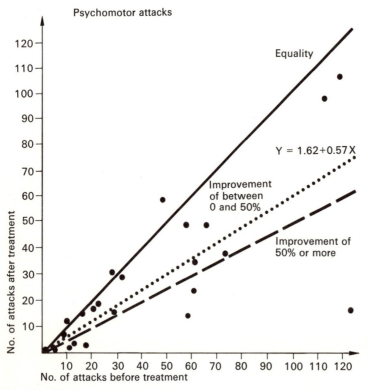

Fig. 2. Comparison of number of psychomotor attacks before and after treatment.

In the present trial only one of the 27 patients showed any significant side effects (Patient No. 1, F.C.). This 29-year-old woman with severe mixed epilepsy due to a porencephalic cyst was given carbamazepine in increasing doses of up to 1,000 mg. daily. A few days after this dose had been achieved, she became extremely confused, ataxic, and drowsy. The dose was reduced to 800 mg. daily, and she rapidly improved. A renewed increase to 1,000 mg. caused the same effects; no further attempt to increase the dosage was made, and the patient remains free from side effects.

I have previously reported on two other patients who displayed side effects that were definitely due to carbamazepine[4]. The first was a boy of ten years whose initial dosage of carbamazepine was 300 mg. daily, increasing to 600 mg. daily on the eighth day. On the 13th day he developed a generalised morbilliform rash with slight pyrexia and a trace of albuminuria. The drug was stopped immediately, chlorpheniramine was given by mouth, and the condition subsided rapidly.

The second case was that of a 71-year-old woman who was started on carbamazepine at a dosage level of 400 mg. daily but stopped the tablets herself on the third day because of symptoms which had started 12 hours after the first dose. She felt generally "awful" and slept badly, waking intermittently in the night not knowing where she was and seeing strange things which she was unable to describe accurately. She would then return to sleep, and the same events recurred in an hour or two. Within 48 hours she became ataxic, nauseated, and confused, and she complained of paraesthesia in the hands and forearms and from the feet to the knees. At this stage she stopped taking carbamazepine, and the symptoms disappeared rapidly. She had never had this experience previously, nor has she since.

Discussion

The results of this trial show a clinically and statistically significant effect of carbamazepine in reducing the frequency of grand mal and psychomotor seizures in a group of 27 people in a residential centre for epilepsy. The effect is particularly encouraging when the nature of the population under study is taken into account. Many of these patients are quite severely handicapped and had already been treated with a variety of anticonvulsants before starting carbamazepine. The fact that the results are better than those in my first trial[4] may be attributable to the use of higher doses of carbamazepine, the mean dose for the present trial being 13.2 mg./kg. as compared with 10.6 mg./kg. in the first, an increase of nearly 25%.

Including the 27 patients reported on here, I now have some 23% of the population at The David Lewis Centre on carbamazepine (34 children, 45 adults), many of whom have shown considerable improvement in response to the drug, and none has suffered any side effects other than those reported above. I agree very much with TAYLOR[5] when he draws attention to what he calls a "negative placebo effect", i.e. to the possibility that a drug may provoke side effects which have no clear-cut relationship with its pharmacological properties.

In addition to my work at The David Lewis Centre, I also hold weekly outpatient epilepsy clinics at Manchester Royal Infirmary and the Royal Manchester Children's Hospital. The patients at these clinics are less handicapped than those at the Centre, but many present considerable epileptic problems. For the last two years I have increasingly been using carbamazepine as the drug of *first* choice in grand mal and psychomotor epilepsy. I fully support some of the conclusions of CEREGHINO et al.[2] who state:

1. Carbamazepine is a major anti-epileptic drug and not merely a supplemental medication.
2. Carbamazepine does not help all patients.
3. Results appear to be best in grand mal and temporal-lobe seizures.
4. Absence seizures are not affected.
5. Initial fears about toxicity seem exaggerated in view of subsequent experience with the drug.
6. A psychotropic effect is probably present.

In conclusion, I would say that carbamazepine is worth trying in *all* cases of grand mal and psychomotor epilepsy, even in severely affected patients. In view of the possible advantages of doses in excess of 1,000 mg. daily, perhaps CIBA-GEIGY might investigate the feasibility of introducing a tablet of 400 or 500 mg.

Summary

A partially controlled trial of carbamazepine in 27 patients resident in a centre for epilepsy is reported. The improvement in grand mal and psychomotor seizure rates was clinically and statistically significant.

Carbamazepine is now the author's drug of first choice for the treatment of these seizures in out-patients.

References

1 BOWER, B.D.: Discussion. In Wink, C.A.S. (Editor): Tegretol in epilepsy, Rep. int. clin. Symp., London 1972, p. 31 (Nicholls, Manchester 1972)
2 CEREGHINO, J.J., BROCK, J.T., VAN METER, J.C., PENRY, J.K., SMITH, L.D., WHITE, B.G.: Carbamazepine for epilepsy. A controlled prospective evaluation. Neurology (Minneap.) *24*, 401 (1974)
3 GAYFORD, J.J., REDPATH, T.H.: The side-effects of carbamazepine. Proc. roy. Soc. Med. *62*, 615 (1969)
4 GRANT, R.H.E.: The use of carbamazepine (Tegretol) in patients with epilepsy and multiple handicaps, loc. cit. [1], p. 16
5 TAYLOR, D.C.: Discussion, loc. cit. [1], p. 122

Preliminary report on a long-term study of the correlations between the therapeutic effects of carbamazepine and the drug's plasma levels

by A. Riccio and F. Monaco*

Introduction

Both the pharmacological and the therapeutic properties of carbamazepine (®Tegretol), a powerful anticonvulsive agent which is chemically related to the iminostilbene derivatives, have already been described in comprehensive studies and reports (see Wink[12] for an extensive review).

Carbamazepine has generally been used in association with other anti-epileptic drugs, mostly barbiturates and diphenylhydantoin[4, 10]. The literature contains only few references to monotherapy with carbamazepine in certain forms of epilepsy[2, 6, 13].

On the other hand, continuous monitoring of the blood levels of anticonvulsive drugs with the aid of methods developed by various authors (e.g. Cereghino et al.[1]; Morselli et al.[8]; Palmér et al.[9]; Troupin et al.[11]) has produced evidence of a strong interaction between carbamazepine and other anticonvulsants; very often, in fact, as a result of competition, or for a variety of unknown reasons, the metabolism of one drug may be inhibited or enhanced by the blood levels of another[3].

The clinical observations we have made over the past two years in more than 250 epileptic patients treated with carbamazepine as the main anticonvulsant have led us to doubt whether multi-drug combinations are really effective[7]. We therefore considered it worthwhile, in collaboration with the Laboratory of Clinical Pharmacology at the "Mario Negri" Institute in Milan, to monitor the blood levels of carbamazepine and/or barbiturates and/or phenytoin in a group of 20 epileptic patients.

Materials and methods

The 20 subjects, all of them male, were selected from among the epileptic patients whom we have been following up in our clinic over the past two years or more. Their ages ranged from six to 35 years, and they had various forms of epilepsy marked by grand mal seizures, psychomotor attacks, or typical and/or atypical absences. In all but three of the subjects, seizures occurred at the rate of at least one a week. The selection of cases for this study was governed in particular by the willingness of the patients to submit to the blood sampling procedures and other clinical examinations required.

* Clinica delle Malattie Nervose e Mentali dell'Università, Turin, Italy.

Of the 20 patients, 15 had secondarily generalised epilepsy, four primarily generalised epilepsy, and one Lennox-Gastaut syndrome (Table 1). The cases of secondarily generalised epilepsy also include four patients with a secondary mixed form in which grand mal seizures alternated with, and preceded, psychomotor attacks[5].

Ten of the patients (Nos 1–10) were hospitalised, while the other ten were followed in the out-patient department. Eight of the 20 subjects had never previously been treated with carbamazepine; the remaining 12 had been receiving the drug, alone or in combination with other anticonvulsants, for periods ranging from a few days to two years. The average daily dosage of carbamazepine was 725 mg. (minimum 400 mg., maximum 1,200 mg.), given in three divided doses at 9 a.m., 12 noon, and 4 p.m. Six patients (Nos 5, 6, 12, 13, 16, and 19) were on monotherapy with carbamazepine.

The duration of the study was 60 days. Blood samples of 5 ml. were taken at 8 a.m. and 6 p.m. on one day a week for nine weeks, and the plasma thus obtained was used for determination of the carbamazepine, phenobarbitone, and diphenylhydantoin levels by means of a routine procedure[8]. Blood counts and E.E.G. examinations were performed prior to treatment and on the 28th and 56th day after the start of medication.

Results and discussion

The study reported on here represents only the preliminary phase of a more extensive longitudinal investigation which will take another ten months to complete. The results available to date relate chiefly to the following points:

1. Clinical course and E.E.G. findings in the group as a whole.
2. Correlation between clinical response and plasma carbamazepine levels in patients receiving monotherapy with carbamazepine.
3. Side effects as determined by clinical examination and laboratory tests.

The effect of carbamazepine, administered alone or in combination with other drugs, on the E.E.G. pattern and on the frequency of epileptic seizures is shown in Figure 1. For the purposes of evaluation we divided the E.E.G. tracings into the following categories:

A. Interseizure record normal.
B. Interseizure record irregular (presence of aspecific slowing up and/or deterioration in background activity).
C. Interseizure record frankly abnormal (presence of spikes, spikes-and-waves, multi-spikes and waves, generalised discharges and/or lateralised discharges and/or focal discharges).

At the commencement of the study, three of our patients could be allotted to Category A, six to Category B, and 11 to Category C. During the period of

Table 1. Data on 20 male epileptic patients receiving for the most part treatment either with carbamazepine alone (Patient Nos in italics) or with carbamazepine in combination with phenobarbitone and/or diphenylhydantoin. S.G.E. = secondarily generalised epilepsy; P.G.E. = primarily generalised epilepsy; G.M. = grand mal; P.M. = petit mal.

Patient No.	Age (years)	Type of epilepsy	Type of seizures	Frequency of seizures	Period of observation	Treatment		
						Carbamazepine (mg./day)	Phenobarbitone (mg./day)	Diphenylhydantoin (mg./day)
1	24	S.G.E.	G.M. + P.M.	Twice weekly	60 days	1,000	100	—
2	19	S.G.E.	G.M. + P.M.	Twice weekly	60 days	800	100	200
3	21	S.G.E.	G.M.	Three times weekly	60 days	600	100	200
4	25	S.G.E.	G.M. + P.M.	Ten times weekly	60 days	400	50	250
5	19	S.G.E.	G.M.	Weekly	60 days	600 (+ 20 mg. phenothiazine)		
6	23	S.G.E.	G.M.	Weekly	60 days	600	100	
7	35	S.G.E.	G.M. + P.M.	Weekly	60 days	600	100	50
8	35	S.G.E.	G.M. + psychomotor attacks	Weekly	60 days	400	100	
9	32	S.G.E.	G.M. + psychomotor attacks	Weekly	60 days	600	100	150
10	18	S.G.E.	G.M.	Weekly	60 days	400	100	100
11	10	P.G.E.	G.M.		60 days + 4 months	800	100	
12	31	P.G.E.	G.M.		60 days + 3 months	400	—	—
13	6	S.G.E.	G.M. + P.M.	Twice weekly	60 days + 1 year	500	—	—
14	22	S.G.E.	G.M. + atypical P.M.	Weekly	60 days + 2 years	1,200	100	200
15	10	P.G.E.	Partial motor secondarily generalised	Weekly	60 days + 1 year	1,000	50	100
16	11	Lennox-Gastaut syndrome	Atypical P.M.		60 days + 2 years	1,000	—	—
17	35	P.G.E.	G.M. + psychomotor attacks	Ten times weekly	60 days + 1 month	600	—	—
18	18	S.G.E.	G.M.	Weekly	60 days + 1 year	600	100	—
19	19	S.G.E.	G.M. + P.M. + psychomotor attacks	Weekly	60 days + 3 years	1,200	—	—
20	32	S.G.E.	G.M. + atypical P.M. + psychomotor attacks	3–4 times weekly	60 days + 1 year	600	100 (+ 600 mg. suc-cinimide)	—

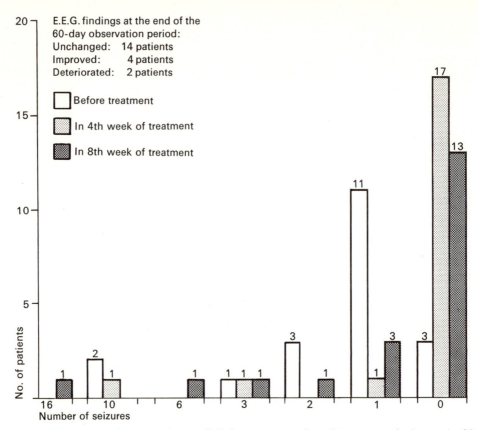

Fig. 1. Effect of carbamazepine on E.E.G. pattern and on frequency of seizures in 20 epileptic patients.

observation the E.E.G. patterns remained unchanged in 14 out of the 20 cases and deteriorated in two.

As regards the effect of treatment on the frequency of seizures, Figure 1 indicates that most of the patients were free of seizures in the fourth and eighth week of therapy, a finding which confirms once again that carbamazepine exerts a therapeutic effect in various forms of epilepsy.

Of interest, however, is the relative discrepancy between clinical response and E.E.G. findings. It is in fact strange that the beneficial clinical effect was accompanied by an improvement in the E.E.G. pattern in only four of the 20 patients, since it tends to be assumed that a favourable clinical situation is always accompanied by regularisation of the E.E.G. pattern.

The relationship between daily dose of carbamazepine administered, plasma levels of the drug, and seizure frequency in the six patients receiving monotherapy with carbamazepine is illustrated in Figures 2–7. This relationship would appear to be rather complex, and it is not possible at the moment to draw any conclusions from the data so far available. The plasma concentration was in fact invariably at or above optimal levels (5–10 mcg./ml.) even in those

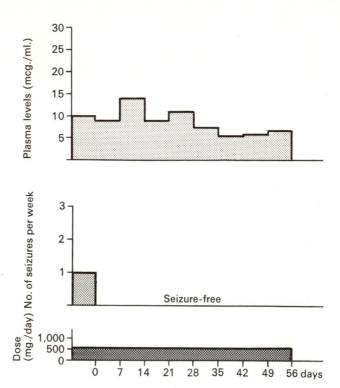

Fig. 2. Relationship between daily dose of carbamazepine administered, plasma levels of the drug, and seizure frequency in Patient No. 5 (cf. Table 1).

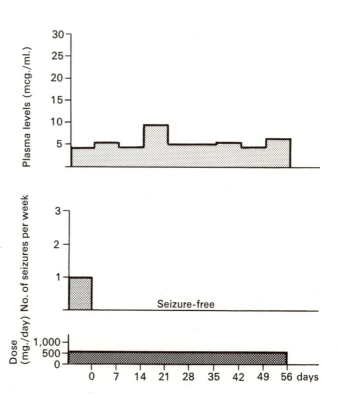

Fig. 3. Relationship between daily dose of carbamazepine administered, plasma levels of the drug, and seizure frequency in Patient No. 6 (cf. Table 1).

115

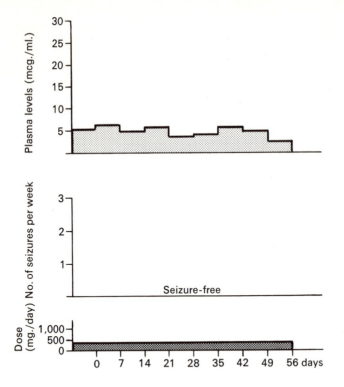

Fig. 4. Relationship between daily dose of carbamazepine administered, plasma levels of the drug, and seizure frequency in Patient No. 12 (cf. Table 1).

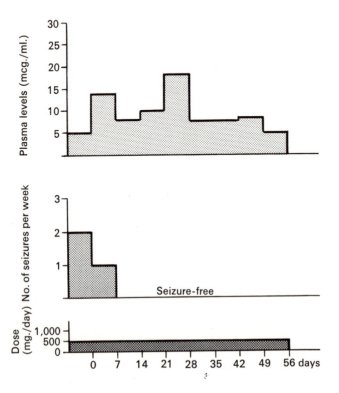

Fig. 5. Relationship between daily dose of carbamazepine administered, plasma levels of the drug, and seizure frequency in Patient No. 13 (cf. Table 1).

116

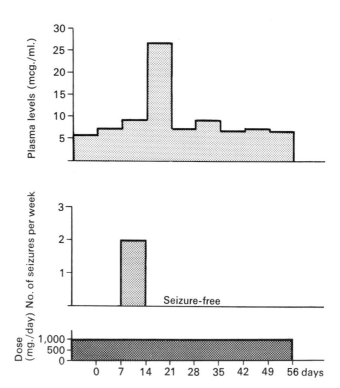

Fig. 6. Relationship between daily dose of carbamazepine administered, plasma levels of the drug, and seizure frequency in Patient No. 16 (cf. Table 1).

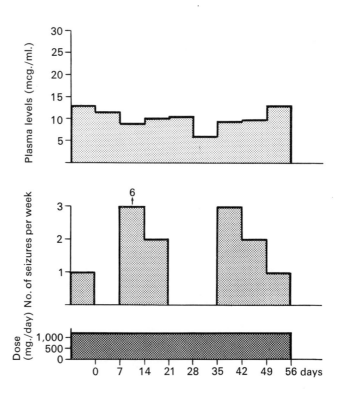

Fig. 7. Relationship between daily dose of carbamazepine administered, plasma levels of the drug, and seizure frequency in Patient No. 19 (cf. Table 1).

Table 2. W.B.C. counts in 20 epileptic patients prior to treatment and 28 and 56 days after the commencement of medication with carbamazepine administered either as monotherapy or in combination with phenobarbitone and/or diphenylhydantoin.

W.B.C. counts		> 5,000	5,000–4,000	< 4,000
	Before treatment*	6 cases	9 cases	3 cases
	On 28th day of treatment	6 cases	4 cases	10 cases
	On 56th day of treatment	6 cases	12 cases	2 cases
Average W.B.C. counts	Before treatment	4,556 ± 1,414		
	On 28th day of treatment	4,150 ± 1,098		
	On 56th day of treatment	4,760 ± 835		
Maximum and minimum W.B.C. counts		Maximum	Minimum	
	Before treatment	7,200	3,800	
	On 28th day of treatment	6,200	3,000	
	On 56th day of treatment	7,000	3,900	

* W.B.C. determined in only 18 cases

patients in whom seizures persisted. We hope that in the further course of our investigation we shall be able to obtain data shedding more light on this problem.

Finally, as regards tolerability, the W.B.C. counts performed on the 28th and 56th day of treatment failed to reveal any consistent changes (Table 2). On the other hand, there was a tendency for the R.B.C. count to decrease. Other known side effects of carbamazepine (drowsiness, gastric disturbances, ataxia, and skin rashes) were not particularly noticeable in our group of patients.

Acknowledgment

The present study was conducted by the medical staff of the Clinic of Nervous and Mental Diseases (Director: Prof. L. BERGAMINI), Turin University Medical School. The authors would like to take this opportunity of thanking their colleagues P. BENNA, A. COVACICH, L. DURELLI, M. FANTINI, P. M. FURLAN, P. GILARDENGO, M. GILLI, and W. TRONI for their assistance.

References

1 CEREGHINO, J. J., VAN METER, J. C., BROCK, J. T., PENRY, J. K., SMITH, L. D., WHITE, B. G.: Preliminary observations of serum carbamazepine concentration in epileptic patients. Neurology (Minneap.) *23*, 357 (1973)
2 DALBY, M. A.: Antiepileptic and psychotropic effect of carbamazepine (Tegretol) in the treatment of psychomotor epilepsy. Epilepsia (Amst.) *12*, 325 (1971)
3 GARATTINI, S., MORSELLI, P. L.: Interazioni tra farmaci (Ferro, Milan 1973)
4 GUPTA, R. K., JOLLY, S. S.: Role of Tegretol in epilepsy. Indian Pract. *25*, 399 (1972)
5 JANZ, D.: Die Epilepsien. Spezielle Pathologie und Therapie (Thieme, Stuttgart 1969)

6 LERMAN, P., KIVITY-EPHRAIM, S.: Carbamazepine as sole anticonvulsant for focal epilepsy of childhood. Epilepsia (Amst.) *15*, 229 (1974)

7 MONACO, F., RICCIO, A., FURLAN, P. M.: Communicazione preliminare sul impiego del Tegretol sciroppo in pazienti epilettici. Riv. Neurol. *44*, 123 (1974)

8 MORSELLI, P. L., GERNA, M., MAIO, D. DE, ZANDA, G., VIANI, F., GARATTINI, S.: Pharmacokinetic studies on carbamazepine in volunteers and in epileptic patients. In Schneider, H., et al. (Editors): Clinical pharmacology of anti-epileptic drugs, Proc. Workshop on the determination of anti-epileptic drugs in body fluids – II, Bethel 1974 (Springer, Berlin/Heidelberg/New York 1975; printing)

9 PALMÉR, L., BERTILSSON, L., COLLSTE, P., RAWLINS, M.: Quantitative determination of carbamazepine in plasma by mass fragmentography. Clin. Pharmacol. Ther. *14*, 827 (1973)

10 SCHEFFNER, D., SCHIEFER, I.: The treatment of epileptic children with carbamazepine. Follow-up studies of clinical course and EEG. Epilepsia (Amst.) *13*, 819 (1972)

11 TROUPIN, A. S., GREEN, J. R., LEVY, R. H.: Carbamazepine as an anticonvulsant: a pilot study. Neurology (Minneap.) *24*, 863 (1974)

12 WINK, C. A. S. (Editor): Tegretol in epilepsy, Rep. int. clin. Symp., London 1972 (Nicholls, Manchester 1972)

13 WULFSOHN, M.: Carbamazepine (Tegretol) in the long-term treatment of grand mal epilepsy. S. Afr. Med. J. *46*, 1091 (1972)

The chemistry of carbamazepine

by A. R. GAGNEUX*

Introduction

For thousands of years epilepsy was treated by sorcery and exorcism. The first
rational therapy was not discovered until the middle of the last century, when
Sir CHARLES LOCOCK[2] introduced the bromides (Table 1). It was thus that in
1857 sodium, potassium, and ammonium bromide became the first and, for
over 50 years, the only anti-epileptic drugs. Then, in 1912, HAUPTMANN[1] discovered the anticonvulsive action of the barbiturate hypnotics. This discovery
opened a gate through which many similar chemical structures have passed
to become, in due course, useful weapons in the anti-epileptic arsenal.

Table 1. Milestones in the chemotherapy of epilepsy.

1857	Sir Charles Locock[2]	Bromides
1912	A. Hauptmann[1]	Barbiturates
1916	E. Wernecke[6]	Hydantoins
1957	W. Schindler[4]	Carbamazepine
1961	L. Sternbach[5]	Benzodiazepines
1964	H. Meunier[3]	Sodium 2-propylvalerate (®Depakine)

Precisely 100 years after LOCOCK introduced his bromides, a novel kind of
anti-epileptic drug was synthesised, namely, carbamazepine (®Tegretol). Because of the unusual structure of carbamazepine, and in view of the papers
which will follow dealing with its biotransformation and pharmacokinetics, it
would appear worthwhile to present here a short review of its chemistry.
I propose first of all to characterise the structure of the carbamazepine molecule, and then to compare it with the structure not only of other polycyclic
drugs but also of other anti-epileptics. Finally, after a brief glance at the
chemical reactivity of carbamazepine, I shall endeavour to illustrate its biological sensitivity to small structural changes.

Structure

The structural elements of the carbamazepine molecule are shown in Figure 1.
They include two benzene rings, one seven-membered (azepine) ring, one

* Research Department, Pharmaceuticals Division, CIBA-GEIGY LIMITED, Basle, Switzerland.

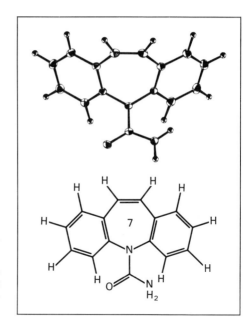

Fig. 1. X-ray picture *(above)* and structural formula *(below)* of carbamazepine. The molecule has two aromatic rings, one seven-membered ring, one double bond, and one amide group. It is a tricyclic amide.

double bond, and one amide group. As some of you may remember, the importance of steric parameters of polycyclic psycho-active drugs was discussed in this very room three years ago[7]. Since we are dealing with a tricyclic structure, it seems appropriate to analyse its topography, in order later to dis-

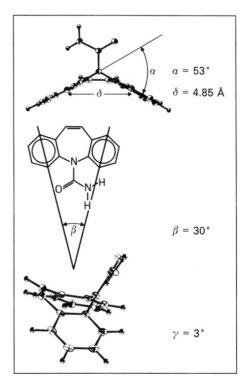

Fig. 2. Three-dimensional structure of carbamazepine as revealed by X-ray diffraction. *Above:* frontal view; *middle:* top view; *below:* side view. Note that the carbamazepine molecule is bent and slightly twisted.

$\alpha = 53°$

$\delta = 4.85$ Å

$\beta = 30°$

$\gamma = 3°$

tinguish it from structurally similar compounds. The three-dimensional structure of carbamazepine as determined by X-ray diffraction (RIHS, G., personal
communication) is presented in Figure 2. The relevant steric parameters are
the angle of flexure α (53°), indicated at the top, and the angle of annellation
β (30°) shown in the centre of the picture. The angle of torsion γ amounts to 3°.
This means that the benzene rings are slightly twisted with respect to each
other. Finally, the distance δ between the centres of the benzene rings measures
4.85 Å.
These values are compared with those of other polycyclic drugs in Figure 3.
The angle of flexure α of carbamazepine resembles those of the antidepressants
maprotiline (®Ludiomil) and imipramine (®Tofranil). The annellation angle
β, on the other hand, approaches only that of imipramine. The value of the

	Angle of flexure α	Angle of annellation β	Angle of torsion γ	Distance δ
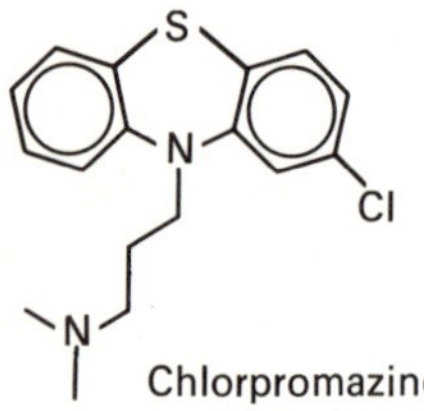 Chlorpromazine	25°	10°	0°	5.1 Å
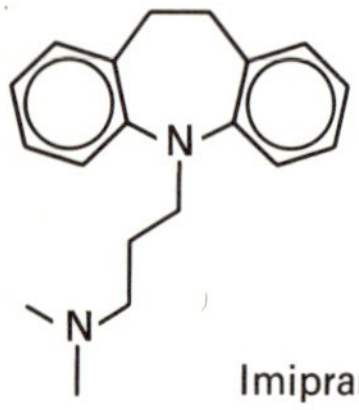 Imipramine	55°	40°	20°	5.1 Å
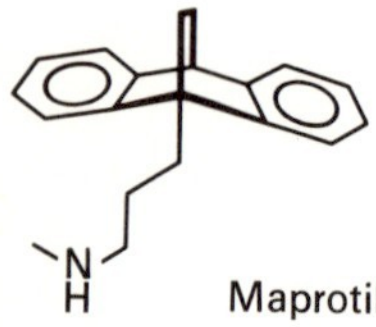 Maprotiline	60°	0°	0°	4.6 Å
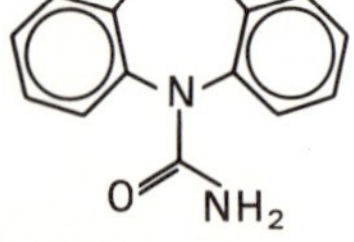 Carbamazepine	53°	30°	3°	4.85 Å

Fig. 3. Structure of carbamazepine compared with that of other polycyclic drugs.

angle γ is 3° for carbamazepine and 0° for maprotiline and chlorpromazine. As far as the distance δ between the benzene rings is concerned, carbamazepine differs from all three comparison compounds by only 5%. It can thus be concluded that the tricyclic skeleton of carbamazepine belongs to the steric family of the polycyclic psycho-active drugs.

Let us now turn to the structure of some other anti-epileptic drugs. Four important types are represented in Figure 4: phenobarbitone, a barbiturate; phensuximide, a cyclic imide; phenytoin, a hydantoin; and clonazepam, a benzodiazepine. Their common structural features are:

1. One saturated carbon atom (i.e. a carbon atom carrying four substituents).
2. An amide group built into the heterocyclic ring.
3. At least one aromatic ring twisted out of the plane of the heterocyclic ring.

When carbamazepine is compared with these structures, the following differences are observed (cf. Figure 1):

1. Carbamazepine *lacks* a saturated carbon atom.
2. The amide group of carbamazepine is *not* part of a heterocyclic ring.
3. Only carbamazepine has a *tricyclic* structure.

As we have seen earlier, the aromatic rings of carbamazepine are slightly twisted in relation to each other. On the other hand, these rings do lie in a plane *different* from that defined by the amide group. In this respect, carbamazepine is *similar* to the four anti-epileptics referred to above.

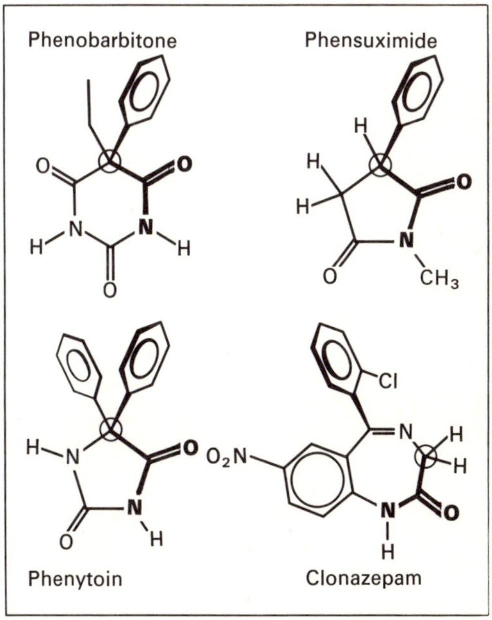

Fig. 4. Structure of four major anti-epileptics. Features common to all four are: a saturated carbon atom (circle), a cyclic amide group (heavy type), and a twisted aromatic ring ("lollipop").

123

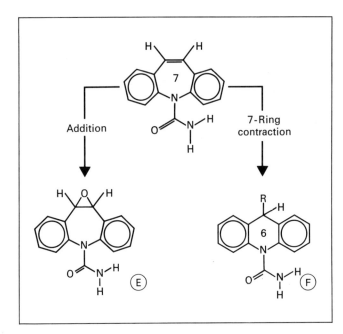

Fig. 5. Diagrammatic representation of the reactivity of carbamazepine. The reactive site of the substance is the C=C double bond. Addition reactions lead, for example, to the epoxide E, while ring contraction gives rise to products such as F.

Reactivity

Let me now comment briefly on the chemical reactivity of carbamazepine (Figure 5). Both chemically and biochemically the most reactive site of the molecule is its carbon-carbon double bond. It undergoes addition reactions, leading, for example, to the epoxide E, which is also a major metabolite. The biosynthesis of metabolite E and its fate in the organism will be discussed by Dr. FAIGLE in the next paper. Another reaction mode of the double bond may result in ring-contracted products, such as F.

Sensitivity

Finally, I shall try to illustrate the biological sensitivity of the carbamazepine structure to minor molecular modifications. This can only be done by reference to a biological parameter. Among various possibilities, the oral ED_{50} for the protection of mice against electroshock was chosen. Details of this test are given in Table 2 (BALTZER, V., personal communication).

Table 2. Biological test for establishing the oral ED_{50} for the protection of mice against electroshock.

1.	Tonic extensor spasms of the hind-legs are induced by electrical stimulation of the brain via corneal electrodes, through which an alternating current of 50 c.p.s. and 16 mA. is passed for 0.2 sec.
2.	Test compounds are administered orally in doses of 2–200 mg./kg. 60 minutes prior to the test.
3.	The ED_{50} is calculated by interpolation (N = 10 animals per dose).

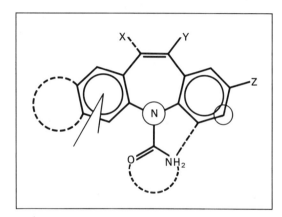

Fig. 6. A few structural
modifications of the carbamazepine parent molecule.

The number of possible structural modifications of the carbamazepine parent
molecule is limited only by the imagination of the chemist. A few of these
variations are indicated in summary fashion in Figure 6. They include:

1. Addition of substituents.
2. Replacement of carbon by hetero-atoms.
3. Various ring closures.
4. Rupture of an aromatic ring.

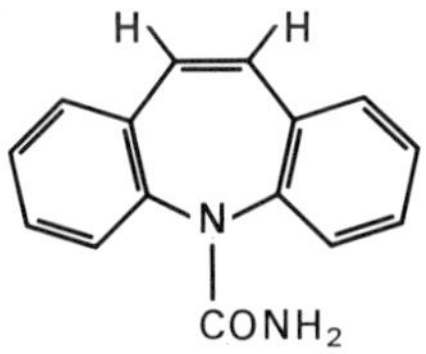	Oral ED_{50} required to protect mice against electroshock (mg./kg.)	Partition coefficient (25 °C.) between n-octanol and water
H, H (CONH₂)		
H, H	10	58
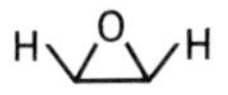 H, O, H	15	7.4
H H, H H	30	66
H, CH₃	60	180
H CH₃, H H	> 200	200
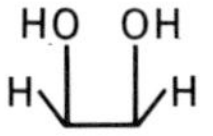 HO OH, H H	> 200	0.63
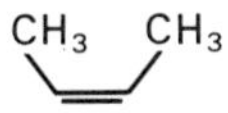 CH₃ CH₃	> 200	600

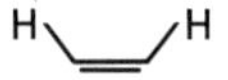

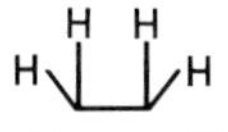

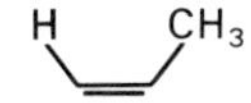

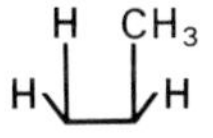

Fig. 7. Derivatives of the carbamazepine parent molecule resulting from modification
of the double-bond substituents.

125

Let us select, as an example, modification of the double-bond substituents. A few of the resulting derivatives are indicated in Figure 7. The modified structural elements are shown on the left and the corresponding ED_{50} values in the middle. On the right, the partition coefficients (MOSER, P., personal communication) have been listed as a measure of the lipophilic character of the various derivatives. From the limited data presented it can only be concluded that the structural changes shown reduce or abolish the protective action against electroshock.

To sum up, carbamazepine possesses singular structural features. It exclusively combines chemical characteristics common to classic anticonvulsants with those of polycyclic psycho-active agents. The uniqueness of the drug's structure is reflected in its remarkable clinical properties.

References

1 HAUPTMANN, A.: Luminal bei Epilepsie. Münch. med. Wschr. *59*, 1907 (1912)
2 LOCOCK, C.: Discussion on Sieveking, E.H.: Analysis of fifty-two cases of epilepsy observed by the author. Lancet *1857/I*, 528
3 MEUNIER, H.E.J.-M.: L'acide dipropylacétique et ses dérivés en tant que nouveaux médicaments dépresseurs du système nerveux central. FR Patent 2.442 M (1964)
4 SCHINDLER, W.: New N-heterocyclic compounds. US Patent 2,948,718 (1960 to Geigy Chemical Corp., Ardsley, N.Y.)
5 STERNBACH, L.H., REEDER, E.: Quinazolines and 1,4-benzodiazepines II. The rearrangement of 6-chloro-2-chloromethyl-4-phenylquinazoline 3-oxide into 2-amino derivatives of 7-chloro-5-phenyl-3H-1,4-benzodiazepine 4-oxide. J. organ. Chem. *26*, 1111 (1961)
6 WERNECKE, E.: Phenyläthylhydantoin (Nirvanol), ein neues Schlaf- und Beruhigungsmittel. Dtsch. med. Wschr. *42*, 1193 (1916)
7 WILHELM, M.: The chemistry of polycyclic psycho-active drugs – serendipity or systematic investigation? In Kielholz, P. (Editor): Depressive illness, Int. Symp., St. Moritz 1972, p. 129 (Huber, Berne/Stuttgart/Vienna 1972)

The biotransformation of carbamazepine

by J. W. FAIGLE*, S. BRECHBÜHLER*, K. F. FELDMANN*, and W. J. RICHTER**

I. Introduction

The term "biotransformation" is applied to the chemical changes which substances undergo in biological systems. Since these changes are almost invariably catalysed by enzymes, the form they take and the rate at which they occur depend on two factors: on the physico-chemical properties of the substance concerned and on the enzymatic complement of the biological system. In the following account of the biotransformation of carbamazepine (®Tegretol), we shall first deal briefly with physico-chemical aspects and then describe in detail the type of chemical transformation which carbamazepine undergoes, as well as the interactions occurring between the active substance itself and the enzymes in question. Although this description will be largely confined to processes taking place in the human organism, reference will also be made to certain supplementary findings from animal experiments.

The structural formula of carbamazepine and the characteristics of its solubility and partition in organic and aqueous media are such that it can be classified as a neutral lipophilic substance (Figure 1). The lipophilism which the molecule displays is attributable to its tricyclic framework, whereas its neutral character can be ascribed to its lack of basic or acid functions. Further details

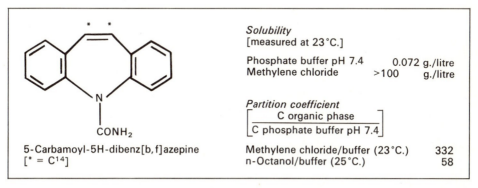

Solubility
[measured at 23 °C.]

Phosphate buffer pH 7.4	0.072 g./litre
Methylene chloride	>100 g./litre

Partition coefficient

$$\left[\frac{C \text{ organic phase}}{C \text{ phosphate buffer pH 7.4}} \right]$$

Methylene chloride/buffer (23 °C.)	332
n-Octanol/buffer (25 °C.)	58

5-Carbamoyl-5H-dibenz[b,f]azepine
[* = C¹⁴]

Fig. 1. The structural formula of carbamazepine, the characteristics of its solubility and partition, and the type and positioning of its radioactive label.

* Research Department, Pharmaceuticals Division, CIBA-GEIGY LIMITED, Basle, Switzerland.
** Physics and Spectroscopy Department, Central Function Research, CIBA-GEIGY LIMITED, Basle, Switzerland.

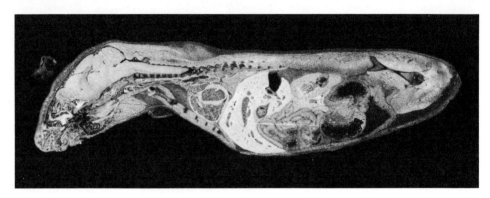

Fig. 2. Distribution of carbamazepine in the mouse one minute after intravenous administration of the C[14]-labelled active substance (dose: 5 mg./kg.; whole-body autoradiography).

on its chemistry have already been given in the paper presented by GA-GNEUX[11].

Since the lipophilism of carbamazepine is a property conducive to diffusion of the active substance through the body's various lipid membranes and barriers, it also facilitates the transport of the drug to its site of action. Illustrated in Figure 2 by reference to the mouse is an example showing just how rapidly these transport processes do in fact occur. This autoradiogram, taken only one minute after administration of an intravenous dose, reveals that carbamazepine has already penetrated into all the animal's tissues and organs. The distribution pattern does not suggest that the drug has any preferential affinity for certain organs in particular. In this autoradiogram of a sagittal section through the mouse, the distribution pattern of carbamazepine has been rendered visible by administering the active substance in C[14]-labelled form. In the negative of the autoradiogram, the radioactivity shows up white. The positioning of the radioactive label is indicated in Figure 1.

The body possesses no mechanism by which exogenous lipophilic substances, including especially those of a neutral character, can be excreted in unchanged form[31]. Such substances therefore first have to be transformed within the organism to more strongly hydrophilic metabolites, with which the kidneys can cope more readily. In the case of carbamazepine, it has been found in man that, when a labelled dose of 400 mg. is administered orally, only about 2% is excreted in the urine in unchanged form and 70% in the form of metabolites[9]. Let us now take a closer look at these metabolites.

II. Chemical aspects of the biotransformation of carbamazepine

1. Methodological problems posed by the isolation of metabolites
Studies dealing with elucidation of the structural formulae of carbamazepine metabolites have been published during recent years by various authors or

groups of authors[1, 3, 5, 6, 8, 10, 15, 17, 22, 23]. Although the structures of approximately a dozen different metabolites are described in these publications, our knowledge of the biotransformation of carbamazepine still cannot be regarded as complete. Firstly, the investigations carried out in man were not based on the use of radioisotopes, and they therefore offer no guarantee that all the metabolites of carbamazepine have been detected. Secondly, some of the methods of isolation employed may involve the production of artefacts. For example, in the case of carbamazepine, acid hydrolysis of conjugated metabolites can easily result in contraction of the seven-membered azepine ring and in the formation of acridine derivatives[2, 4].

2. New findings relating to the structure of carbamazepine metabolites

With a view to obtaining more reliable data, we have attempted in our own laboratories to arrive at as complete a picture as possible of the metabolites excreted in the urine by administering radioactively labelled carbamazepine to human subjects in an oral dose of 400 mg. For this purpose, the individual metabolites were isolated on a preparative scale using a high-resolution liquid chromatographic technique; where necessary, a gentle enzymatic cleavage process was resorted to, but care was taken not to employ any aggressive chemical hydrolysing agents. The structure of the metabolites was elucidated by means of spectroscopic methods, independently of which inverse isotope-dilution analysis was also used in order either to confirm or to disprove those structural formulae that appeared doubtful. Inverse isotope-dilution analysis can be carried out directly on unmodified urine: following the addition of an excess of non-radioactive synthetic carrier material having the same structure as the compound to be determined, the latter is re-isolated in isotopically diluted form and its radioactivity measured; this method eliminates all possibility of subsequent artefact formation.

Initial findings from this study have already been published elsewhere[9]. Meanwhile, the work has been largely, but not entirely, completed. A summary review of the data thus far obtained is given in Table 1; listed in the last column of this table are the reference numbers for papers in which the structural formulae of the metabolites in question have already been either described or proposed. In this connection, it is interesting to note that we have been unable to confirm the occurrence of the acridine derivatives XI and XII which several authors have postulated. The formation of artefacts, to which reference has already been made, might well provide an explanation for these discrepancies. Much the same applies to the iminostilbene metabolite X. As for the acridone compound XIII, although we were able to isolate this metabolite preparatively, isotope-dilution analysis revealed that the quantity present in the urine was equivalent at the most to only 0.1% of the dose administered.

3. Pathways involved in the biotransformation of carbamazepine

From the data presented in Table 1 it is possible to discern two different pathways for the biotransformation of carbamazepine, the first starting from epoxi-

Table 1. Compounds whose presence in human urine as metabolites of carbamazepine has been either confirmed or excluded by studies reported upon in the present paper.

Structure No.	Designation of compound	Method of assay	Quantity*	References
I	Carbamazepine	Isolation, I.D.A.**	+	5, 6, 9, 22
II	10,11-Epoxycarbamazepine	Isolation, I.D.A.	+	5, 9, 10, 17, 22
III	2-OH-Carbamazepine	Isolation, I.D.A.	++***	22
IV	3-OH-Carbamazepine	Isolation, I.D.A.	++***	–
V	1-OH-Carbamazepine	Isolation	++***	–
VI	Trans-10,11-di-OH-10,11-di-H-carbamazepine	Isolation, I.D.A.	+++***	9 (see also 5, 15)
VII	Cis-10,11-di-OH-10,11-di-H-carbamazepine	I.D.A.	○	1
VIII	10-OH-10,11-di-H-carbamazepine	I.D.A.	○	1, 5, 22
IX	9-Hydroxymethyl-10-carbamoyl acridan	Isolation, I.D.A.	++***	–
X	Iminostilbene	I.D.A.	○	5, 8, 23
XI	Acridine	I.D.A.	○	6
XII	9-Methylacridine	I.D.A.	○	3, 5, 6
XIII	Acridone	Isolation, I.D.A.	(+)	6

* Calculated or estimated in % of the dose administered: ○ (≤0.1%), + (0.1–2%), ++ (2–10%), +++ (10–30%)
** Inverse isotope-dilution analysis (sensitivity of the method: <0.1% of the dose administered)
*** Excreted partly or mostly in glucuronide form

dation of position 10, 11 in the molecule, and the second from hydroxylation in one of the aromatic rings. The two reaction sequences are outlined in Figures 3 and 4, respectively.

The data in Table 1 indicating in percent the amounts of the various metabolites recovered in the urine suggest that the epoxidation pathway (Figure 3) is quantitatively the more important of the two. Hardly any of the resultant epoxycarbamazepine, however, is excreted from the body as such, the reason being that opening of its oxirane ring leads to the formation of the transdiol VI. In the light of what is known about such reactions in general, it would appear that both steps, i.e. epoxidation and opening of the oxirane ring, are catalysed by enzymes from the endoplasmic reticulum of the liver – the epoxidation by mono-oxygenases[16] and the ring opening by an epoxide-hydrase[24]. Mammalian epoxide-hydrase is known to have the effect of producing diols of trans-configuration, a fact which is consonant with the configuration displayed by metabolite VI[9]. It is still a matter of speculation, however, whether contraction of the ring – which probably starts in metabolite II or VI and leads, via unknown intermediate steps, to product IX – occurs spontaneously or in response to enzymatic activity. In this particular instance, the possibility of

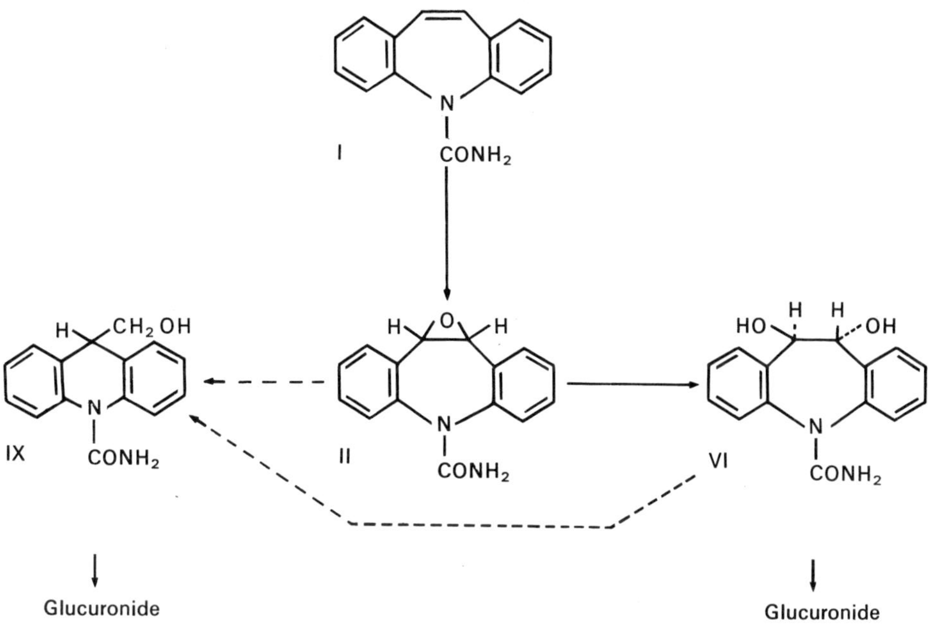

Fig. 3. Biotransformation of carbamazepine via epoxidation of the 10,11 double bond.

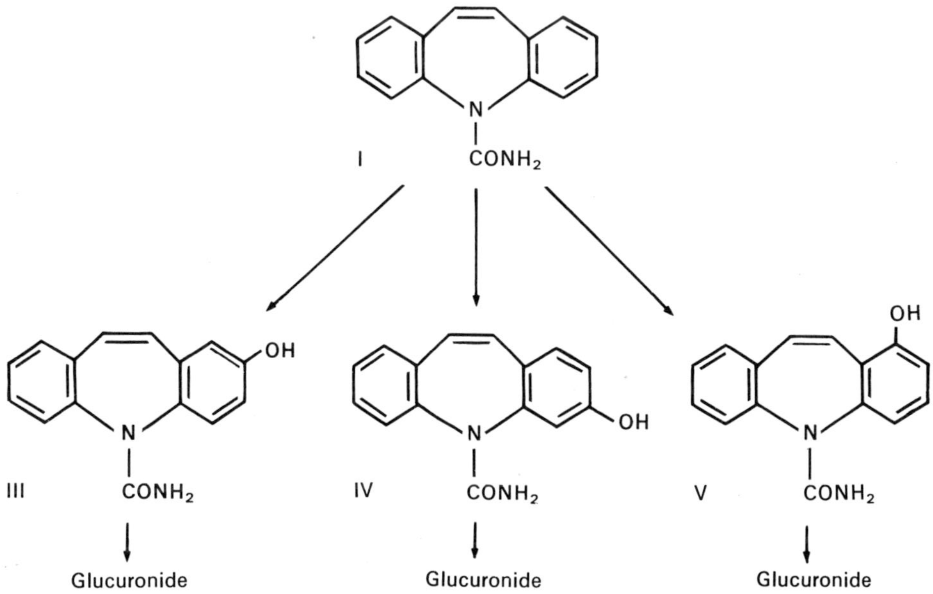

Fig. 4. Biotransformation of carbamazepine via aromatic hydroxylation.

an artefact being formed during the working-up process can be excluded, because the product in question was first isolated in glucuronide form and only then gently liberated with the aid of glucuronidase. Moreover, the presence of product IX was confirmed by isotope-dilution analysis.

131

From what is generally known, it may be concluded that production of the phenolic metabolites (Figure 4) is catalysed by hepatic oxygenases[14]. The resultant metabolites III, IV, and V are excreted chiefly in conjugated form. The possibility that other reaction pathways, besides those outlined in Figures 3 and 4, may also be involved, is one that cannot yet be excluded with certainty. There are, in fact, some metabolites, including strongly polar products containing no glucuronide, which have still to be elucidated. The findings obtained to date nevertheless do indicate that little if any formation of acridine derivatives or iminostilbenes occurs.

III. Pharmacokinetic aspects of the biotransformation of carbamazepine

1. Kinetics of metabolites in relation to the unchanged drug following single and repeated doses

In animal experiments, the epoxycarbamazepine metabolite II has been found to display anticonvulsive activity similar to that of carbamazepine itself[11, 23]. There is thus reason to suppose that in man this metabolite contributes to the therapeutic effect of carbamazepine. The significance of this epoxide, as compared with the intact active substance and the other metabolites, will therefore now be discussed by reference to the respective blood concentration patterns.

Presented in Figure 5 are the results of an experiment in which labelled carbamazepine was administered to two healthy subjects in a single oral dose

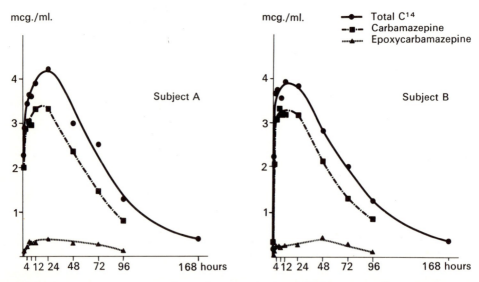

Fig. 5. Concentration curves for carbamazepine and 10,11-epoxycarbamazepine, as well as for the sum of all radioactive substances, in the plasma of man following a single oral dose of 400 mg. C[14]-labelled carbamazepine (values obtained in two subjects).

of 400 mg. This figure shows the plasma concentration curves (based on measurements yielded by isotope-dilution analysis) plotted for the unchanged substance and for the epoxide, as well as for the total radioactivity[9]. From these curves it can be seen that the concentration of intact active substance in the plasma is higher than that of all the metabolites together. Calculated on the basis of the area under the concentration-time curve between 0 and 96 hours, carbamazepine accounts for about 75% of the radioactivity measured, epoxycarbamazepine for 10%, and the sum of all the other metabolites for only 15%. The maximum concentration attained is approximately 3.3 mcg. per ml. for the unchanged substance and 0.39 mcg./ml. for the epoxide.

In another experiment, the pattern of the plasma concentrations was determined in six healthy subjects receiving repeated doses of 200 mg. daily. For this purpose, unlabelled carbamazepine was employed, and the carbamazepine and epoxycarbamazepine concentrations were therefore measured by a densitometric method involving the use of thin-layer plates and an internal standard (BRECHBÜHLER, S., publication in preparation). In each of the six subjects, kinetic data relating to a single 200 mg. dose were first obtained over a four-day period. The concentration patterns in response to daily doses of 200 mg. were then recorded during and after 14 days of treatment (extended in one case to 17 days)*.

The results of this experiment are given in Figure 6 in the form of curves plotted for the mean values in respect of the five subjects treated for 14 days. As was to be expected, the plasma concentration both of carbamazepine and

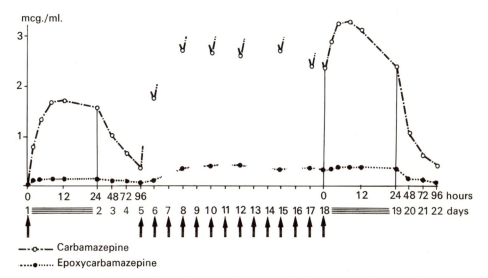

—··o··— Carbamazepine

····•······ Epoxycarbamazepine

Fig. 6. Concentrations of carbamazepine and 10,11-epoxycarbamazepine in the plasma of man following single and repeated oral doses of 200 mg. carbamazepine daily (mean values for five subjects; ▬▬▬ = time scale elongated; the arrows at the bottom indicate the days on which treatment was administered).

---

* Aliquots of the same plasma samples were assayed for carbamazepine independently by GÉRARDIN and HIRTZ[13] using gas-liquid chromatography.

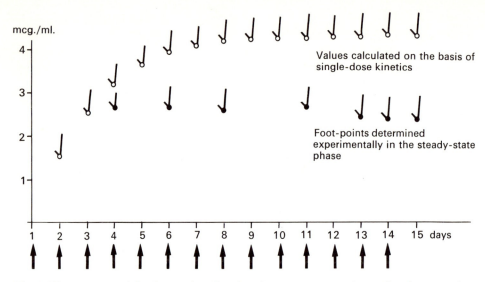

mcg./ml.

Values calculated on the basis of
single-dose kinetics

Foot-points determined
experimentally in the steady-state
phase

Fig. 7. Time course of the foot-points for the plasma concentrations of carbamazepine in man over a 14-day period of treatment with oral doses of 200 mg. daily (mean values for five subjects; the arrows at the bottom indicate the days on which treatment was administered).

of epoxycarbamazepine rose following repeated doses. In the case of carbamazepine, the concentrations recorded in the steady state were lower than the anticipated concentrations calculated from the single-dose kinetics by the method of WAGNER[30]; a graphic comparison between the calculated and the measured values is given in Figure 7. For the epoxy metabolite it is impossible to calculate the anticipated concentration exactly, because the elimination rate constant cannot be determined under these experimental conditions. From a rough estimate, however, it would appear that the steady-state concentration of the epoxide either approximates to the anticipated value or is somewhat lower.

2. Does carbamazepine stimulate its own degradation?

MORSELLI et al.[23] and SCHNEIDER and STENZEL[28] have suggested that, by inducing drug-metabolising enzymes, carbamazepine may accelerate its own biotransformation – a phenomenon referred to as auto-induction. The difference between the measured and the anticipated steady-state concentration of carbamazepine, to which reference has just been made, might certainly be accountable for in terms of auto-induction, but it could equally well be due to diminished absorption.

If enzyme induction does take place, it should be reflected in a shortening of the half-life of carbamazepine. An analysis of the data on the plasma concentrations recorded in all six of the above-mentioned subjects reveals that the half-life was 36.9 ± 3.2 hours $(\bar{x} \pm s_{\bar{x}})$ following a single dose and 27.9 ± 1.9 hours following repeated doses. This decrease occurred in each of the subjects tested and was statistically significant $(P < 0.05)$, a finding which can be taken

Table 2. Pharmacokinetic data on carbamazepine, determined from the time course of the plasma concentration in six subjects following single and repeated oral doses of 200 mg. carbamazepine daily.

Subject No.	Single dose			14th dose of a two-week period of treatment		
	$t_{max.}$ [*] (hr)	$C_{max.}$ [**] (mcg./ml.)	$t_{1/2}$ [***] (hr)	$t_{max.}$ [*] (hr)	$C_{max.}$ [**] (mcg./ml.)	$t_{1/2}$ [***] (hr)
1	24	1.5	36.5	12	3.2	27.7
2	8	1.9	36.5	8 [****]	3.1 [****]	23.1 [****]
3	12	1.6	28.9	4	3.6	27.7
4	12	2.0	40.8	8	4.3	36.5
5	8	1.8	28.9	8	2.9	24.8
6	4	1.9	49.5	4	3.0	27.7
$\bar{x}$	11.3	1.8	36.9	7.3	3.4	27.9
$S_{\bar{x}}$	2.8	0.08	3.2	1.2	0.21	1.9

   [*] Time at which maximum plasma concentration was measured
  [**] Maximum plasma concentration measured
 [***] Half-life
[****] 17th dose in Subject No. 2 (see text)

as proof that auto-induction does indeed occur (for individual values, see Table 2).

In this connection, it should perhaps be added that, with only a few exceptions, the individual half-life values for carbamazepine following a single dose are reported in the literature as ranging from 20 to 50 hours [9, 12, 13, 21, 23, 26], the overall average being 37 hours. In one paper, extreme values of 9 and 95 hours are quoted, but without any accompanying data on the concentrations measured [18]. KAUKO and TAMMISTO [20] claim to have obtained differing half-life values following administration of two different carbamazepine preparations; these findings, however, are open to doubt, also in view of the unspecific nature of the method of analysis employed by these authors.

It has already been mentioned that the acceleration of the biotransformation of carbamazepine resulting from auto-induction does not lead to any demonstrable rise in the plasma concentration of epoxycarbamazepine. According to CHRISTIANSEN [7] and SCHNEIDER [27], under the conditions of combined therapy – such as is commonly resorted to in the treatment of epilepsy – the degradation of carbamazepine is likely to be further accelerated by a process of hetero-induction. In this case, however, the diminution in the steady-state concentration of carbamazepine is alleged to be accompanied by a significant rise in the epoxycarbamazepine level. SCHNEIDER and STENZEL [28] state that in patients receiving not only carbamazepine but also phenobarbitone, diphenylhydantoin, and/or primidone, the half-life of carbamazepine is only 4–26 hours. Similar evidence of induction has also been reported by STRANDJORD and JOHANNESSEN [29] and JOHANNESSEN and STRANDJORD [19].

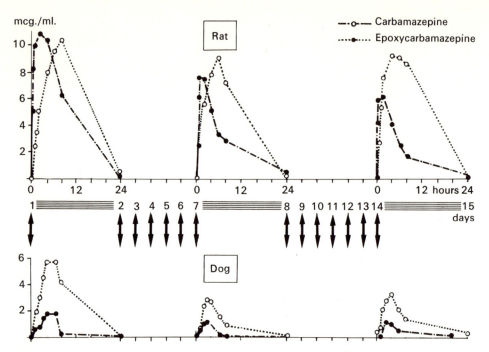

Fig. 8. Concentrations of carbamazepine and 10,11-epoxycarbamazepine in the plasma of rats (N = 5) and dogs (N = 3) during treatment with carbamazepine given in repeated oral doses of 50 mg./kg. daily (▬▬▬ = time scale elongated; the arrows indicate the days on which treatment was administered).

Further research will be necessary before any final conclusions can be reached with regard to the phenomenon of hetero-induction. There is an element of uncertainty, for example, about the half-life values reported by SCHNEIDER and STENZEL, which were obtained using an unspecific method of analysis. In connection with the therapeutic effect of carbamazepine, it will also be necessary to determine to what extent the decrease in the plasma carbamazepine concentration is offset by an increase in the epoxide concentration.

3. Which enzymes are induced by carbamazepine?

Animal experiments have yielded certain findings shedding light on the question of the enzymes that are induced by carbamazepine.

In the first place, it has been demonstrated that rats and dogs likewise exhibit signs of enzyme induction when given carbamazepine in repeated oral doses of 50 mg./kg. daily. As can be seen from Figure 8, showing the plasma concentration patterns recorded on the first, seventh, and 14th day, the concentration integral in respect of carbamazepine progressively diminishes with time. The epoxycarbamazepine integral either remains unchanged or also tends to diminish. Neither of these two animal species attains a steady state, because they excrete the drug at a much faster rate than man.

Independently of these findings, it has also been discovered in rats that after seven days of treatment with oral doses of 200 mg./kg. daily the liver displays

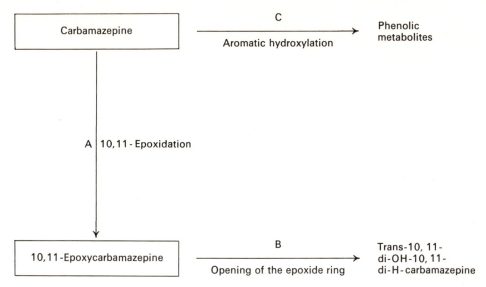

Fig. 9. Reactions controlling the degradation of carbamazepine and 10,11-epoxy-carbamazepine.

enhanced cytochrome P-450 and N.A.D.P.H. (nicotinamide-adenine-di-nucleotide phosphate) cytochrome c-reductase activity, and that after 14 days the values for N-demethylase activity show an increase as well (HESS, R., et al., unpublished findings). These effects are reversible.

The data which have already been presented in the section of this paper headed "Chemical aspects of the biotransformation of carbamazepine" indicate that the concentrations of carbamazepine and epoxycarbamazepine depend on the rate at which three different, experimentally confirmed, transformation reactions occur. These three reactions are outlined diagrammatically in Figure 9. Two of them (A and C) are catalysed by mono-oxygenases – of which cytochrome P-450, mentioned above, is an important representative – whereas the third reaction (B) is catalysed by an epoxide hydrase. The induction of oxygenases by carbamazepine may be regarded as proven; and, though it has not been confirmed experimentally that carbamazepine is also able to induce epoxide hydrase, other substrates exist which are known to be capable of so doing[25].

The phenomena of auto-induction that have been observed in animals and man – involving acceleration of the degradation of carbamazepine unaccompanied by any demonstrable increase in the epoxide concentration – may be attributable either solely to stimulation of phenol production (C) or to a simultaneous stimulation of epoxide formation (A) and epoxide cleavage (B) or, alternatively, to a combination of A, B, and C. If the phenomena of hetero-induction as described in man – entailing a decrease in the steady-state concentration of carbamazepine together with a simultaneous increase in the epoxide concentration – were to be confirmed, a likely explanation would be the additional and preferential stimulation of reaction A.

137

It will require further experimentation, however, before a final answer to this whole question is forthcoming.

IV. Conclusions

From the work which has been reviewed here the following conclusions can be drawn:

Carbamazepine undergoes extensive biotransformation in the body, the most important primary reactions being epoxidation of the 10, 11 double bond and hydroxylation of the aromatic ring.

The enzymes participating in the primary reactions are inducible by carbamazepine itself, as well as by substances such as phenobarbitone, diphenylhydantoin, and primidone. As a result of such induction, the half-life of carbamazepine is shortened.

It is probable that 10,11-epoxycarbamazepine, the most prominent of the primary metabolites, contributes to the anti-epileptic activity of carbamazepine. Though it is believed to exert little influence where carbamazepine is given alone, it may play a bigger role in combined drug regimens.

From the purely metabolic standpoint, it is preferable to administer carbamazepine alone rather than in combination with other medication, because in the case of monotherapy one can gain a better insight into the processes of induction.

When monitoring plasma concentrations for clinical purposes, it is advisable to measure the carbamazepine and epoxycarbamazepine levels simultaneously.

References

1 BAKER, K. M., CSETENYI, J., FRIGERIO, A., MORSELLI, P. L., PARRAVICINI, F., PFIFFERI, G.: 10,11-Dihydro-10,11-dihydroxy-5H-dibenz[b,f]azepine-5-carboxamide, a metabolite of carbamazepine isolated from human and rat urine. J. med. Chem. *16*, 703 (1973)

2 BAKER, K. M., FRIGERIO, A., MORSELLI, P. L., PFIFFERI, G.: Identification of a rearranged degradation product from carbamazepine-10,11-epoxide. J. pharm. Sci. *62*, 475 (1973)

3 BEYER, K.-H., BREDENSTEIN, O.: Chemie und Analytik des Carbamazepins (Tegretal). Dtsch. Apoth.-Ztg *109*, 1581 (1969)

4 BEYER, K.-H., BREDENSTEIN, O., SCHENCK, G.: Isolierung und Identifizierung eines Carbamazepin-Reaktionsproduktes. Arzneimittel-Forsch. (Drug Res.) *21*, 1033 (1971)

5 BRAZIER, J. L.: Dosage de la carbamazepine. Etude de son métabolisme chez l'homme. Thesis, Lyons 1973

6 BREDENSTEIN, O.: Analytik einiger therapeutisch angewandter Dibenzazepinderivate und Metabolismus des 5-Carbamoyl-5H-dibenzo[b,f]azepin (INN: Carbamazepin; Tegretal). Thesis, Berlin 1972

7 CHRISTIANSEN, J.: Drug interaction in epileptic patients. In Schneider, H., et al. (Editors): Clinical pharmacology of anti-epileptic drugs, Proc. Workshop on the determination of anti-epileptic drugs in body fluids – II, Bethel 1974 (Springer, Berlin/Heidelberg/New York 1975; printing)

8 Csetenyi, J., Baker, K. M., Frigerio, A., Morselli, P. L.: Iminostilbene – a metabolite of carbamazepine isolated from rat urine. J. Pharm. Pharmacol. 25, 340 (1973)

9 Faigle, J. W., Feldmann, K. F.: Pharmacokinetic data of carbamazepine and its major metabolites in man, loc. cit. [7]

10 Frigerio, A., Fanelli, R., Biandrate, P., Passerini, G., Morselli, P. L., Garattini, S.: Mass spectrometric characterization of carbamazepine-10,11-epoxide, a carbamazepine metabolite isolated from human urine. J. pharm. Sci. 61, 1144 (1972)

11 Gagneux, A. R.: The chemistry of carbamazepine. In Birkmayer, W. (Editor): Epileptic seizures – behaviour – pain, Int. Symp., St. Moritz 1975, p. 120 (Huber, Berne/Stuttgart/Vienna 1975)

12 Gauchel, G., Gauchel, F. D., Birkofer, L.: A micromethod for the determination of carbamazepine in blood by high speed liquid chromatography. Z. klin. Chem. 11, 459 (1973)

13 Gérardin, A., Hirtz, J.: The quantitative assay of carbamazepine in biological material and its application to basic pharmacokinetic studies, loc. cit. [11], p. 151

14 Gillette, J. R., Davis, D. C., Sasame, H. A.: Cytochrome P-450 and its role in drug metabolism. Ann. Rev. Pharmacol. 12, 57 (1972)

15 Goenechea, S., Hecke-Seibicke, E.: Beitrag zum Stoffwechsel von Carbamazepin. Z. klin. Chem. 10, 112 (1972)

16 Grover, P. L.: K-region epoxides of polycyclic hydrocarbons: formation and further metabolism by rat-lung preparations. Biochem. Pharmacol. 23, 333 (1974)

17 Herrmann, B.: Determination of carbamazepine in biological specimens. In: Plasmakoncentrationsbestämningar av antiepileptika: metodologiska och kliniska aspekter, Konf. Lidingö, Sweden, 1971, p. 15; abstract of paper

18 Hooper, W. D., DuBetz, D. K., Eadie, M. J., Tyrer, J. H.: Preliminary observations on the clinical pharmacology of carbamazepine ("Tegretol"). Paper presented at Meet. Aust. Ass. Neurol., 1974

19 Johannessen, S. I., Strandjord, R. E.: The influence of phenobarbital and diphenylhydantoin on carbamazepine serum levels, loc. cit. [7]

20 Kauko, K., Tammisto, P.: Comparison of two generically equivalent carbamazepine preparations. Ann. clin. Res. 6, Suppl. 11: 21 (1974)

21 Kupferberg, H. J.: quoted in Cereghino, J. J., Van Meter, J. C., Brock, J. T., Penry, J. K., Smith, L. D., White, B. G.: Preliminary observations of serum carbamazepine concentration in epileptic patients. Neurology (Minneap.) 23, 357 (1973)

22 Morselli, P. L., Gerna, M., Frigerio, A., Zanda, G., Nadai, F. de: Metabolic aspects of carbamazepine in animals and man. In: Abstr. Vth World Congr. Psychiat., Ciudad de México 1971, p. 439 (Prensa Médica Mexicana, Mexico 1971)

23 Morselli, P. L., Gerna, M., Maio, D. de, Zanda, G., Viani, F., Garattini, S.: Pharmacokinetic studies on carbamazepine in volunteers and in epileptic patients, loc. cit. [7]

24 Oesch, F.: Mammalian epoxide hydrases: inducible enzymes catalysing the inactivation of carcinogenic and cytotoxic metabolites derived from aromatic and olefinic compounds. Xenobiotica 3, 305 (1973)

25 Oesch, F.: Monooxygenase and epoxide hydratase. Dissociation of the biosynthesis of the two tightly coupled systems. Paper presented at IVth Europ. Workshop Drug Metab., Mainz 1974

26 Palmér, L., Bertilsson, L., Collste, P., Rawlins, M.: Quantitative determination of carbamazepine in plasma by mass fragmentography. Clin. Pharmacol. Ther. 14, 827 (1973)

27 Schneider, H.: Carbamazepine: the influence of other anticonvulsant drugs on its serum level; first results, loc. cit. [7]

28 SCHNEIDER, H., STENZEL, E.: Carbamazepin: Tageszeitlicher Verlauf des Serum-Spiegels unter Langzeitmedikation. Paper presented at XVIth Ann. Meet. Dtsch. Sekt. Int. Liga Epilepsie, Berlin 1974

29 STRANDJORD, R. E., JOHANNESSEN, S. I.: A preliminary study of serum carbamazepine levels in healthy subjects and in patients with epilepsy, loc. cit. [7]

30 WAGNER, J. G.: Relevant pharmacokinetics of antimicrobial drugs. Med. Clin. N. Amer. *58*, 479 (1974)

31 WEINER, I. M.: Mechanisms of drug absorption and excretion. The renal excretion of drugs and related compounds. Ann. Rev. Pharmacol. *7*, 39 (1967)

Pharmacokinetic studies with carbamazepine in epileptic patients

by P. L. Morselli*, L. Bossi**, and M. Gerna*

Introduction

Knowledge of the pharmacokinetic profile of a given drug is nowadays considered essential for rational therapy, since it has become evident that the intensity and the duration of a drug's therapeutic and toxic effects are very often closely related to its biological availability and disposition. In addition, it has also been shown on many occasions that kinetic parameters derived from studies in normal volunteers given a single dose do not apply to patients subjected to chronic treatment with higher dosages. This is well known to be the case with, for example, diphenylhydantoin[5,7] and propranolol[17,18].

In patients, moreover, different drugs are very often administered concomitantly, and we know today that possible drug interactions are so numerous that data obtained following a single dose of a single drug cannot be applied with any degree of reliability to the situation occurring in patients receiving chronic treatment with two or more drugs[14].

In view of these considerations it is obvious that more extensive and accurate studies must be carried out in patients in order to define more clearly the different variables capable of modifying a drug's plasma levels and, therefore, its therapeutic and toxic effects. In the field of the anticonvulsive agents a great deal of work has been done on diphenylhydantoin and phenobarbitone, with the result that much more is now known about their toxic and therapeutic thresholds as well as about their mutual interactions[10,11,20]. On the other hand, very few data are available on the pharmacokinetics of carbamazepine (®Tegretol) following chronic treatment with this drug. In previous studies we described its pharmacokinetic profile[12,15,16], as well as its metabolic degradation[1,4], in healthy volunteers. In the present study we shall report some observations made in epileptics (adults and children) which shed more light on the pharmacokinetics of carbamazepine during chronic treatment.

Materials and methods

a) Observations in epileptic patients
Longitudinal monitoring of plasma carbamazepine and carbamazepine-10,11-epoxide levels during chronic treatment was carried out in epileptic patients

* Laboratorio di Farmacologia Clinica, Istituto di Ricerche Farmacologiche "M. Negri", Milan, Italy.
** Istituto Neurologico "C. Besta", Milan, Italy.

(adults and children) receiving carbamazepine alone or combined with other anti-epileptic drugs (phenobarbitone, diphenylhydantoin, diazepam, or clonazepam).

Plasma sampling was performed in most cases at weekly intervals, immediately before and 5–6 hours after drug administration (at 7 a.m., 1 p.m., and 7 p.m.). In a few cases it was possible to determine the carbamazepine concentrations in the cerebrospinal fluid at the same time as the plasma levels.

The apparent plasma disappearance rate of carbamazepine after discontinuation of chronic treatment was ascertained in four patients. The apparent plasma half-life of carbamazepine-10,11-epoxide was also evaluated in these cases.

In five cases of meningioma the brain concentrations were assayed in the course of surgery.

b) Analytical methods

Quantitative determination of carbamazepine and carbamazepine-10,11-epoxide in body fluids and tissues was performed by gas-liquid chromatography, using a method previously described[13].

Results

a) Relationships between plasma carbamazepine levels and daily drug intake

No clear-cut relationship appeared to exist between the daily intake of carbamazepine (expressed in mg./kg. body weight) and the plasma levels measured after at least two weeks of uninterrupted treatment in 41 patients receiving the drug in combination with other anti-epileptic compounds (Figure 1).

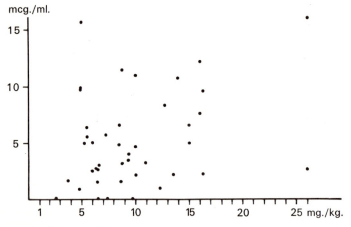

Fig. 1. Relationship between the daily intake (mg./kg.) of carbamazepine and the steady-state plasma levels (mcg./ml.) in 41 adult epileptic patients receiving the drug in combination with other anticonvulsive agents.

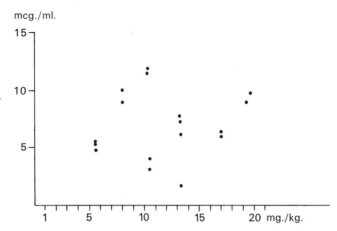

Fig. 2. Relationship between the daily intake (mg./kg.) of carbamazepine and the steady-state plasma levels (mcg./ml.) in ten adult epileptic patients receiving only carbamazepine. In seven of these patients the plasma levels were determined twice, the second occasion being after modification of the daily dose.

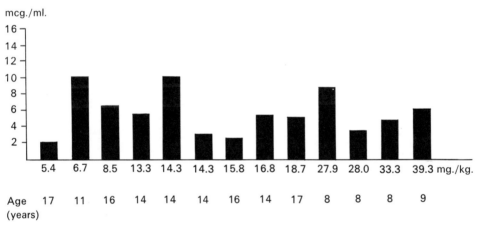

Fig. 3. Relationship between the daily intake (mg./kg.) of carbamazepine in 13 children and the steady-state plasma levels (mcg./ml.). In these cases other drugs were administered in addition to carbamazepine.

The same lack of relationship was evident in ten cases in which carbamazepine was given alone (Figure 2). In children, too, as shown in Figure 3, we could find no relationship between daily dose and plasma levels. This lack of correlation between daily dose per kg. body weight and steady-state plasma level underlines the need to monitor the plasma levels during chronic therapy. Another point worth stressing is the remarkable fluctuation which can be observed in some patients during long-term monitoring and which in most cases is indicative of a poor compliance. An example in point is given in Figure 4, which shows the time course of the plasma carbamazepine levels monitored at weekly intervals over a period of 12 weeks in institutionalised adult patients receiving the drug together with diphenylhydantoin and phenobarbitone.

143

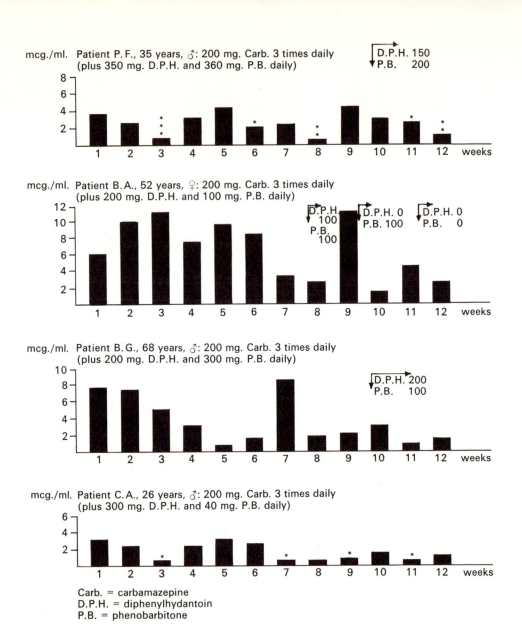

Carb. = carbamazepine
D.P.H. = diphenylhydantoin
P.B. = phenobarbitone

Fig. 4. Plasma levels of carbamazepine (mcg./ml.) monitored at weekly intervals over a period of 12 weeks in four non-cooperating institutionalised epileptic patients. The asterisks indicate occurrence of seizures.

b) Plasma levels of carbamazepine-10,11-epoxide in epileptic patients undergoing chronic treatment

The plasma concentrations of carbamazepine and of carbamazepine-10,11-epoxide monitored over a period of 20 days in six adult patients receiving carbamazepine alone are indicated in Table 1.

The plasma levels ranged from 1.78 to 20.3 mcg./ml. for carbamazepine and from zero to 4.2 mcg./ml. for carbamazepine-10,11-epoxide. The ratio between

Table 1. Plasma concentrations (mcg./ml.) of carbamazepine (Carb.) and of carbamazepine-10,11-epoxide (Carb.-epox.) in six epileptic patients during chronic treatment with carbamazepine only.

Patient	Age (years)	Sex	Dose (mg./kg.)	Compound determined in plasma	Days of treatment					Effect
					2	5	10	15	20	
G.C.	36	M	15.0	Carb.	8.2	n.p.	12.5	10.9	14.00	Good
				Carb.-epox.	n.p.	n.p.	n.p.	n.p.	n.p.	
V.V.	35	F	10.3	Carb.	2.1	2.0	n.p.	1.78	3.00	None
				Carb.-epox.	n.p.	n.p.	n.p.	n.p.	n.p.	
P.E.	21	F	11.9	Carb.	12.9	10.3	11.3	8.8	n.p.	Good
				Carb.-epox.	n.d.	1.8	2.1	1.8	n.p.	
R.E.	34	F	9.7	Carb.	11.0	12.6	8.3	11.0	n.p.	Good
				Carb.-epox.	n.d.	1.8	1.6	2.5	n.p.	
Z.P.	57	M	11.7	Carb.	n.p.	20.3	18.6	n.p.	n.p.	Good
				Carb.-epox.	n.p.	4.2	2.5	n.p.	n.p.	
B.R.	15	M	14.0	Carb.	n.p.	7.0	11.6	n.p.	10.8	Moderate
				Carb.-epox.	n.p.	2.5	1.8	n.p.	2.1	

n.p. = not performed
n.d. = not detectable

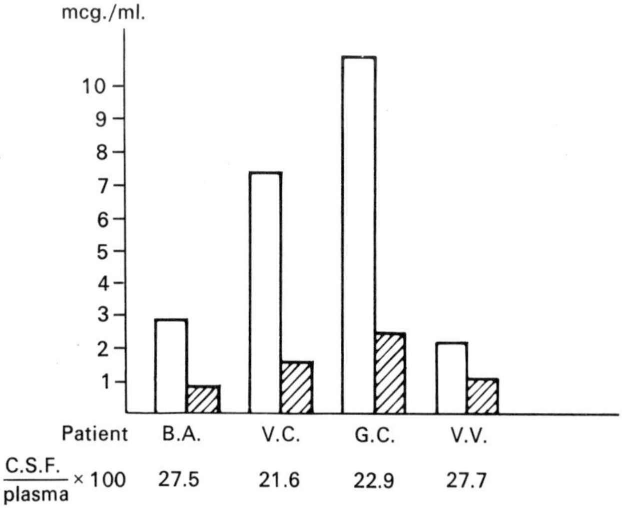

Fig. 5. Plasma levels (plain columns) and cerebrospinal fluid concentrations (hatched columns) of carbamazepine in four adult epileptic patients.

Patient	B.A.	V.C.	G.C.	V.V.
$\frac{C.S.F.}{plasma} \times 100$	27.5	21.6	22.9	27.7

the metabolite and the parent compound was not constant, and the levels of the epoxide did not seem to be related to those of carbamazepine itself.

It may be interesting to note that a complete lack of effect was observed only in Patient V.V., whose plasma carbamazepine levels were considerably lower than those of the other five subjects.

In two of these patients and in two others the C.S.F. levels of carbamazepine were determined at the same time as the plasma concentrations. The results of these determinations are shown in Figure 5. The C.S.F./plasma ratio exhibits a good measure of agreement with the plasma protein-binding data obtained in volunteers[2,16].

Table 2. Plasma concentrations (mcg./ml.) of carbamazepine (Carb.), carbamazepine-10,11-epoxide (Carb.-epox.), diphenylhydantoin (D.P.H.), and phenobarbitone (P.B.) in four epileptic children during combined treatment.

Patient	Age (years)	Sex	Body weight (kg.)	Treat- ment	Dose (mg./kg.)	Compound determined in plasma	Weeks of treatment				
							1	2	3	4	5
L. E.	8	M	43	P.B.	3.4	P.B.	38.0	57.0	30.2	42.8	35.0
				Carb.	27.9	Carb.	8.7	8.1	7.5	3.6	3.0
						Carb.-epox.	2.4	1.8	2.4	0.4	n.d.
D. L. P.	14	M	60	P.B.	4.1	P.B.	29.0	36.0	22.8	36.0	34.2
				D.P.H.	3.3	D.P.H.	2.6	1.0	2.3	4.5	5.0
				Carb.	16.6	Carb.	5.8	6.4	5.6	2.5	5.4
						Carb.-epox.	2.0	2.2	2.2	0.6	0.4
B. D.	8	M	18	P.B.	8.3	P.B.	24.6	46.4	45.0	49.0	42.7
				Carb.	33.3	Carb.	9.6	6.8	4.6	4.2	5.0
						Carb.-epox.	2.0	2.4	1.8	2.6	2.4
N. R.	16	F	47	P.B.	5.1 → 4.2*	P.B.	68.5	63.0	49.7	44.0	n.p.
				D.P.H.	4.2 → 6.3*	D.P.H.	3.8	5.3	8.1	11.4	n.p.
				Carb.	8.5	Carb.	5.1	6.4	6.9	9.4	n.p.
						Carb.-epox.	n.d.	1.2	2.3	n.d.	n.p.

* The dose of P.B. was reduced and that of D.P.H. increased after the second week of treatment.
n.p. = not performed
n.d. = not detectable

Comparable data with regard to plasma levels were obtained over a five-week period in four hospitalised epileptic children receiving carbamazepine in combination with diphenylhydantoin and/or phenobarbitone (Table 2). Here, too, no fixed ratio was apparent between the carbamazepine-10,11-epoxide levels and the carbamazepine concentrations. In two cases (Patients L. E. and B. D.) there was a progressive drop in the plasma carbamazepine levels in the course of time, while in Patient N.R. a rise in the carbamazepine concentrations and a fall in the epoxide levels were observed concomitantly with an increase in the plasma diphenylhydantoin levels.

c) Apparent plasma half-life of carbamazepine and of carbamazepine-10,11-epoxide following repeated administration of carbamazepine
In four patients the apparent plasma half-life of carbamazepine and of carbamazepine-10,11-epoxide was evaluated following repeated administration of carbamazepine for 15–20 days.
Data relating to three of these cases are presented in Figure 6. In these three cases the apparent plasma half-life of carbamazepine was significantly shorter than that previously observed in normal volunteers following a single administration, which suggests that either an auto-induction phenomenon or a residual effect from previous drug treatment may have been involved. The apparent plasma half-life of carbamazepine-10,11-epoxide was found to be much shorter than that of the parent compound in two cases (it amounted to eight hours in Patient R. E. and to six hours in Patient P. E.), whereas the shortening was less marked in Patient P. L. (14 hours).

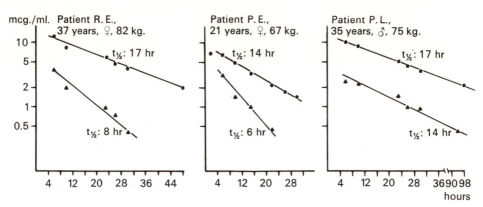

Fig. 6. Apparent half-life ($t_{\frac{1}{2}}$) of carbamazepine (•) and carbamazepine-10,11-epoxide (▲) after repeated administration of carbamazepine in three epileptic patients.

Table 3. Brain and plasma concentrations of carbamazepine in five neurosurgical patients, all of whom received the drug for at least three days prior to surgery.

Patient	Age (years)	Sex	Diagnosis	Dose of carbamazepine		Plasma levels (mcg./ml.)	Brain levels (mcg./g.)	Brain/ plasma ratio
				(mg. daily)	(mg./kg.)			
B.G.	50	F	Meningioma of lesser wing	400	4.6	8.7	9.7	1.1
B.C.	45	F	Meningioma of olfactory sulcus	600	7.5	3.6	8.1	2.25
C.P.	41	F	Meningioma of olfactory sulcus	600	8.65	8.7	9.6	1.1
L.F.	52	M	Parieto-occipital meningioma	600	8.8	5.1	10.5	2.05
M.G.	63	F	Meningioma of olfactory sulcus	600	9.5	4.4	4.8	1.09

In the fourth case, in which the treatment had to be discontinued because of severe side effects (nystagmus, ataxia, vomiting, diplopia), the apparent plasma half-life of carbamazepine was 119 hours and no traces of epoxide could be found in the plasma.

d) Brain levels of carbamazepine
Brain and plasma levels of carbamazepine were measured in five patients suffering from meningioma. In these cases the drug was administered prophylactically for 3–4 days prior to surgery.
The findings in respect of the brain and plasma concentrations are listed in Table 3, together with other essential data on the patients. It can be seen that the brain/plasma ratios, observed in our cases about 13 hours after the last dose of the drug, were of the same order of magnitude as the values previously obtained in animals[15]. No attempt was made on this occasion to separate the levels in grey matter from those in white matter.

In previous studies it was observed that in normal healthy volunteers the apparent plasma half-life ranged from 30 to 50 hours while the apparent volume of distribution was relatively constant ($\simeq 0.95$ litre/kg.) [16, 19].

The finding that the apparent plasma half-life of carbamazepine was significantly shorter in three epileptic patients than in normal volunteers indicates that this factor should be taken into account in the assessment of dosage schedules. Carbamazepine is a known metabolic inducer[6], and the possibility of auto-induction during repeated treatments cannot be excluded. A definite auto-induction phenomenon has in fact been observed in the rat[3, 12]. Our observations on the C.S.F. concentration of the drug in epileptic patients are in good agreement with the binding of 74–76% found for carbamazepine in normal volunteers[2], and they confirm previous data reported by JOHANNESSEN and STRANDJORD[8, 9]. Other anticonvulsive drugs do not seem to have any significant displacing effect on carbamazepine[16].

Monitoring of plasma drug levels in poorly cooperating institutionalised patients over a period of 12 weeks revealed that the plasma concentration of carbamazepine in one and the same patient varied to a remarkable extent.

This observation highlights the problem of drug compliance in cases of poor patient cooperation and emphasises the difficulties of evaluating the efficacy of a given treatment without monitoring the plasma levels of the drug concerned. Variations attributed to induction phenomena or to other drug interactions may, in fact, be sustained by poor drug compliance.

Monitoring of the plasma levels of carbamazepine-10,11-epoxide showed that this compound is usually present after a few days of treatment, and that it may account for about 15–45% of the parent drug. The percentage, however, varies greatly not only from one subject to another but also in one and the same subject at different points in time. This is understandable, since, in three of the cases in which it was measured, the apparent plasma half-life of the epoxide seemed to be shorter than that of carbamazepine. In rats, the epoxide, administered intraperitoneally in doses of 25, 50, and 100 mg./kg., affords clearcut protection against convulsions induced by maximal electrical stimulation; following the 100 mg./kg. dose, this protection may last for up to 6–8 hours (GERNA and MORSELLI, unpublished data). Whether the epoxide also displays this property in man, is not yet known. However, the observation that the epoxide has a relatively short half-life in humans casts some doubt on the ability of this metabolite to exert a relevant anti-epileptic effect in man.

In general, subjects whose plasma carbamazepine levels were between 7 and 12 mcg./ml. tended to display a better therapeutic response. When given in combination with other anti-epileptic drugs, carbamazepine seemed to attain plasma levels which were lower than those reached with monotherapy.

An example of the relationships between the plasma levels of carbamazepine and the drug's therapeutic effect is illustrated in Figure 7. It is evident from this figure that good control of symptomatology was achieved with levels of about 8–10 mcg./ml. Following the discontinuation of therapy, the clinical

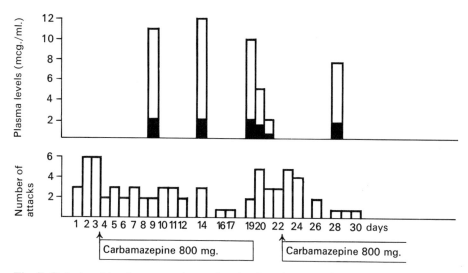

Fig. 7. Relationships between plasma levels of carbamazepine *(above,* plain columns) and of carbamazepine-10,11-epoxide *(above,* black columns) and therapeutic effect *(below)* in one epileptic patient.

picture clearly deteriorated as soon as the plasma levels dropped below 6 mcg. per ml. The resumption of treatment led once again to normalisation of the symptomatology at plasma levels of about 8 mcg./ml.

In conclusion, the findings presented here indicate that the plasma half-life of carbamazepine may be significantly shorter in epileptic patients than it is in normal volunteers; they also show that carbamazepine-10,11-epoxide is present in the plasma during repeated administration of carbamazepine, and they suggest that pharmacokinetic data obtained in volunteers may not be relevant to the assessment of dosage schedules in patients.

These facts and the remarkable between-patient and within-patient variability observed in the plasma levels of carbamazepine underline the need for more long-term monitoring of plasma drug levels in epileptic patients, so as to ensure that dosage schedules and therapeutic effectiveness can be assessed with a greater degree of accuracy.

References

1 BAKER, K.M., CSETENYI, J., FRIGERIO, A., MORSELLI, P.L., PARRAVICINI, F., PFIFFERI, G.: 10,11-Dihydro-10,11-dihydroxy-5H-dibenz[b,f]azepine-5-carbox-amide, a metabolite of carbamazepine isolated from human and rat urine. J.med. Chem. *16*, 703 (1973)

2 DI SALLE, E., PACIFICI, G. M., MORSELLI, P. L.: Studies on plasma protein binding of carbamazepine. Pharmacol. Res. Commun. *6*, 193 (1974)

3 FARGHALI-HASSAN, ASSAEL, B. M., GERNA, M., GARATTINI, S., MORSELLI, P.L.: Carbamazepine pharmacokinetics in young adult and pregnant rats. Relationships with the pharmacologic effect. Europ. J. Pharmacol. (submitted for publication)

4 FRIGERIO, A., FANELLI, R., BIANDRATE, P., PASSERINI, G., MORSELLI, P. L., GAR-
ATTINI, S.: Mass spectrometric characterization of carbamazepine-10,11-epoxide,
a carbamazepine metabolite isolated from human urine. J. pharm. Sci. *61*, 1144
(1972)

5 GLAZKO, A. J., CHANG, T.: Diphenylhydantoin. Absorption, distribution, excretion, loc. cit. [20], p. 127

6 HANSEN, J. M., SIERSBAEK-NIELSEN, K., SKOVSTED, L.: Carbamazepine-induced
acceleration of diphenylhydantoin and warfarin metabolism in man. Clin. Pharmacol. Ther. *12*, 539 (1971)

7 HOUGHTON, G. W., RICHENS, A.: Rate of elimination of tracer doses of phenytoin
at different steady-state serum phenytoin concentrations in epileptic patients.
Brit. J. clin. Pharmacol. *1*, 155 (1974)

8 JOHANNESSEN, S. I., STRANDJORD, R. E.: The concentration of carbamazepine
(Tegretol) in serum and in cerebrospinal fluid in patients with epilepsy. Acta
neurol. scand. *48*, Suppl. 51:445 (1972)

9 JOHANNESSEN, S. I., STRANDJORD, R. E.: Concentration of carbamazepine (Tegretol)
in serum and in cerebrospinal fluid in patients with epilepsy. Epilepsia (Amst.)
14, 373 (1973)

10 KUTT, H.: Pharmacodynamic and pharmacokinetic measurements of antiepileptic
drugs. Clin. Pharmacol. Ther. *16*, 243 (1974)

11 MORSELLI, P. L.: Significato ed importanza della misura e del controllo delle con-
centrazioni plasmatiche dei farmaci nella terapia dell'epilessia. Prospett. Pediat.
12, 523 (1973)

12 MORSELLI, P. L., BIANDRATE, P., FRIGERIO, A., GARATTINI, S.: Pharmacokinetics
of carbamazepine in rats and humans. Europ. J. clin. Invest. *2*, 297 (1972); abstract
of paper

13 MORSELLI, P. L., BIANDRATE, P., FRIGERIO, A., GERNA, M., TOGNONI, G.: Gas
chromatographic determination of carbamazepine and carbamazepine-10-11-
epoxide in human body fluids. In Meijer, J. W. A., et al. (Editors): Methods of
analysis of anti-epileptic drugs, Proc. Workshop on the determination of anti-
epileptic drugs in body fluids, Noordwijkerhout, The Netherlands 1972, p. 169,
Int. Congr. Ser. No. 286 (Excerpta Medica, Amsterdam/American Elsevier, New
York 1973)

14 MORSELLI, P. L., GARATTINI, S., COHEN, S. N. (Editors): Drug interactions (Raven
Press, New York 1974)

15 MORSELLI, P. L., GERNA, M., GARATTINI, S.: Carbamazepine plasma and tissue
levels in the rat. Biochem. Pharmacol. *20*, 2043 (1971)

16 MORSELLI, P. L., GERNA, M., MAIO, D. DE, ZANDA, G., VIANI, F., GARATTINI, S.:
Pharmacokinetic studies on carbamazepine in volunteers and in epileptic patients.
In Schneider, H., et al. (Editors): Clinical pharmacology of anti-epileptic drugs,
Proc. Workshop on the determination of anti-epileptic drugs in body fluids – II,
Bethel 1974 (Springer, Berlin/Heidelberg/New York 1975; printing)

17 MORSELLI, P. L., MORGANTI, A., BIANCHETTI, G., DI SALLE, E., LEONETTI, G.,
CHIDSEY, C. A., ZANCHETTI, A.: Plasma levels and pharmacokinetic studies of
propranolol during chronic treatment in hypertensive patients. Europ. J. clin.
Invest. *4*, 347 (1974); abstract of paper

18 SHAND, D. G.: Pharmacokinetic properties of the β-adrenergic receptor blocking
drugs. Drugs *7*, 39 (1974)

19 STRANDJORD, R. E., JOHANNESSEN, S. I.: A preliminary study of serum carbamazepine levels in healthy subjects and in patients with epilepsy, loc. cit. [16]

20 WOODBURY, D. M., PENRY, J. K., SCHMIDT, R. P. (Editors): Antiepileptic drugs
(Raven Press, New York 1972)

The quantitative assay of carbamazepine in biological material and its application to basic pharmacokinetic studies

by A. Gérardin and J. Hirtz*

Introduction

The quantitative assay of carbamazepine in blood or plasma is extremely important both for the monitoring of blood levels in the course of long-term treatment and because of the light it can shed on the drug's pharmacokinetics. Unfortunately, such assays are not easy to perform. The purpose of the present paper is to describe a new method of assaying carbamazepine in biological material and to report on the application of this method to a basic pharmacokinetic study.

Quantitative assay of carbamazepine

Numerous methods for the quantitative determination of carbamazepine have already been described. The optical methods (Table 1) are based on the ab-

Table 1. Optical methods for the assay of carbamazepine.

Authors	Method	Material studied	Limit of detection	Specificity
Führ[10]	Absorption of carbamazepine itself (290 mμ)	Blood, urine	Approx. 4 mcg./ml.	Low
Beyer and Klinge[1]	Heating with HCl. Absorption of the corresponding methylacridine (255 mμ)	Water	At least 1 mcg./ml.	Nil
Frey and Yrjänä[8]	HNO$_3$/NO$_2$. Absorption of the resultant dye (400 mμ)	Serum	Not indicated	Relatively good. Diol not measured, and the epoxide only to the extent of 20%
Nielsen and Remmer[26]	HNO$_3$/NO$_2$. Absorption of the resultant dye (400 mμ)	Serum	Not indicated	Partial
Gruska et al.[14]	Heating with HCl. Absorption of the corresponding methylacridine (255 mμ)	Blood, urine, dialysis fluid	Approx. 1 mcg./ml.	Nil
Morselli et al.[25]	Absorption of carbamazepine itself (290 mμ)	Plasma	0.5 mcg./ml.	Said to be good
Johannessen and Strandjord[15]	Modification of the method described by Nielsen and Remmer[26]	Serum, C.S.F.	?	?

* Centre de Recherche Biopharmaceutique CIBA-GEIGY, Rueil Malmaison, France.

Table 2. Methods based on thin-layer chromatography.

Authors	Method	Material studied	Limit of detection	Specificity
Braunhofer and Zicha [3]	Not described	C.S.F., blood, bile, duodenal juice	0.01 mcg./ml. (?)	?
Scheiffarth et al.[30]	Separation and scratching, measurement of fluorescence following treatment with an acid	C.S.F., bile, urine, serum	0.02 mcg./ml.	Possibly good, but bad solvent system
Schmidt et al.[31]	Qualitative method (including gas chromatography, infrared and ultraviolet absorption)	–	–	Determination performed in the presence of other drugs. Separation of metabolites not studied
Weist and Schmid [34]	Fluorescence	Gastric juice, urine	Qualitative	Ditto
Lauffer et al.[19]	Direct measurement of fluorescence on the plates following treatment with perchloric acid	Gastric juice, urine	10–20 ng.	Measurement performed in the presence of other drugs. Separation of metabolites not studied
Gardner-Thorpe et al.[12]	Visual comparison on the plates (semiquantitative)	–	<1 mcg.	Ditto
Christiansen [4]	Measurement performed on the plates with Vitatron	Plasma	Approx. 10 ng.	Good
Christiansen [5]	Measurement performed on the plates with Vitatron	Plasma	?	Good
Faber and Man in't Veld [7]	Determination of fluorescence following treatment with perchloric acid. Measurement performed on the plates with Vitatron	Plasma	10 ng.	Good

sorption of carbamazepine or of one of its derivatives in the ultraviolet or visible spectrum, and they are not very specific. The methods employing thin-layer chromatography (Table 2) are both specific and sensitive, but they call for equipment (i.e. a densitometer) which is still seldom used, especially in hospital laboratories. With the aid of gas chromatography (Table 3) it is apparently possible to make a precise and specific quantitative assay of carbamazepine, but the substance is not very stable at the temperatures required to volatilise it. Depending on the conditions of the experiment, it invariably

Table 3. Methods based on gas chromatography.

Authors	Method	Material studied	Limit of detection	Specificity
Larsen et al.[18]	Direct	Serum	?	?
Meijer and Meinardi[22]	?	Blood	?	?
Bohn[2]	–	Serum	Approx. 1 mcg./ml.	?
Meijer[21]	Direct. Internal standard. Combined with thin-layer chromatography	Serum, C.S.F.	1 mcg./ml.	Good when combined with thin-layer chromatography
Gardner-Thorpe et al.[11]	Direct	Plasma	1 ng.	No data. Separation of other anti-epileptics
Kupferberg[16]	Trimethylsilyl derivative	Plasma	0.5 mcg./ml.	Separation of metabolites not described
Toseland et al.[32]	Direct. Internal standard	Plasma	2 mcg./ml.	Separation of metabolites not described
Larsen et al.[17]	Direct. Internal standard	Serum	1 mcg./ml.	Separation of metabolites not described
Morselli et al.[23]	No details given, paper presented at a congress			
Morselli et al.[24]	Direct. Internal standard	Plasma	0.5 mcg./ml.	Good ?
Palmér et al.[27]	Gas chromatography and mass-spectrometry	Plasma	Approx. 50 ng./ml.	Internal standard: 10,11-dihydro-carbamazepine
Friel and Green[9]	Direct. Internal standard	Serum	0.5 mcg./ml.	No data. Separation of other anti-epileptics
Roger et al.[29]	Derivative obtained prior to gas-liquid chromatography	Plasma	0.5 mcg./ml.	?
Cremers and Verheesen[6]	Derivative obtained prior to gas-liquid chromatography. No internal standard	Serum	Not indicated	No data
Perchalski and Wilder[28]	Derivative obtained prior to gas-liquid chromatography	Plasma	0.2 mcg./ml.	?
Mashford et al.[20]	Direct. Internal standard. Alkaline flame ionisation detector	Plasma	Approx. 1 mcg./ml.	No data

disintegrates to a more or less marked degree, this disintegration resulting in iminostilbene:

Some authors, however, have succeeded in reducing the extent of the disintegration to a point where it produces only a negligible error in the quantitative assay, but the methods they employ are difficult to perform with different equipment or even in another laboratory.

We have found[13] that a stable derivative of carbamazepine (I) can be obtained by dehydrating the amide group to cyanide, which gives carbamazepine cyanamide (II):

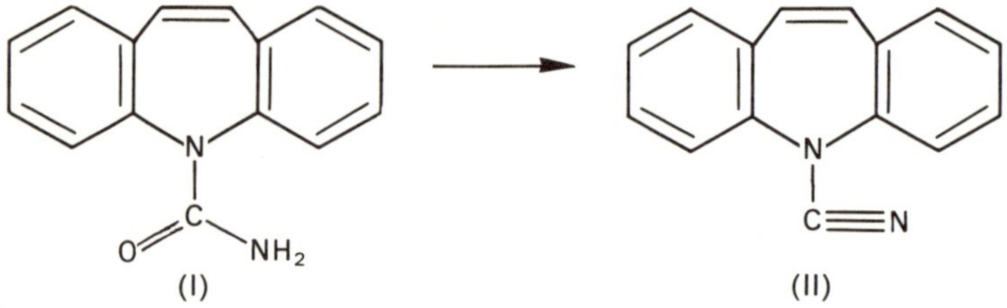

This derivative is perfectly stable and does not yield iminostilbene at the temperatures required for gas chromatography.

Method

Reagents

All solvents must be of analytical reagent grade. Carbon disulphide and methylene chloride are employed as they are, but all the other solvents are redistilled prior to use. Trifluoroacetic anhydride and triethylamine are used in the form of 10% solutions v/v in methylene chloride, which are freshly prepared each day; 10-methoxycarbamazepine is employed as an internal standard. A stock solution containing 2.5 mcg./ml. in methylene chloride is prepared and stored at +4°C.

Equipment

The chromatographic determinations are carried out with a gas chromatograph equipped with a flame ionisation detector. The glass columns, two metres in length, are filled with Chromosorb W (90/115 mesh) which has been treated with hexamethyldisilazane and impregnated with 5% cyanopropylphenylmethyl silicon. The operating temperature is 270°C. The retention time for the carbamazepine derivative (II) is approximately five minutes; its retention volume relative to the internal standard is 0.62 (Figure 1).

The glassware is washed in the usual manner and then subjected to ultrasonic treatment for 15 minutes in a chloroform bath. The columns used in the purification stage are made from Pasteur pipettes, the capillary ends of which have been cut off; these columns are filled to a level of 3 cm. with adsorption chromatography silica gel of Grade 2 activity. They are immersed in a 1:1 mixture of ethyl ether and pentane and the air bubbles are removed by suction. Once they are ready for use, the columns are stored at a temperature of less than 22°C.

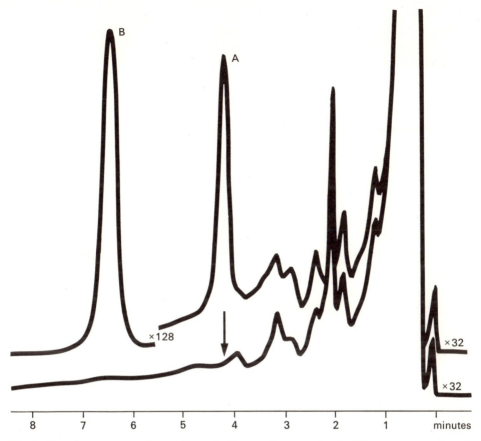

Fig. 1. Gas chromatography performed after carbamazepine had been extracted and the derivative obtained (see text).
Lower curve: normal human plasma (the arrow indicates the position of carbamazepine).
Upper curve: human plasma containing 250 ng. carbamazepine per ml. A: carbamazepine in the form of the derivative (II); B: internal standard (10-methoxycarbamazepine).

Experimental procedure

1 ml. plasma or urine, 2 ml. ethyl ether, 1 ml. internal standard solution, and 0.25 ml. of a 30% sodium hydroxide solution are placed into a 10 ml. glass centrifuge tube with ground-glass stopper. The mixture is shaken for five minutes and centrifuged. The organic phase is collected and evaporated to dryness under a nitrogen flow.

The residue is dissolved in 200 mcl. of a 1:1 mixture of ethyl ether and pentane and introduced into a small column filled with silica gel (see above); 4 ml. of a 1:1 mixture of ethyl ether and pentane is passed through the column and discarded; this is followed by 4 ml. of acetone, which is collected in a 10 ml. glass centrifuge tube and evaporated to dryness under nitrogen. The residue is dissolved in 100 mcl. of the triethylamine solution; 50 mcl. of the trifluoroacetic anhydride solution is added. The stoppered tube is left to stand for ten

155

Table 4. Comparison of results obtained in the plasma and urine of a subject given 400 mg. C[14]-labelled carbamazepine by mouth.

Plasma			Urine		
Time (hr)	Isotope dilution (mcg./ml.)	Gas-liquid chromatography (mcg./ml.)	Time (hr)	Isotope dilution (mcg./ml.)	Gas-liquid chromatography (mcg./ml.)
24	4.28	4.01	0–24	1.28	1.28
48	2.85	3.05	24–48	1.00	1.02
72	2.21	2.25	48–76	0.71	0.72

minutes, whereupon 2 ml. ethyl ether and 1 ml. of 0.25 M sodium hydroxide solution are added. The mixture is shaken for three minutes and centrifuged. The organic phase is transferred to a glass tube with a conical bottom and evaporated under nitrogen. The residue is dissolved in 100 mcl. carbon disulphide, and 1–5 mcl. is injected into the gas chromatograph.

The concentrations are determined by reference to a calibration curve, which is prepared from methylene chloride solutions containing known quantities of carbamazepine (I) and the same quantity of the internal standard as that used for the unknown samples. These solutions are evaporated to dryness under nitrogen, and the residues are treated as described above.

This method has been compared with assays based on isotope dilution following oral administration of C[14]-labelled carbamazepine to a volunteer. The results of this comparison, shown in Table 4, demonstrate that the specificity of the proposed method of assay is satisfactory.

Pharmacokinetics of carbamazepine following administration of single oral doses

Six healthy male subjects aged between 31 and 49 years, who had not taken any drug for at least one week prior to the experiment, were each given single oral doses of 100, 200, and 600 mg. carbamazepine. The experiment was divided into three parts so that each subject received each of the three doses. The sequence in which they were given the various doses was randomised, and an interval of one month was allowed to elapse between one part of the experiment and the next. No other drugs were taken.

Carbamazepine was administered in the form of ®Tegretol tablets of 200 mg. The doses were all given in the morning before the subjects had had anything to eat or drink. They received a light breakfast one hour later. Blood samples were collected in heparinised tubes immediately before administration of the drug and 1, 2, 4, 7, 10, 24, 48, 72, 96, and 168 hours afterwards. The plasma was separated by centrifugation and stored at a temperature of −20°C. until assay.

Plasma concentration/time curves were determined with the aid of a Wang 702 computer, using a special programme which made it possible to obtain the multi-exponential equation giving optimal adjustment to the experimental data. The computer also plotted the curve relating to the equation established in this way, and supplied the following calculated values:

β: absolute value of the slope of the last log.-linear segment of the curve from which the half-life $(t_{1/2})$ can be calculated.

A_∞:   area under the plasma concentration curve, calculated on the basis of the multi-exponential equation and extrapolated to infinite time.

$C_{max.}$: maximum plasma concentration, calculated from the equation.

$t_{max.}$: time corresponding to $C_{max.}$.

The mean values and 95% confidence limits for these different pharmacokinetic parameters are given in Table 5. The average plasma concentration curves for the three doses are shown in Figure 2.

As the dose administered increases, the mean values for $t_{max.}$ and β also increase, but the differences between the three values of each of these parameters are not statistically significant. Hence, a mean value for β can be calculated for all the subjects and all the doses, and this mean value can then be used to calculate the mean half-life, which amounts to 37.5 ± 5.5 hours ($P = 0.05$).

The maximum plasma concentration $(C_{max.})$ increases linearly as a function of the dose administered. Although the corresponding regression line does not pass through the origin of the graph, a statistical test shows that the distance between the intercept on the plasma concentration axis and the origin is not significantly different from zero.

The values for A_∞ are likewise proportional to the dose administered. Nevertheless, the corresponding regression line does not pass through the origin of the graph. By using the values of the product of β times W times A_∞ (W being the subjects' body weight), errors due to between-patient and within-patient variations in β and W can largely be eliminated. Under these conditions, a linear relationship is obtained, and the regression line passes through the origin (Figure 3). For doses of between 100 and 600 mg., therefore, the amount absorbed is independent of the dose administered.

The average plasma concentration curves reflect a mono-exponential decrease for doses of 200 and 600 mg. For the dose of 100 mg., on the other hand, a bi-exponential decrease is observed. It is thus impossible, on the basis of our results, to define the pharmacokinetic model of carbamazepine. However, with

Table 5. Pharmacokinetic parameters of carbamazepine following administration of a single dose. Mean values and 95% confidence limits for six subjects.

Dose administered	$C_{max.}$ (mcg./ml.)	$t_{max.}$ (hr)	β (hr^{-1})	$t_{1/2}$ (hr)	A_∞ (mcg.·hr/ml.)
100	0.97 ± 0.17	7.84 ± 1.37	0.0175 ± 0.0066	43.6 ± 14.7	67.63 ± 26.73
200	1.65 ± 0.16	9.60 ± 3.32	0.0199 ± 0.007	37.6 ± 11.2	113.70 ± 35.51
600	4.30 ± 0.79	12.53 ± 4.03	0.0227 ± 0.0033	30.9 ± 4.4	279.15 ± 76.27

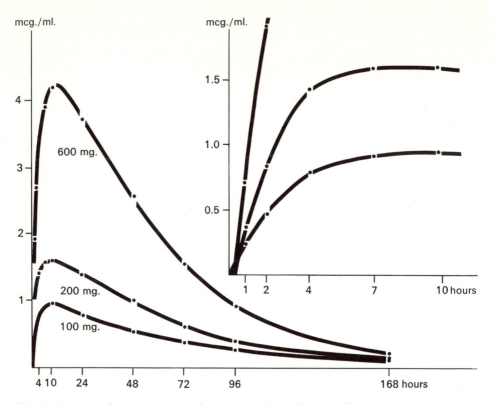

Fig. 2. Average plasma concentration curves (six subjects) following oral administration of 100, 200, and 600 mg. carbamazepine. Abscissa: time in hours; ordinate: plasma concentrations expressed in mcg. carbamazepine per ml. plasma. The inset shows the plasma concentrations during the first ten hours plotted on a larger scale.

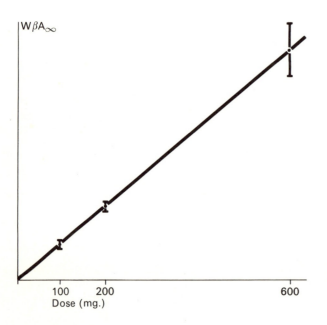

Fig. 3. Relationship between dose administered and product of W times β times A_∞ (W = subject's body weight, β = slope of the last log.-linear segment of the plasma concentration curve, and A_∞ = area under the plasma concentration curve extrapolated to infinite time).

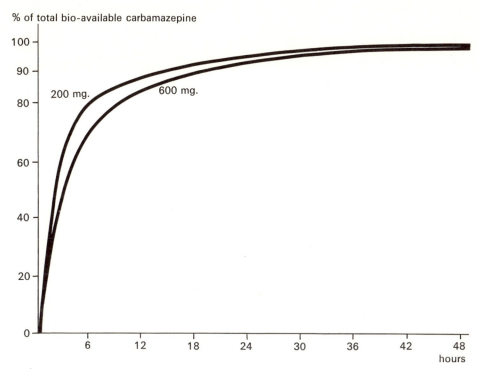

% of total bio-available carbamazepine

200 mg.   600 mg.

Fig. 4. Relative amounts of bio-available carbamazepine, expressed in percent of the total bio-available amount following oral doses of 200 and 600 mg.

the aid of the WAGNER-NELSON equation[33], the rate of appearance of carbamazepine in the plasma can be calculated for doses corresponding to a single-compartment model (Figure 4). The curves obtained show that 95% of the bio-available carbamazepine appears in the plasma within approximately 24 hours. It therefore seems that some other factor must be responsible for making absorption appear to be slower than it is in reality.

Pharmacokinetics of carbamazepine following administration of repeated oral doses

Six healthy male subjects aged between 31 and 48 years, who had not taken any drug for at least one week prior to the experiment, were each given a single oral dose of 200 mg. carbamazepine on the first day of the study; this dose was then repeated daily from the fifth to the 18th day.
Carbamazepine was administered in the form of Tegretol tablets of 200 mg. The dose was invariably given at about 8 o'clock in the morning before the subjects had had anything to eat or drink. They received a light breakfast two hours afterwards and a light lunch four hours afterwards.
Blood samples were collected in heparinised tubes so that complete plasma concentration/time curves could be plotted for the first and 18th days. From the fifth to the 18th day a second series of blood samples was taken immedi-   159

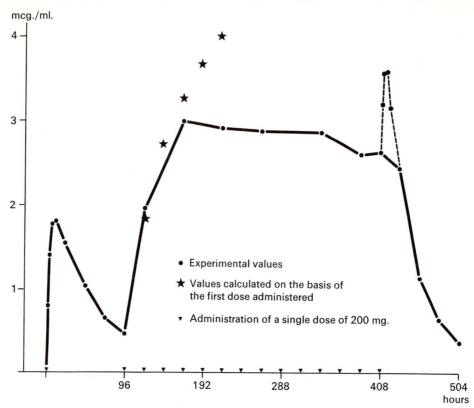

Fig. 5. Plasma concentrations of carbamazepine during repeated administration of the drug. Abscissa: time in hours; ordinate: plasma concentrations expressed in mcg. carbamazepine per ml. plasma.

ately before administration of the daily dose so that the pattern of the minimal concentration (foot-points) could be studied.

The average values for the six subjects are indicated in Figure 5. It should be noted that the individual values showed a wide scatter, that the minimum plasma concentrations during the period of repeated drug administration were not constant, and that their pattern differed from one subject to another. Figure 5 reveals, however, that a more or less steady state was attained after about seven days of repeated administration. It is not possible to say whether the plasma carbamazepine levels remained stable subsequently, or whether, as the curve for the average values seems to indicate, they tended to diminish; the apparent decrease at the end of treatment might be due to individual variations.

We determined the theoretical values for the minimal concentrations on the basis of the half-life calculated from the concentration/time curve (Day 1). As Figure 5 shows, these theoretical values quickly exceeded the experimental values, which indicates that the apparent overall rate of elimination increases (i.e. that the half-life decreases) during repeated administration of the drug; this phenomenon occurred very early on, inasmuch as it was already visible

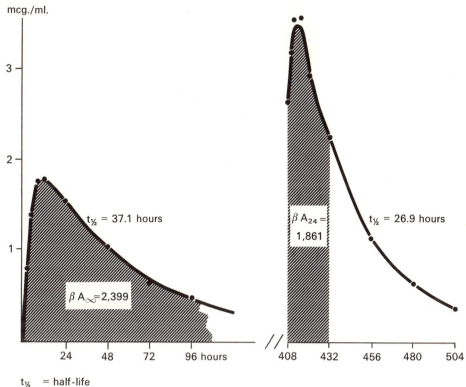

mcg./ml.

$t_{1/2} = 37.1$ hours

$\beta A_{24} = 1,861$

$t_{1/2} = 26.9$ hours

$\beta A_{\infty} = 2,399$

24   48   72   96 hours   408   432   456   480   504

$t_{1/2}$ = half-life
A_{∞} = area under the plasma concentration curve extrapolated to infinite time
A_{24} = area under the plasma concentration curve in the interval of 24 hours following
          administration of the previous dose
β = apparent rate of elimination constant

Fig. 6. Comparison of the plasma concentration curves of carbamazepine for Days 1 and 18.

on the second day of repeated treatment. It is probably due to an enzyme induction process which progressively accelerates the metabolism of carbamazepine. Support for this assumption is provided by a comparison of the half-lives calculated from the plasma concentration curves on Days 1 and 18 (Figure 6): the half-life calculated on the basis of the mean values for six subjects decreased from 37.1 to 26.9 hours.

It is also interesting to compare the areas under these two plasma concentration curves. If there had been no change in half-life, the area under the first curve, extrapolated to infinite time, should have been equal to the area under the second curve measured in the interval of 24 hours between two doses. In fact, however, the half-life did vary, and this has to be taken into account by multiplying the values for the area under the curve A by the apparent elimination rate constant β (calculated from the mean values of the six subjects). The results indicated in Figure 6 reveal that the product of β times A in the two instances differs, the difference amounting to 25% of the mean value of the two products. This would seem to suggest that the amount of carbamazepine absorbed decreases slightly during repeated administration of the drug. Nevertheless, owing to the wide variations observed from one subject to another, this hypothesis cannot be confirmed on the basis of the present data and will require to be tested further.

Conclusions

The experimental results obtained in our study show that the pharmacokinetics of carbamazepine raise several problems which cannot be solved by investigations based on oral administration of the drug. In particular, the question of whether the distribution of carbamazepine follows a single-compartment or a multi-compartment model still remains unanswered.

Acknowledgments

The authors' thanks are due to Dr. S. BRECHBÜHLER for preparing Tables 1–3 and to Dr. W. THEOBALD for conducting the clinical experiments.

References

1 BEYER, K.-H., KLINGE, D.: Zum spektrophotometrischen Nachweis von Carbamazepin. Arzneimittel-Forsch. (Drug. Res.) *19*, 1759 (1969)
2 BOHN, L.: Gaskromatografi i klinisk kemi med henblik på kvalitativ og kvantitativ laegemiddelpåvisning (Gas chromatography in clinical chemistry with a view to qualitative and quantitative determination of drugs). Nord. Med. *83*, 48 (1970)
3 BRAUNHOFER, J., ZICHA, L.: Eröffnet Tegretal neue Therapiemöglichkeiten bei bestimmten neurologischen und endokrinen Krankheitsbildern? Eine klinische, elektroenzephalographische und dünnschichtchromatographische Studie. Med. Welt (Stuttg.) *17* (N.F.), 1875 (1966)
4 CHRISTIANSEN, J.: Assay of drugs and their metabolites in capillary blood. Scand. J. clin. Lab. Invest. *27*, Suppl. 118: 67 (1971)
5 CHRISTIANSEN, J.: Quantitation of drugs and their metabolites in blood and tissues by thin-layer chromatography utilizing in situ scanning. Scand. J. clin. Lab. Invest. *29*, Suppl. 126: Abstr. 13.10 (1972)
6 CREMERS, H. M. H. G., VERHEESEN, P. E.: A rapid method for the estimation of anti-epileptic drugs in blood serum by gas-liquid chromatography. Clin. chim. Acta *48*, 413 (1973)
7 FABER, D. B., MAN IN 'T VELD, W. A.: A thin-layer chromatographic method for determining carbamazepine in blood. J. Chromatogr. *93*, 238 (1974)
8 FREY, H., YRJÄNÄ, T.: Carbamazepine titers of epileptic patients. Scand. J. clin. Lab. Invest. *25*, Suppl. 113: 90 (1970); abstract of paper
9 FRIEL, P., GREEN, J. R.: Quantitative assay for carbamazepine serum levels by gas-liquid chromatography. Clin. chim. Acta *43*, 69 (1973)
10 FÜHR, J.: Untersuchungen über die Verträglichkeit und Ausscheidung eines neuartigen Antiepilepticums. Arzneimittel-Forsch. (Drug Res.) *14*, 74 (1964)
11 GARDNER-THORPE, C., PARSONAGE, M. J., SMETHURST, P. F., TOOTHILL, C.: A comprehensive gas chromatographic scheme for the estimation of antiepileptic drugs. Clin. chim. Acta *36*, 223 (1972)

162

12 GARDNER-THORPE, C., PARSONAGE, M.J., TOOTHILL, C.: A comprehensive scheme for the evaluation of anticonvulsant concentrations in blood using thin-layer chromatography. Clin. chim. Acta *35*, 39 (1971)

13 GÉRARDIN, A.: A GLC determination of carbamazepine suitable for pharmacokinetic studies. J. pharm. Sci. (printing)

14 GRUSKA, H., BEYER, K.-H., KUBICKI, S., SCHNEIDER, H.: Klinik, Toxikologie und Therapie einer schweren Carbamazepin-Vergiftung. Arch. Toxikol. *27*, 193 (1971)

15 JOHANNESSEN, S.I., STRANDJORD, R.E.: The concentration of carbamazepine (Tegretol) in serum and in cerebrospinal fluid in patients with epilepsy. Acta neurol. scand. *48*, Suppl. 51: 445 (1972)

16 KUPFERBERG, H.J.: GLC determination of carbamazepine in plasma. J. pharm. Sci. *61*, 284 (1972)

17 LARSEN, N.-E., NAESTOFT, J., HVIDBERG, E.: Rapid routine determination of some anti-epileptic drugs in serum by gas chromatography. Clin. chim. Acta *40*, 171 (1972)

18 LARSEN, N.-E., WENDELBOE, J., BOHN, L.: Determination of carbamazepine (Tegretol) by gas chromatography. Scand. J. clin. Lab. Invest. *23*, Suppl. 110: 35 (1969); abstract of paper

19 LAUFFER, S., SCHMID, E., WEIST, F.: Dünnschichtchromatographische Trennung und spektrophoto-fluorometrischer Nachweis psychotroper Pharmaka. Arzneimittel-Forsch. (Drug Res.) *19*, 1965 (1969)

20 MASHFORD, M.L., RYAN, P.L., THOMSON, W.A.: Determination of carbamazepine in plasma. J. Chromatogr. *89*, 11 (1974)

21 MEIJER, J.W.A.: Simultaneous quantitative determination of anti-epileptic drugs, including carbamazepine, in body fluids. Epilepsia (Amst.) *12*, 341 (1971)

22 MEIJER, J.W.A., MEINARDI, H.: The separation, identification and quantitative estimation of commonly used antiepileptic drugs in body fluids. In Drake, C.G., Duvoisin, R. (Editors): IVth Int. Congr. neurol. Surg., IXth Int. Congr. Neurol., New York 1969, Abstr. 711, p. 251; Int. Congr. Ser. No. 193 (Excerpta Medica Foundation, Amsterdam etc. 1969)

23 MORSELLI, P.L., BIANDRATE, P., FRIGERIO, A., GARATTINI, S.: Pharmacokinetics of carbamazepine in rats and humans. Europ. J. clin. Invest. *2*, 297 (1972); abstract of paper

24 MORSELLI, P.L., BIANDRATE, P., FRIGERIO, A., GERNA, M., TOGNONI, G.: Gas chromatographic determination of carbamazepine and carbamazepine-10,11-epoxide in human body fluids. In Meijer, J.W.A., et al. (Editors): Methods of analysis of anti-epileptic drugs, Proc. Workshop on the determination of anti-epileptic drugs in body fluids, Noordwijkerhout, The Netherlands 1972, p. 169, Int. Congr. Ser. No. 286 (Excerpta Medica, Amsterdam/American Elsevier, New York 1973)

25 MORSELLI, P.L., GERNA, M., GARATTINI, S.: Carbamazepine plasma and tissue levels in the rat. Biochem. Pharmacol. *20*, 2043 (1971)

26 NIELSEN, H.R., REMMER, H.: Kvantitativ bestemmelse af karbamazepin (Tegretol) i serum (Quantitative determination of Tegretol in the serum). Ugeskr. Laeg. *131*, 2200 (1969)

27 PALMÉR, L., BERTILSSON, L., COLLSTE, P., RAWLINS, M.: Quantitative determination of carbamazepine in plasma by mass fragmentography. Clin. Pharmacol. Ther. *14*, 827 (1973)

28 PERCHALSKI, R.J., WILDER, B.J.: Rapid gas-liquid chromatographic determination of carbamazepine in plasma. Clin. Chem. *20*, 492 (1974)

29 ROGER, J.-C., RODGERS, G., Jr., SOO, A.: Simultaneous determination of carbamazepine ("Tegretol") and other anticonvulsants in human plasma by gas-liquid chromatography. Clin. Chem. *19*, 590 (1973)

30 SCHEIFFARTH, F., WEIST, F., ZICHA, L.: Zum Nachweis von 5-Carbamyl-5H-dibenzo[b,f]azepin im Liquor cerebrospinalis mittels Dünnschichtchromatographie. Z. klin. Chem. *4*, 68 (1966)

31 SCHMIDT, G., BÖSCHE, J., KEDING, H.: Nachweis von Antiepileptica in Blut und Harn. Akt. Probl. Verkehrsmed. *3*, 45 (1966)

32 TOSELAND, P.A., GROVE, J., BERRY, D.J.: An isothermal GLC determination of the plasma levels of carbamazepine, diphenylhydantoin, phenobarbitone and primidone. Clin. chim. Acta *38*, 321 (1972)

33 WAGNER, J.G., NELSON, E.: Per cent absorbed time plots derived from blood level and/or urinary excretion data. J. pharm. Sci. *52*, 610 (1963)

34 WEIST, F., SCHMID, E.: Dünnschichtchromatographischer Schnellnachweis von Tranquilizern der Benzodiazepin-Reihe und von thymoleptischen Medikamenten. Med. Welt (Stuttg.) *20* (N.F.), 369 (1969)

Preliminary report on serum carbamazepine determinations and their application to the treatment of epilepsy

by L. Oller Ferrer-Vidal*, J. Sabater-Tobella**, and
L. Oller-Daurella***

Introduction

The anticonvulsive effects of carbamazepine (®Tegretol), an iminostilbene derivative prepared by synthesis, have been amply demonstrated over the past 15 years in studies carried out by Theobald and Kunz[29], Lorgé[20], Hernández-Peón[12], Gardner-Thorpe et al.[10], Bonduelle et al.[2], Gamstorp[9], Bird et al.[1], Pryse-Phillips and Jeavons[25], Janz[13], Subirana et al.[27], Dobrescu and Coeugniet[7], Grant[11], Wolf[30], Dalby[6], and many others. Thanks to the techniques devised by Larsen et al.[18], Frey and Yrjänä[8], Meijer[21], and Kupferberg[16], it has been possible in the last five years to assay the blood levels of this substance with a high degree of accuracy. The first clinico-analytical studies on the drug – by Johannessen and Strandjord[14] and Cereghino et al.[4,5] – are of more recent date.

Carbamazepine, which has a molecular weight of 236.26, presents the following principal characteristics: it is rapidly absorbed from the gastro-intestinal tract, as is shown by the fact that maximum blood levels are reached only two and a half hours after ingestion of the drug[22,29]. Plasma protein-binding influences its ability to cross the blood-brain barrier, the C.S.F./plasma quotient being 0.22[15]. It has a half-life of about 30 hours[26]. Its therapeutic and toxic blood levels are, on the average, 1.7–4.9 and 10 mcg./ml., respectively, but it must be pointed out that these levels vary widely from one subject to another. The drug is eliminated mainly via the kidneys, approximately 60% of the dose administered being excreted within 24 hours[23].

Methods

Fifty patients were selected who were undergoing regular treatment with carbamazepine, either as monotherapy (five cases) or in combination with phenobarbitone, diphenylhydantoin, succinimides, or benzodiazepines. All were receiving carbamazepine in three daily doses, with an interval of eight hours between doses. Their ages ranged from four to 61 years; 28 (56%) were males. In the case of patients who were being given phenobarbitone in combination with carbamazepine, the regularity with which the medication was actually

* Centro Antiepiléptico de PENEPA, Barcelona, Spain.
** Cátedra de Bioquímica de la Universidad Autónoma de Barcelona, Spain.
*** Centro de Lucha Antiepiléptica de Barcelona, Spain.

taken was tested by calculating the theoretical serum levels of phenobarbitone with the aid of equations devised by Svensmark and Buchthal[28]. Eight patients originally selected for the trial were subsequently discarded, because the results of this test suggested that they were not taking their drugs regularly.

With regard to the type of seizures from which they were suffering, the patients could be divided into two groups: the first group comprised 40 patients with seizures generally regarded as being responsive to carbamazepine (partial seizures of simple or complex symptomatology, primarily generalised seizures, myoclonic attacks, and secondarily generalised seizures), while the second group consisted of ten patients with other types of seizure.

Gas chromatography was invariably employed to assay the serum levels of phenobarbitone and carbamazepine. For phenobarbitone we used the technique of Larsen et al.[17], as modified by one of us (Sabater-Tobella), and for carbamazepine the method described by Larsen et al.[18], about which we had been personally informed in Copenhagen.

No assays were performed until sufficient time had passed for the substance administered to reach a steady-state level. Blood samples were taken at 6.30 p.m., approximately four hours after the second dose of the day. As tests carried out in a number of patients revealed, the findings did not differ significantly whether the blood samples were taken in the morning or in the evening.

Results and discussion

1. Correlation between serum carbamazepine levels and dose administered

Firstly, we analysed the correlations between the serum levels of phenobarbitone and carbamazepine and the doses administered per kg. body weight (Figures 1 and 2). The results of this analysis showed that in the case of phenobarbitone there was a good correlation between daily dose in mg./kg. and serum levels, the regression line being approximately the same as that obtained in preliminary experiments with 500 cases[24]. As regards carbamazepine, the scatter was more pronounced. This difference may be due to the fact that with phenobarbitone the fraction eliminated in 24 hours was very constant and largely identical for all the patients, whereas with carbamazepine it varied considerably from one individual to another.

Our 50 cases were divided into two subgroups depending on whether they weighed more or less than 60 kg. The regression lines obtained were similar to those we had found in previous experiments[24].

Patients who developed signs and symptoms of toxicity have been represented by triangles in Figures 1 and 2. In the case of phenobarbitone, these side effects, taking the form of drowsiness, ataxia, etc., occurred as a rule at serum levels of 30 mcg./ml. or more.

In two instances the serum phenobarbitone levels were above the theoretical maximum. These were two obese patients who had a great deal of panniculus adiposus. When calculating the distribution volume of the drug, it must be

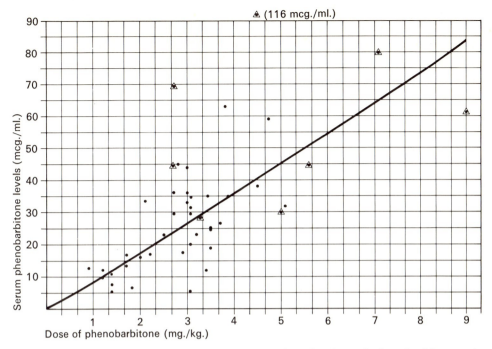

Fig. 1. Serum phenobarbitone levels plotted against the dose of phenobarbitone administered in 45 epileptic patients. The triangles indicate cases in which side effects occurred.

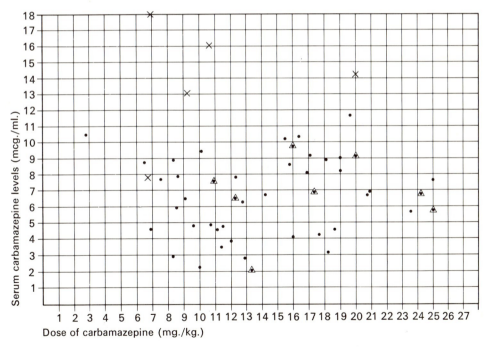

Fig. 2. Serum carbamazepine levels plotted against the dose of carbamazepine administered in 50 epileptic patients. The triangles indicate cases in which side effects occurred and the crosses patients receiving monotherapy with carbamazepine.

167

remembered that the substance is taken up to a lesser extent by adipose tissue than by other organs and tissues and that the dose in mg./kg. was higher than if it had been calculated on the basis of effective body mass (i.e. without adipose tissue). Similar observations have been described by other authors[28]. Concerning carbamazepine, two points should be made:

1. We found, on the whole, no obvious relationship between the side effects recorded and the serum carbamazepine levels. We therefore attribute these side effects to the medication with which carbamazepine was combined.

2. Five of our patients were receiving monotherapy with carbamazepine. In these cases the serum levels were very much higher than we had expected on the basis of the daily dose. The possible influence exerted by additional drugs, especially phenobarbitone, on the serum levels of carbamazepine will be discussed later on. In one of their cases, JOHANNESSEN and STRANDJORD[14] obtained results similar to those recorded in our five patients.

Although our findings differ somewhat from those reported by JOHANNESSEN and STRANDJORD[14], the discrepancy disappears once we exclude the five of our patients who received carbamazepine alone.

2. Serum levels and control of seizures

The clinical studies of BONDUELLE et al.[2], SUBIRANA et al.[27], HERNÁNDEZ-PEÓN[12], BIRD et al.[1], LIVINGSTON et al.[19], etc. have shown that carbamazepine is indicated chiefly in certain particular types of seizure. Included among these are partial seizures of simple and complex symptomatology, primarily generalised seizures, myoclonic attacks, and secondarily generalised seizures. Not included are, for example, typical and atypical absences, predominantly unilateral seizures, and atonic seizures. As already mentioned, we divided our 50 patients into two groups on the basis of the type of seizure they displayed. When each of these groups was split up into patients whose seizures were controlled by the medication and patients whose seizures were not controlled, two interesting points emerged:

1. Firstly, taking the sample as a whole, the average phenobarbitone levels were higher in the patients whose seizures were not completely controlled. This difference might be explained by the fact that in these cases the dosage of phenobarbitone was successively and repeatedly increased in an attempt to eliminate the seizures (Table 1).

2. In Group A (i.e. the group with seizures generally considered to be responsive to carbamazepine) the average phenobarbitone levels were more or less the same whether the seizures were controlled or not, whereas the average carbamazepine levels were some 25% lower in the only partially controlled cases than in the completely controlled ones. In these partially controlled patients, therefore, the doses of carbamazepine administered do not seem to have been high enough to produce effective serum levels.

In Group B (i.e. the group with seizures regarded as being only slightly sensitive to carbamazepine), on the other hand, the phenobarbitone levels were

Table 1. Correlations between serum levels of phenobarbitone and carbamazepine and control of seizures in 50 epileptic patients.

	No. of cases	Mean serum levels (mcg./ml.)	
		Phenobarbitone	Carbamazepine
Groups A and B together			
Seizures completely controlled	32	24.48	7.96
Seizures partially controlled	18	42.47	6.26
Group A (partial seizures, grand mal, myoclonic attacks, and secondarily generalised seizures) : 40 cases			
Seizures completely controlled	32	25.63	8.02
Seizures partially controlled	8	26.80	6.03
Group B (absences and other types of seizure): 10 cases			
Seizures completely controlled	–	–	–
Seizures partially controlled	10	54.44	7.58

very high, the average figure being 54.44 mcg./ml. Since these were usually very refractory cases, the dosage of phenobarbitone had – perhaps mistakenly – been increased. As regards the average serum levels of carbamazepine in this group, it is noteworthy that these levels (7.58 mcg./ml.) were practically the same as in the completely controlled cases of Group A (8.02 mcg./ml.). The difference in clinical effect between the two groups – i.e. the fact that in Group B the seizures were only partially controlled, whereas in those patients of Group A whose serum carbamazepine levels averaged out at 8.02 mcg./ml. they were completely controlled – suggests that a serum carbamazepine level of approximately 8 mcg./ml. exerts a therapeutic effect only in seizures responsive to the drug.

3. Serum levels of carbamazepine in monotherapy and combined therapy
The serum carbamazepine levels were also analysed on the basis of whether or not the patients were receiving supplementary medication. In the 45 patients who were given carbamazepine in combination with other anticonvulsants,

Table 2. Serum carbamazepine levels in combined therapy as compared with monotherapy.

	No. of cases	Mean daily dose of carbamazepine (mg./kg.)	Mean serum carbamazepine levels (mcg./ml.)	Ratio between dose and serum levels
Combined therapy (carbamazepine plus phenobarbitone, diphenyl-hydantoin, succinimides, or benzodiazepines)	45	14.80	6.59	2.24
Monotherapy	5	10.68	13.88	0.76

169

the ratio between the dose administered (in mg./kg.) and the serum levels was 2.24. In the five patients receiving carbamazepine alone it was 0.76 (Table 2). This may be interpreted as indicating that patients receiving monotherapy with carbamazepine show much higher serum levels of this drug than do patients given carbamazepine in combination with other substances. In other words, to attain a serum level of 1 mcg./ml., patients on monotherapy require a dose of only 0.76 mg./kg., whereas those on combined therapy require one of 2.24 mg./kg. Perhaps the explanation is to be sought in the hypothesis that other anticonvulsants, including phenobarbitone, stimulate the biotransformation of carbamazepine in the hepatocytes.

The present tendency of many epileptologists, including ourselves, is to commence anticonvulsive therapy with a single drug, and the findings reported above may support the contention that a certain very restricted group of seizures should be treated with carbamazepine alone. If, in cases where this treatment proves ineffective, drugs such as phenobarbitone or diphenylhydantoin have subsequently to be added to the regimen, the dose of carbamazepine would have to be increased at the same time in order to ensure that the serum carbamazepine levels remain similar to those recorded prior to the addition of other drugs to the regimen.

4. Correlation between E.E.G. background activity and the serum levels of carbamazepine and phenobarbitone

In the context of this preliminary analysis we also tried to correlate the serum levels with the E.E.G. background activity. This electro-encephalographic parameter was selected as an index of cortical function, because some authors have implied that certain anticonvulsants may have a negative influence on – i.e. may slow down – cerebral bio-electrical activity. Our own findings may indeed provide support for this view.

E.E.G. background activity was evaluated in patients treated with phenobarbitone and/or carbamazepine, and the evaluation was performed on the

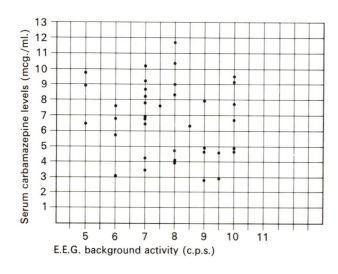

Fig. 3. Serum carbamazepine levels plotted against E.E.G. background activity in 38 epileptic patients.

same days as the serum-level determinations. From our original group of 50 patients we excluded those aged less than 12 years, so that normal E.E.G. background activity ranged between 8.5 and 12 c.p.s.

In a first series of 38 patients (Figure 3), there seemed to be no correlation between the serum levels of carbamazepine and slowing down of the background activity. But in a second group of 100 patients, which included the 38 from the first series, high serum levels of phenobarbitone did appear to go hand in hand with lower E.E.G. background activity, while serum phenobarbitone levels of less than 30 mcg./ml. were for the most part associated with normal E.E.G. background activity of above 8.5 c.p.s. (Figure 4 and Table 3).

Conclusions

In our opinion, the most important findings emerging from our preliminary study, which of course require corroboration in a further, more detailed analysis, are as follows:

1. The serum levels of carbamazepine were appreciably higher when the drug was used as monotherapy than when it was given in combination with other anticonvulsants.

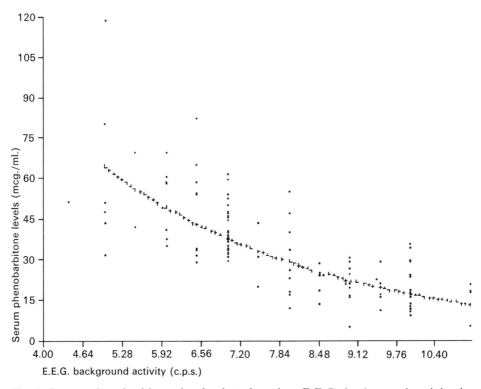

Fig. 4. Serum phenobarbitone levels plotted against E.E.G. background activity in 100 epileptic patients.

Table 3. Analysis (performed with the aid of the IBM Call/360 curve-fitting programme) of the correlation between serum phenobarbitone levels and E.E.G. background activity in 100 epileptic patients.

Curve	Correlation coefficient	A	B
1 Y = A + B*X Straight line	−.7348	+1.0090 E+02	−8.4063 E+00
2 Y = A*EXP (B*X) Simple exponential	−.7556	+2.4153 E+02	−2.6571 E−01
3 Y = A*X**B Simple power	−.7493	+1.8584 E+03	−2.0247 E+00
4 Y = A + B/X Hyperbola	.7428	−2.8948 E+01	+4.7883 E+02
5 Y = 1/(A + B*X) Hyperbola	.6042	−4.8167 E−02	+1.1258 E−02
6 Y = X/(B + A*X) Simple rational	−.5612	+1.1880 E−01	−5.8925 E−01
7 Y = K + A*B**X Modified exponential	n.a.		
8 Y = K*A**(B**X) Gompertz	n.a.		
9 1/Y = K + A*B**X Logistic	n.a.		
10 Y = A[1−E(−B*X)] Growth curve	.3853	−1.3333 E+03	−3.2697 E−03

$$Y = 0.024153 \; e \, (-2.6571 \, X)$$

n.a. = not applicable, i.e. curve cannot be fitted

2. There seemed to be a certain correlation between the serum levels of phenobarbitone and E.E.G. background activity. A similar correlation was not found in the case of carbamazepine.

Summary

The results of preliminary studies on the application of serum carbamazepine determinations to the treatment of epilepsy are described. The serum levels of carbamazepine and phenobarbitone were analysed with respect to the following parameters: dose administered, control of seizures, and background activity in the E.E.G. This paper is a preliminary report and marks a first step in a more extensive study which is already under way.

References

1 BIRD, C. A. K., GRIFFIN, B. P., MIKLASZEWSKA, J. M., GALBRAITH, A. W.: Tegretol (carbamazepine): a controlled trial of a new anti-convulsant. Brit. J. Psychiat. *112*, 737 (1966)

2 BONDUELLE, M., BOUYGUES, P., SALLOU, C., GROBUIS, S.: Expérimentation clinique de l'anti-épileptique G 32883 (Tégrétol). Résultats portant sur 100 cas observés en trois ans. Rev. neurol. *110*, 209 (1964)

3 BUCHTHAL, F., LENNOX-BUCHTHAL, M.A.: Relation of serum concentration to control of seizures. In Woodbury, D.M., et al. (Editors): Antiepileptic drugs, p. 335 (Raven Press, New York 1972)

4 CEREGHINO, J.J., BROCK, J.T., VAN METER, J.C., PENRY, J.K., SMITH, L.D., WHITE, B.G.: Carbamazepine for epilepsy. A controlled prospective evaluation. Neurology (Minneap.) *24*, 401 (1974)

5 CEREGHINO, J.J., VAN METER, J.C., BROCK, J.T., PENRY, J.K., SMITH, L.D., WHITE, B.G.: Preliminary observations of serum carbamazepine concentration in epileptic patients. Neurology (Minneap.) *23*, 357 (1973)

6 DALBY, M.A.: Antiepileptic and psychotropic effect of carbamazepine (Tegretol) in the treatment of psychomotor epilepsy. Epilepsia (Amst.) *12*, 325 (1971)

7 DOBRESCU, D., COEUGNIET, E.: L'action anticonvulsivante de l'imipramine et de l'amitriptyline associées au phénobarbital, à la phénytoïne et au diazépam. Rev. neurol. *132*, 135 (1970)

8 FREY, H., YRJÄNÄ, T.: Carbamazepine titers of epileptic patients. Scand. J. clin. Lab. Invest. *25*, Suppl. 113: 90 (1970); abstract of paper

9 GAMSTORP, I.: A clinical trial of Tegretol in children with severe epilepsy. Develop. Med. Child Neurol. *8*, 296 (1966)

10 GARDNER-THORPE, C., PARSONAGE, M.J., TOOTHILL, C.: A comprehensive scheme for the evaluation of anticonvulsant concentrations in blood using thin-layer chromatography. Clin. chim. Acta *35*, 39 (1971)

11 GRANT, R.H.E.: The use of carbamazepine (Tegretol) in patients with epilepsy and multiple handicaps. In Wink, C.A.S. (Editor): Tegretol in epilepsy, Rep. int. clin. Symp., London 1972, p. 16 (Nicholls, Manchester 1972)

12 HERNÁNDEZ-PEÓN, R.: Anticonvulsive action of G. 32883. In Bradley, P.B., et al. (Editors): Neuro-Psychopharmacology, Vol. III, Proc. IIIrd Meet. Coll. int. neuro-psychopharmacol., Munich 1962, p. 303 (Elsevier, Amsterdam/London/New York 1964)

13 JANZ, D.: Terapia medica dell'epilessia infantile. In: Simp. "L'epilessia nell'infanzia", Milan 1968, p. 67

14 JOHANNESSEN, S.I., STRANDJORD, R.E.: Concentration of carbamazepine (Tegretol) in serum and in cerebrospinal fluid in patients with epilepsy. Epilepsia (Amst.) *14*, 373 (1973)

15 JOHANNESSEN, S.I., STRANDJORD, R.E.: Absorption and distribution between serum and cerebrospinal fluid of certain antiepileptic drugs. In Subirana, A., et al. (Editors): Abstr. Xth Int. Congr. Neurol., Barcelona 1973, p. 162; Int. Congr. Ser. No. 296 (Excerpta Medica, Amsterdam etc. 1973)

16 KUPFERBERG, H.J.: GLC determination of carbamazepine in plasma. J. pharm. Sci. *61*, 284 (1972)

17 LARSEN, N.-E., NAESTOFT, J., HVIDBERG, E.: Rapid routine determination of some anti-epileptic drugs in serum by gas chromatography. Clin. chim. Acta *40*, 171 (1972)

18 LARSEN, N.-E., WENDELBOE, J., BOHN, L.: Determination of carbamazepine (Tegretol) by gas chromatography. Scand. J. clin. Lab. Invest. *23*, Suppl. 110: 35 (1969); abstract of paper

19 LIVINGSTON, S., VILLAMATER, C., SAKATA, Y., PAULI, L.L.: Use of carbamazepine in epilepsy: results in 87 patients. J. Amer. med. Ass. *200*, 204 (1967)

20 LORGÉ, M.: Klinische Erfahrungen mit einem neuen Antiepilepticum, Tegretol (G. 32883), mit besonderer Wirkung auf die epileptische Wesensveränderung. Schweiz. med. Wschr. *93*, 1042 (1963)

21 MEIJER, J.W.A.: Simultaneous quantitative determination of anti-epileptic drugs, including carbamazepine, in body fluids. Epilepsia (Amst.) *12*, 341 (1971)

22 Meinardi, H.: Applications pratiques du dosage des médicaments. Cah. Epilepsie No. 4: 135 (1971)

23 Meinardi, H.: Carbamazepine, loc. cit. [3], p. 487

24 Oller F.-V., L., Oller-Daurella, L.: Resultados del análisis mediante ordenador de 500 casos de determinaciones plasmáticas de anticonvulsivantes. In preparation

25 Pryse-Phillips, W. E. M., Jeavons, P. M.: Effect of carbamazepine (Tegretol) on the electroencephalograph and ward behaviour of patients with chronic epilepsy. Epilepsia (Amst.) *11*, 263 (1970)

26 Strandjord, R. E., Johannessen, S. I.: Several doses a day of antiepileptic drugs? loc. cit. [15], p. 236

27 Subirana, A., Oller-Daurella, L., Chillón, D.: Dos años de experiencia del tratamiento de la epilepsia con Tegretol. Rev. clín. esp. *104*, 336 (1967)

28 Svensmark, O., Buchthal, F.: Accumulation of phenobarbital in man. Epilepsia (Amst.) *4*, 199 (1963)

29 Theobald, W., Kunz, H. A.: Zur Pharmakologie des Antiepilepticums 5-Carbamyl-5H-dibenzo[b,f]azepin. Arzneimittel-Forsch. (Drug Res.) *13*, 122 (1963)

30 Wolf, P.: Tegretol in grand mal epilepsy, loc. cit. [11], p. 95

Reversible psychic disorders in epileptic patients

by H. Helmchen*

1. Introduction

An epileptic can react psychically to stress in just the same way as any other human being; that is to say, his psychic reactions may be normal or they may be abnormal, taking the form, for instance, of pathological developments or neuroses. On the other hand, they may possibly be secondary to the epilepsy itself – for example, in cases where the patient's experience of epilepsy as a chronic disease with all its attendant circumstances is processed in a pathogenic manner, or in cases where psychic disorders of cerebral origin that are correlated with the epilepsy, such as personality changes or mood disorders, influence not only the way in which the abnormal processing of the experience occurs but also the resultant manifestations. Although little systematic investigation has yet been done in this field and many questions still remain unanswered, it nevertheless seems that here, too, the well-known rules governing psychodynamic and sociomedical diagnosis and treatment are applicable. In this paper, therefore, I should like to concentrate on psychic disorders which are a direct and specific manifestation or consequence of an epileptic disturbance in cerebral function[14], and I shall confine myself in this connection to the diagnosis and treatment of those psychic disorders that are reversible.

2. Description of syndromes

The reversible psychic disorders encountered in epileptics can be classified under the general heading of psychic disorders assignable to somatic causes. Depending on the prominence of their axial symptom, which is a disturbance of consciousness, these reversible disorders are divided into transient syndromes[30, 36] and reactions of an acute exogenous type[2].

The transient syndromes include episodic mood disorders and productive psychotic episodes, whereas twilight states constitute an acute exogenous reaction. Typical of the reversible syndromes is their abrupt onset and their, as a rule, equally rapid disappearance. Though they may last for only minutes or hours, they mostly persist for days or weeks, and in rare cases even for months.

2.1. Episodic mood disorders

These disorders are characterised by a usually unmotivated and sudden shift in basic mood. In the majority of cases, the patient becomes dysphoric, irritable,

---

* Psychiatrische Klinik der Freien Universität, Berlin.

dejected, cross, and subdepressive. His field of affective awareness is narrowed down, sometimes to such an extent that a single type of affect predominates – be it anxiety, mistrust, aimless wandering ("poriomania"), or even, though only seldom, an enhanced sense of vitality. The patient's range of thought is also constricted, and his thought processes become more sluggish and sometimes less clear; pronounced disorders of orientation, on the other hand, cannot be demonstrated. He frequently complains of physical symptoms of an autonomic nervous type, such as sweating, muzziness, and tiredness.

2.2. Episodic psychoses

The episodic mood disorders mentioned above must be differentiated from episodic psychoses. The latter, which often used to be simply included under the general heading of "twilight states", are now subdivided into at least two groups, the first comprising twilight states and other "organic" syndromes and the second productive psychotic episodes (Table 1a).

2.2.1. Twilight states

Where the syndrome is dominated by disturbances in drive and in consciousness marked by a decrease in alertness or by disorientation, it resembles, in its more severe forms, "epileptic" stupor or "epileptic" delirium. In cases of stupor, the patient lapses into a state of apathetic muzziness and mental sluggishness, his reactions are delayed, and he shows a tendency towards perseveration. If the condition is not very severe, it may merely give the impression of being an "organic" syndrome. In cases of delirium, on the other hand, the patient displays pronounced motor excitation and disorientation, experiences vivid visual and auditory hallucinations, and may be completely dominated by chaotic delusions. Far more frequently, however, twilight states fall between these two extremes: a certain degree of motor restlessness is present, and the patient in his mentally clouded, dream-like condition often experiences his momentary situation as something more or less appreciably different from what it actually is. This experience of dream-like unreality carries strong affective overtones and, in combination with explosive increases in drive, may give rise to dangerously irresponsible actions of forensic import. For example, if the

Table 1a. Psychopathological syndromes.

General classification of psychic disorders assignable to somatic causes	Individual psychopathological syndromes

Transient syndromes	Reversible syndromes
	   Episodic mood disorders
	   Episodic psychoses
	      Productive psychotic episodes
	      Stupor
	      Twilight states

Reactions of the acute exogenous type	Other "organic" syndromes

patient's experience is coloured by anxiety or suspicion, and if he feels himself threatened, he may react by becoming violent or even by committing suicide. In rare cases, twilight states may also be characterised by a joyous, ecstatic experience. It is frequently possible to establish contact with these patients, even though the contact may be only superficial and fragmentary. Uncomplicated thought processes may appear to be unaffected, but differentiated thinking becomes impossible. Disturbances of memory, ranging up to and including complete amnesia for the duration of the twilight state, are usually present. Patients whose memory is thus impaired may be difficult to assess in cases where their remembrance of concrete experiences is restricted by the presence of broad areas in which their recollections are blurred, vague, or even non-existent.

2.2.2. Productive psychotic episodes

The less prominent these disturbances of consciousness are and the better orientated the patient appears, the more readily understandable are his patterns of experience, even though they are almost invariably falsified by delusions. Conditions of this kind have also been referred to as "orientated", "collected", or even "organised" twilight states. Such designations, however, are not merely contradictions in terms, but also inaccurate, because – as GRUHLE[12] rightly pointed out as long ago as 1936 – these patients are not really suffering from a twilight state at all. Here, the purely descriptive term "productive psychotic episode" is therefore preferable. These conditions may be associated with the development of systematised forms of delusion, which usually disappear again after the affective disorder invariably responsible for them has subsided. In cases where the delusions are accompanied by visual and, in particular, auditory hallucinations, it is no longer possible, if orientation is unaffected, to distinguish the often profuse symptoms of productive psychoses from the symptoms of some cases of schizophrenia, despite the fact that attempts are repeatedly made to differentiate psychopathologically between these schizophrenia-like psychoses associated with epilepsy and the "endogenous" schizophrenias. It is claimed, for example, that a tendency for the content of the delusion to have religious, mystic, or cosmic connotations, and also the presence of faint signs indicating an "enechetic" personality change, occasionally render it possible to distinguish different psychopathological syndromes[19]. On the other hand, SLATER and BEARD[33] found this type of content in only 14% of cases. It must be borne in mind, too, that the themes underlying the delusions are also to some extent dependent on the spirit of the times[23]. In 1953 SELBACH[31] mentioned a report by HACKEBÛS and FUNDYLER, according to which "epileptic piousness" and delusions of a religious nature in epileptics had largely disappeared in the Soviet Union by as early as 1930. TELLENBACH[34] pointed out in particular that in his 12 patients the delusions remained unsystematic even where the psychosis persisted for some considerable time, whereas SLATER and BEARD[33] actually claim to have observed long-term systematisation of delusions among their 69 patients. Productive psychotic episodes seem to be most frequently associated with an "epileptic" personality change; SLATER and BEARD,

177

for example, noted an association of this kind in 55 of their 69 cases. One essential point appears to be that in these productive psychotic episodes the affective warmth of the personality is retained more often than it is in process schizophrenias, and features indicative of an organic personality change rather than of a typical schizophrenic end-state tend to develop eventually[32].

In this connection, it should be noted that many studies on psychoses, especially on schizophrenia-like psychoses occurring in association with epilepsy, fail to draw a sufficiently clear distinction between psychotic episodes lasting for hours or days and chronic psychoses persisting for months or years. The *chronic psychoses associated with epilepsy* apparently occupy a position midway between the definitely reversible and the mainly irreversible syndromes. This statement should perhaps be qualified by pointing out that whether or not the syndrome should be regarded as irreversible will also depend, of course, on the therapeutic measures undertaken and the period of observation. In the light of his finding that over a follow-up period of 1–3 years the schizophrenia-like symptoms which had been present for 2–25 years disappeared in approximately one-third of his 69 patients and showed a marked improvement in an additional one-third, SLATER[32] was convinced that the schizophrenia-like states were only a phase in the overall course of epilepsy and that the disease became in fact increasingly organic and less typically schizophrenic.

Finally, attention should also be drawn to the fact that phasic psychoses classifiable upon clinical examination as apparently belonging to the pure endogenous type are very seldom observed in epileptics[1, 18, 29, 35].

3. Syndrome pathogenesis

Information on the circumstances under which reversible syndromes manifest themselves can be obtained not only from clinical classifications, but also from

Table 1b. Clues to the pathogenesis of the various syndromes.

Individual psycho-pathological syndromes	Clinical correlatives (not obligatory)	E.E.G. correlatives (not obligatory)
Reversible syndromes		
Episodic mood disorders	More usually pre-paroxysmal	More usually forced normalisation
Episodic psychoses		
Productive psychotic episodes	More usually pre-paroxysmal	More usually forced normalisation
Stupor	Petit mal status	(Ir)regular spike-and-wave patterns
Twilight states	Status psychomotoricus (seldom)	More usually temporal delta and theta waves and sharp waves
	More usually post-paroxysmal	More usually generalised pathological activity, spike-and-wave patterns, spikes, sharp waves, paroxysmal dysrhythmia
Other "organic" syndromes	E.g. drug poisoning	Generalised pathological activity, beta waves

paraclinical findings, including in particular those yielded by electro-encephalography (Table 1b). On the basis of these classifications and findings, reversible psychopathological syndromes fall into three groups:

1. They may be a direct manifestation of the paroxysmal epileptic disorder of
   cerebral function.
2. They may be initiated or terminated by epileptic seizures.
3. They may have no recognisable connection with epileptic seizures.

The longer the duration of the epilepsy and the greater the variety of seizures
experienced by the patient, the more likely he is to display a reversible psychopathological syndrome.

3.1. Psychopathological manifestations of epileptic seizures or of status epilepticus

Direct psychopathological manifestations of an epileptic disturbance in cerebral function are petit mal status, which clinically takes the form of
stupor[11,17,24,28], and status psychomotoricus (or certain other rare forms of
focal attack) appearing as a twilight state or as a productive psychosis followed
by amnesia[6,16,20,21,37]. In the E.E.G. tracings, petit mal status is characterised
by regular or irregular spike-and-wave patterns occurring continuously or with
brief interruptions, whereas status psychomotoricus can be recognised by the
presence – chiefly in the temporal region – of usually continuous, irregular
theta and delta waves, intermingled with sharp waves.

It is surprising that status psychomotoricus was not described at all until a few
years ago, since when only very few reports have been published on it[6,37]. This
may be due to the fact that these psychopathological syndromes are seen chiefly
by psychiatrists, who tend simply to attribute them to a transient organic psychosis of obscure origin; where an attempt is nevertheless made to establish a
more exact diagnosis, the necessary electro-encephalographic confirmation
may be impossible to obtain for a variety of reasons – e.g. transient nature of
the syndrome, refusal of the patient to allow an E.E.G. record to be taken, or
technical difficulties. Consequently, status psychomotoricus may quite often
pass unrecognised. JUNG[20] postulates that temporal-lobe status epilepticus can
also be subsumed under the heading of LANDOLT's twilight states of an "organic
type" accompanied by slow, dysrhythmic E.E.G. patterns.

3.2. Psychopathological precursors and sequelae of epileptic seizures

Psychopathological manifestations of the disturbance occurring in cerebral
function immediately before or immediately after an epileptic seizure can be
termed pre-paroxysmal or post-paroxysmal psychopathological syndromes.
Those syndromes that are suddenly terminated by a seizure more frequently
take the form of mood disorders or paranoid psychoses (i.e. psychoses marked
by hallucinations) without any accompanying disturbance of consciousness,
whereas the syndromes which immediately follow a single seizure, a series of
seizures, or status epilepticus are generally twilight states associated with a
disturbance of consciousness. As far back as 1923 KRAEPELIN[22] drew attention

179

to these clear-cut psychopathological differences between pre-paroxysmal and post-paroxysmal syndromes. This clinical distinction is matched by corresponding differences in the E.E.G. tracings. Short-lived pre-paroxysmal psychic disorders in particular quite often correlate with an improvement in the E.E.G. findings, i.e. with a partial or even complete "forced" normalisation. Short-lived post-paroxysmal psychic disorders, on the other hand, are as a rule accompanied in the E.E.G. record by a gradually subsiding generalised pathological activity and often also by paroxysmal dysrhythmia, spike-and-wave patterns, spikes, or sharp waves.

3.3. Psychic disorders having no recognisable connection with epileptic seizures

The syndromes described so far display obvious links with the paroxysmal disturbance of cerebral function that occurs in epilepsy or with the precursors or sequelae of this disturbance. The same cannot be said, or at least not without reservations, of those psychopathological syndromes which develop independently of epileptic seizures. These syndromes may be marked by an impairment of affect and drive, or by loss of memory, associated with fluctuations in alertness. Alternatively, they may take the form of mood disturbances or of psychoses in which there is no disturbance of consciousness. These psychoses, which are predominantly of the paranoid, hallucinatory type, may occur episodically or they may be chronic. In cases where syndromes of the apparently "organic" type, as well as "free-floating" twilight states unconnected with seizures, develop in patients who are not suffering from status psychomotoricus, the first possibility to be borne in mind is that of a psychic disorder due to transient drug poisoning[27]. It should be stressed in this connection that the manifestations of toxic psychoses may also resemble those of profuse excitatory reactions of the acute exogenous type[3]. "Free-floating" mood disorders and episodic psychoses unaccompanied by disturbances of consciousness cannot be distinguished clinically from the pre-paroxysmal syndromes already described. Occasionally, they are also indirectly associated with a seizure, as one of our own observations has shown (Case-record No. 556/60): in this patient a twilight state – which followed a series of seven major seizures and was accompanied by disorientation – persisted initially for four days; its subsequent course, marked by phasic fluctuations in the degree to which consciousness was disturbed, culminated in a psychosis of the paranoid (hallucinatory) type lasting two days and involving no disorientation whatsoever. Hence, as more and more time elapsed since the termination of the patient's seizures, a reaction of the acute exogenous type changed into a transient syndrome.

In view of the special importance attaching to the E.E.G. as an aid in differentiating between these psychopathological syndromes from the pathogenetic standpoint, it should be mentioned that the transformation in the psychopathological syndrome seems to be paralleled by certain pathophysiological shifts. These shifts can occasionally be followed in the E.E.G. tracings, in which they may be reflected, for example, in the fact that generalised pathological activity may tend to become normalised, possibly after a phase of marked fluctuations. Although it may seem a logical step to correlate E.E.G.

findings with the various reversible psychopathological syndromes in an endeavour to obtain more accurate information on the underlying disturbances in cerebral function, the fact remains that the results obtained to date by this approach are open to many different interpretations. In a study based on data supplied by 75 participants at a colloquium held in Marseilles in 1956, DONGIER[5] carried out a statistical evaluation of the clinical and electroencephalographic manifestations of 536 psychotic episodes in 516 epileptic patients. The main conclusions yielded by this study were as follows: predominantly short-lived confusional states accompanied by clouding of consciousness – i.e. reactions of the acute exogenous type – occur as a rule immediately following a seizure, are associated with generalised pathological E.E.G. activity, and display correlations with "centrencephalic" epilepsy. On the other hand, mood disorders of usually longer duration and psychotic episodes accompanied by either no definite decrease in consciousness or only a fluctuating decrease – i.e. conditions which can be subsumed under the heading of transient syndromes – often develop prior to a seizure, are associated with variable E.E.G. findings, and tend to display links with psychomotor epilepsy. In the latter group of disorders, the interseizure E.E.G. records taken during the psychotic episode reveal either no changes at all or an increase in epileptic discharges in the temporal region without any alteration in background activity. A third possibility is that E.E.G. tracings which were pathological prior to the episode may become normalised during it – a phenomenon described by LANDOLT[25, 26] in 1953 as "forced normalisation". Other investigators[9, 10, 13, 20] have concluded that no consistent correlations between psychopathological syndromes in epileptics and E.E.G. findings have yet been demonstrated.

4. Treatment

If we base our concept of psychic diseases on the assumption that they are conditioned by a plurality of phenomena, we are implying that several factors – e.g. of a cerebral, psychodynamic, and sociosituational nature – are invariably operative in the pathogenesis of any psychopathological syndrome, even though their relative importance may differ markedly from one case to another. This difference in relative importance must be taken into account when drawing up an overall treatment plan for each patient. Although in such a plan close attention should of course be paid to therapeutic measures directed against psychic disorders of primarily psychological or social origin, I shall confine myself here, for the reasons outlined in the introduction to this paper, to the treatment of psychic disorders of primarily cerebral origin. In these disorders the approach to treatment is mainly governed by three factors[4]:

1. The wide variety of psychopathological syndromes falling into this category.
2. The large gaps in our knowledge of their pathogenesis.
3. The high proportion of cases in which reversible and irreversible syndromes are intermingled and by no means easy to separate.

Table 1c. Treatment. The drugs printed in italics possess anticonvulsive properties.

Individual psycho-pathological syndromes	Treatment	
	Drug therapy	Other measures
Reversible syndromes	*Tegretol,* levomepromazine, amitriptyline	
Episodic mood disorders	*Diazepam*	
Episodic psychoses		
Productive psychotic episodes	Haloperidol, levomepromazine	Reduction of anti-convulsive medication
Stupor	*Diazepam (clonazepam)* i.v.	
Twilight states	*Phenytoin* i.v.	Hospitalisation
	(Haloperidol)	
Other "organic" syndromes		Reduction of medication

Let me try to illustrate what I mean by reference to a few examples[4, 15] (Table 1c).

4.1. Mood disorders and productive psychotic episodes

Depending on the clinical classification of their target symptoms, mood disorders can be treated with anxiolytic minor tranquillisers such as diazepam, with mood-enhancing psycho-active drugs such as ®Tegretol (carbamazepine) or amitriptyline, or with neuroleptics of the sedating type such as levomepromazine. Worth noting in this connection is that amitriptyline and levomepromazine, in contrast to diazepam and Tegretol, do not possess any anticonvulsive properties; on the contrary, in common with many other tricyclic psycho-active agents, they may even possibly lower the convulsive threshold. Tricyclic drugs are therefore indicated in episodic mood disorders accompanied by forced normalisation of the E.E.G. findings, because, in cases where the development of a mood disorder or an episodic psychosis is linked with the disappearance of seizures and with an at least partial normalisation of the E.E.G. tracings, the aim of therapy must be to lower the convulsive threshold – albeit, if possible, to only a subclinical degree. This "pathologisation" of the E.E.G. can be achieved in a number of ways. First of all, the anticonvulsive medication should be reduced slowly and carefully. The convulsive threshold can then be further lowered by adding neuroleptics to the regimen. This second method may be particularly useful in cases where a psychotic excitation state has to be brought under control quickly. For this purpose, haloperidol (administered orally in the form of drops, or intravenously) or levomepromazine can be employed.

4.2. Stupor

Cases of stupor associated with petit mal status and marked by intermittent or continuous spike-and-wave patterns in the E.E.G. can as a rule be inter-

rupted within a matter of minutes by giving the patient a very slow intravenous injection of diazepam. It is reported that petit mal status of this type
can be even more effectively terminated with the aid of clonazepam, a drug,
however, which is at present available only in Switzerland and France, where
it is marketed under the name ®Rivotril[7, 8].

4.3. Twilight states

As already mentioned earlier on in this paper, twilight states associated with
a fairly marked narrowing of consciousness and, at the same time, with disturbances of orientation may be manifestations of widely differing disorders of
cerebral function:

1. They occur most frequently following a seizure and subside spontaneously
   after a few hours or days. Careful surveillance of the patient, to ensure that
   he does not commit an irresponsible act, is sometimes sufficient in itself.
   Often, however, the risk is too great and the patient will have to be admitted to a psychiatric clinic.
2. On the other hand, in cases where the twilight state is a manifestation of
   prolonged focal epileptic excitation, such as occurs in status psychomotoricus, an attempt should first of all be made to interrupt this status in the
   usual way by administering high doses of phenytoin (1–2 ampoules i.v., 1 ampoule i.m.). If this proves of no avail and the status persists for a period of
   days, one can try combining the anticonvulsant with a non-sedative neuroleptic.
3. Finally, it should be borne in mind that twilight states, including especially
   those displaying overtones of amentia and occasionally also those characterised by very profuse expansive symptoms, may also be a manifestation
   of drug poisoning. It goes without saying that appropriate treatment in
   these instances consists in carefully reducing the medication to a suitable
   level.

5. Summary

By way of recapitulation, the most important aspects of the diagnosis and
treatment of reversible psychic disorders of primarily cerebral origin in epileptics are summarised in Table 2.
In this summary table, the syndromes are differentiated in the first place
from the psychopathological standpoint. A comparison of these syndromes
with those encountered in the presence of psychic disorders assignable to
somatic causes provides the first clues to their pathogenesis. This pathogenetic
aspect is then analysed in greater detail by considering the clinical and
electro-encephalographic correlations obtaining between these disorders, on
the one hand, and epileptic seizures, on the other. Finally, it is upon this
pathogenetic analysis, as well as upon the psychopathological target symptoms,
that the choice of treatment depends.

Table 2. Summary review indicating the most important aspects of the diagnosis and treatment of reversible psychic disorders of primarily cerebral origin in epileptics.

General classification of psychic disorders assignable to somatic causes	Individual psycho-pathological syndromes	Clinical correlatives (not obligatory)	E.E.G. correlatives (not obligatory)	Treatment	
				Drug therapy	Other measures
	Reversible syndromes				
Transient syndromes	Episodic mood disorders	More usually pre-paroxysmal	More usually forced normalisation	*Tegretol,* levomepromazine, amitriptyline *Diazepam*	
	Episodic psychoses				
	Productive psychotic episodes	More usually pre-paroxysmal	More usually forced normalisation	Haloperidol, levomepromazine	Reduction of anticonvulsive medication
	Stupor	Petit mal status	(Ir)regular spike-and-wave patterns	*Diazepam (clonazepam)* i.v.	
	Twilight states	Status psychomotoricus (seldom)	More usually temporal delta and theta waves and sharp waves	*Phenytoin* i.v.	Hospitalisation
		More usually post-paroxysmal	More usually generalised pathological activity, spike-and-wave patterns, spikes, sharp waves, paroxysmal dysrhythmia	(Haloperidol)	
Reactions of the acute exogenous type	Other "organic" syndromes	E.g. drug poisoning	Generalised pathological activity, beta waves		Reduction of medication

1 BECHTHOLD, H.-G., SCHOTTKY, A.: Phasische Verstimmung und Epilepsie. Zwei polare Fälle. Nervenarzt *42*, 539 (1971)

2 BONHOEFFER, K.: Die exogenen Reaktionstypen. Arch. Psychiat. Nervenkr. *58*, 58 (1917)

3 DIEHL, L.: Psychische Wirkungen von Antiepileptika. Paper presented at XVIth Ann. Meet. Dtsch. Sekt. Int. Liga Epilepsie, Berlin 1974

4 DIEHL, L., HELMCHEN, H.: Therapie epileptischer Psychosen und Verstimmungen. In Penin, H. (Editor): Psychische Störungen bei Epilepsie. Psychosen, Verstimmungen, Persönlichkeitsveränderungen, XIVth Ann. Meet. Dtsch. Sekt. Int. Liga Epilepsie, Bonn 1972, p. 193 (Schattauer, Stuttgart/New York 1973)

5 DONGIER, S.: Statistical study of clinical and electroencephalographic manifestations of 536 psychotic episodes occurring in 516 epileptics between clinical seizures. Epilepsia (Amst.) *1*, 117 (1959/60)

6 DREYER, R.: Zur Frage des Status epilepticus mit psychomotorischen Anfällen. Ein Beitrag zum temporalen Status epilepticus und zu atypischen Dämmerzuständen und Verstimmungen. Nervenarzt *36*, 221 (1965)

7 DREYER, R.: Die Pharmakotherapie der Epilepsien. In Kisker, K.P., et al. (Editors): Psychiatrie der Gegenwart, Vol. II/Part 2, 2nd Ed., p. 713 (Springer, Berlin/Heidelberg/New York 1972)

8 GASTAUT, H., COURJON, J., POIRÉ, R., WEBER, M.: Treatment of status epilepticus with a new benzodiazepine more active than diazepam. Epilepsia (Amst.) *12*, 197 (1971)

9 GLASER, G.H.: The problem of psychosis in psychomotor temporal lobe epileptics. Epilepsia (Amst.) *5*, 271 (1964)

10 GLASER, G.H., NEWMAN, R.J., SCHAFER, R.: Interictal psychosis in psychomotor temporal lobe epilepsy. In Glaser, G.H. (Editor): EEG and behavior, p. 345 (Basic Books, New York 1963)

11 GRÜNEBERG, F., HELMCHEN, H.: Impulsiv-Petit mal-status und paranoide Psychose. Nervenarzt *40*, 381 (1969)

12 GRUHLE, H.W.: Über den Wahn bei Epilepsie. Z. ges. Neurol. Psychiat. *154*, 395 (1936)

13 HEDENSTRÖM, I. von, SCHORSCH, G.: EEG-Befunde bei epileptischen Dämmer- und Verstimmungszuständen. Arch. Psychiat. Nervenkr. *199*, 311 (1959)

14 HELMCHEN, H.: Zerebrale Bedingungskonstellationen psychopathologischer Syndrome bei Epileptikern. In Helmchen, H., Hippius, H. (Editors): Entwicklungstendenzen biologischer Psychiatrie (Thieme, Stuttgart 1975; printing)

15 HELMCHEN, H.: Therapeutische Probleme komplizierter Epilepsien des Erwachsenen. Med. Welt (Stuttg.) *26*, 499 (1975)

16 HELMCHEN, H., HOFFMANN, I., KANOWSKI, S.: Dämmerzustand oder Status fokaler sensorischer Anfälle? Nervenarzt *40*, 389 (1969)

17 HESS, R., SCOLLO-LAVIZZARI, G., WYSS, F.E.: Borderline cases of petit mal status. Europ. Neurol. (Basle) *5*, 137 (1971)

18 JANZ, D.: Discussion, loc. cit. [4], p. 78

19 JANZARIK, W.: Der Wahn schizophrener Prägung in den psychotischen Episoden der Epileptiker und die schizophrene Wahnwahrnehmung. Fortschr. Neurol. Psychiat. *23*, 533 (1955)

20 JUNG, R.: Neurophysiologie und Psychiatrie. In Gruhle, H.W., et al. (Editors): Psychiatrie der Gegenwart, Vol. I/1 A, p. 325 (Springer, Berlin/Heidelberg/New York 1967)

21 KISKER, K.P.: Sprachliche Stereotypien bei Temporallappen-Epilepsie (Ein Beitrag zur Konstitution verbaler Sprachanteile). Nervenarzt *28*, 366 (1957)

22 KRAEPELIN, E.: Psychiatrie, 8th Ed. (new, unrevised edition), Vol. III, p. 1040 (Barth, Leipzig 1923)

23 Kranz, H.: Das Thema des Wahns im Wandel der Zeit. Fortschr. Neurol. Psychiat. *23*, 58 (1955)

24 Kruse, R.: Hypsarrhythmie, Spike-wave-Variant und Petit mal-Status im Kindes-alter. Zbl. ges. Neurol. Psychiat. *194*, 219 (1968); abstract of paper

25 Landolt, H.: Einige klinisch-elektroencephalographische Korrelationen bei epi-leptischen Dämmerzuständen. Nervenarzt *24*, 479 (1953); abstract of paper

26 Landolt, H.: Über Verstimmungen, Dämmerzustände und schizophrene Zu-standsbilder bei Epilepsie. Schweiz. Arch. Neurol. Psychiat. *76*, 313 (1955)

27 Müller, J., Müller, D.: Hirnelektrische Korrelate bei Überdosierung von anti-konvulsiven Medikamenten. Nervenarzt *43*, 270 (1972)

28 Niedermeyer, E., Khalifeh, R.: Petit mal status ("spike-wave-stupor"). An electro-clinical appraisal. Epilepsia (Amst.) *6*, 250 (1965)

29 Peters, U.H.: Discussion, loc. cit. [4], p. 79

30 Scheid, W.: Lehrbuch der Neurologie, 2nd Ed. (Thieme, Stuttgart 1966)

31 Selbach, H.: Die cerebralen Anfallsleiden: Genuine Epilepsie, symptomatische Hirnkrämpfe und die Narkolepsie. In Bergmann, G. von, et al. (Editors): Hand-buch der inneren Medizin, 4th Ed., Vol. V/3, Neurologie, p. 1082 (Springer, Berlin/Göttingen/Heidelberg 1953)

32 Slater, E.: The schizophrenia-like illnesses of epilepsy. In Herrington, R.N. (Editor): Current problems in neuropsychiatry. Brit. J. Psychiat., Special Publ. No. 4, p. 77 (Headley Brothers, Ashford, Kent 1969)

33 Slater, E., Beard, A.W.: Schizophrenia-like psychoses of epilepsy. Brit. J. Psy-chiat. *109*, 95 (1963)

34 Tellenbach, H.: Epilepsie als Anfallsleiden und als Psychose. Über alternative Psychosen paranoider Prägung bei «forcierter Normalisierung» (Landolt) des Elektroencephalogramms Epileptischer. Nervenarzt *36*, 190 (1965)

35 Weitbrecht, H.J.: Discussion, loc. cit. [4], p. 80

36 Wieck, H.H.: Zur klinischen Stellung des Durchgangs-Syndroms. Schweiz. Arch. Neurol. Neurochir. Psychiat. *88*, 409 (1961)

37 Wolf, P.: Zur Klinik und Psychopathologie des Status psychomotoricus. Nerven-arzt *41*, 603 (1970)

Discussion

P. KIELHOLZ: Having listened to Dr. HELMCHEN's excellent paper in which he systematically reviewed the various types of psychic disturbance encountered in epileptic patients, I should merely like to supplement and elaborate on what he had to say about episodic mood disorders.

It was MANFRED BLEULER* who stressed that particular importance attaches to epileptic mood disorders, because they are almost always present in epilepsy and constitute one of the commonest indications for admission of such patients to psychiatric clinics. They develop without any apparent reason – or, at least, without the patient having experienced any event which might satisfactorily explain them – and they can be subdivided according to their incidence and phenomenology into four groups:

1. Mood disorders marked by dysphoria and irritability.
2. Depressive mood disorders.
3. Mood disorders marked by depression and anxiety.
4. Mood disorders marked by euphoria and manic symptoms.

These mood disorders may occur immediately before or after a grand mal or psychomotor seizure, but they are also liable to be encountered in the intervals between attacks. They last for periods of time ranging from a few hours to several days and are frequently terminated by a seizure. They are due to a combination of many different factors, including pre-morbid personality structure, sequelae of disturbances in cerebral function, developmental anomalies, and environmental circumstances.

By far the commonest episodic mood disorders are the ones characterised by *dysphoria and irritability*, in which the patients suddenly become irritable or aggressive without any apparent motive, or else display an inordinate degree of irritability or aggressiveness in response to even the mildest stimulus. This inevitably brings them into conflict with their environment.

Next in order of frequency are the *depressive mood disorders* with or without overtones of anxiety; these disorders closely resemble endogenous depression, but are relatively seldom accompanied by suicidal impulses.

According to the large-scale study conducted by DONGIER**, to which Dr. HELMCHEN referred, *manic mood disorders* are observed in only 5% of epileptics and thus represent the rarest type of episodic mood disorder encountered in such patients. They are marked by an enhanced feeling of vitality, the patient very often imagining that he has finally recovered from his epilepsy or experiencing states akin to religious ecstasy. Unlike the manic disturbances occurring in the course of bipolar depression, the euphoric episodes met with in epileptics are not associated with flight of ideas.

Little is known about what happens in the brain during these various mood disorders. Analysis of E.E.G. records taken during an episodic mood disorder commonly reveals a slow, diffuse delta activity which is sometimes bisynchronous and sometimes not. As reported by various authors***, however, the most striking feature of the E.E.G.

---

* BLEULER, E.: Lehrbuch der Psychiatrie, 12th Ed. (revised by Bleuler, M.), p. 364 (Springer, Berlin/Heidelberg/New York 1972)

**DONGIER, S.: Statistical study of clinical and electroencephalographic manifestations of 536 psychotic episodes occurring in 516 epileptics between clinical seizures. Epilepsia (Amst.) *1*, 117 (1959/60)

*** LANDOLT, H.: Petit mal; Temporallappenepilepsie; epileptische Dämmerzustände und Verstimmungen. In: Schulte, W.: Epilepsie und ihre Randgebiete in Klinik und Praxis, p. 33 (Lehmanns, Munich 1964)

HESS, R.: Elektrische Hirnaktivität und Psychopathologie. Schweiz. med. Wschr. *93*, 102 (1963)

LOEB, C., GIBERTI, F.: Considerazioni cliniche ed elettroencefalografiche a proposito di sindromi psicosiche in soggetti epilettici. Sist. nerv. *9*, 219 (1957)

tracings is the tendency for the pattern to become normalised and for focal changes and paroxysmal dysfunctions to regress.

In line with their multifactorial origin, epileptic mood disorders may be amenable to a wide variety of psychotherapeutic measures. The aim of these measures, whether carried out on an individual, group, or family basis, is to achieve greater harmony between the patient and his home or occupational environment, to improve his interpersonal relationships, and to neutralise conflict situations.

As far as the use of drugs is concerned, epileptic mood disorders should be treated by reference to their psychopathological target symptoms. There is a tendency, when selecting drugs, to pay too little attention to the fact that episodes marked by dysphoria and irritability really belong to the category of depressive mood disorders. Crossness and irritability are simply very mild signs of a shift in basic mood towards depression. For example, irritability is often observed in cases of endogenous depression when the patient is just emerging from a depressive phase and his aggressiveness is becoming directed once again at his environment. Hence, in mood disorders characterised by dysphoria and depression it is advisable to resort to basic therapy with ®Tegretol (carbamazepine), which has a drive-enhancing and a slight mood-brightening effect. In cases where the epileptic mood disorder displays clear-cut overtones of anxiety and depression or, in particular, of crossness and irritability, treatment with Tegretol should be supplemented with an antidepressant possessing primarily anxiolytic and relaxing properties.

Of the antidepressants displaying primarily mood-brightening and anxiolytic properties, the most effective have proved to be ®Ludiomil (maprotiline), which is especially useful in severe mood disorders with overtones of anxiety – and amitriptyline. Possessing as it does a broad spectrum of activity (Figure 1), Ludiomil has the advantage that it is also indicated in mixed forms of episodic mood disorder, i.e. mood disorders marked by varying degrees of both irritability and depression. By supplementing antiepileptic medication with an antidepressant whose various effects are in a judiciously balanced ratio to one another, it is possible largely to avoid those unpredictable drug interactions which are an ever-present risk of any combined therapy.

W. BIRKMAYER: The clear account Dr. KIELHOLZ has just given us of the clinical features of the various types of episodic mood disorder encountered in epileptic patients provides yet another illustration of the differing angles from which psychiatrists and neurologists view such cases. The neurologist is rarely, if ever, confronted with the symptoms Dr. KIELHOLZ has described, and he wouldn't even recognise them if he were! A concrete example in point springs to my mind in this connection: SCHALTENBRAND, an eminent specialist in the field of research on multiple sclerosis, published a number of years ago a voluminous manual* in which he gave a detailed description of all the signs and symptoms of multiple sclerosis except for the psychic manifestations of the disease; these he omitted, not because of an oversight, but because in his opinion they simply didn't occur in patients with multiple sclerosis. Later, when he happened to be paying a visit to my department, I showed him some 200 cases of multiple sclerosis in which the disease was complicated by what – for us at least – was a clearly recognisable psychic component. Precisely because, in severe neurological disorders, the psychiatrist sees things which often escape the notice of the neurologist, I consider it absolutely essential that contact should be maintained between the two disciplines of neurology and psychiatry – and by this I mean maintained not only at congresses and symposia but also at the hospital bedside.

H. PETSCHE: I should like to comment briefly on the phenomenon of so-called "forced normalisation" to which Dr. HELMCHEN referred in his paper. When LANDOLT first propounded the thesis in which he coined this term, we were very surprised at the idea that epileptic-psychotic episodes presenting a manifestly severe clinical picture

---

188   * SCHALTENBRAND, G.: Die multiple Sklerose des Menschen (Thieme, Leipzig 1943)

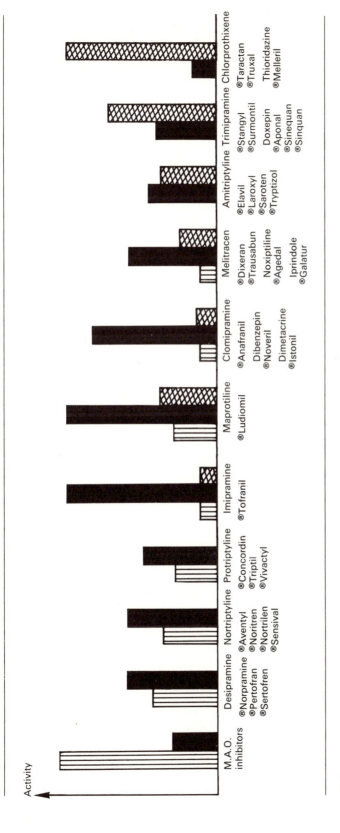

Activity

M.A.O. inhibitors	Desipramine	Nortriptyline	Protriptyline	Imipramine	Maprotiline	Clomipramine	Melitracen	Amitriptyline	Trimipramine	Chlorprothixene
	®Norpramin	®Aventyl	®Concordin	®Tofranil	®Ludiomil	®Anafranil	®Dixeran	®Elavil	®Stangyl	®Taractan
	®Pertofran	®Noritren	®Triptil			Dibenzepin	®Trausabun	®Laroxyl	®Surmontil	®Truxal
	®Sertofren	®Nortrilen	®Vivactyl			®Noveril	Noxiptiline	®Saroten		Thioridazine
		®Sensival				Dimetacrine	®Agedal	®Tryptizol	Doxepin	®Melleril
						®Istonil	Iprindole		®Aponal	
							®Galatur		®Sinequan	
									®Sinquan	

▭ Drive-enhancing (disinhibiting)

■ Depression-relieving (mood-brightening)

▨ Anxiety-reducing (anxiolytic)

Fig. 1. Diagrammatic representation of the activity patterns of antidepressive agents.

189

could be associated with normalisation of the E.E.G. patterns. Dr. HELMCHEN has now drawn attention in his paper to one important fact, namely, that forced normalisation of the E.E.G. tends to occur mainly prior to seizures, whereas after the seizures the E.E.G. tracings are usually found to be markedly pathological for some considerable time, during which more or less clear-cut psychic changes may also be discerned. Here, there would seem to be some similarity with the electro-encephalographic findings obtained in patients subject to psychomotor attacks, which are also frequently preceded by a brief phase of normalisation characterised by a transient decrease in the voltage and an increase in the frequency of the waves.

We know very much more about correlations between the E.E.G. patterns and the psychic manifestations of epilepsy since BANCAUD et al.* published the results of detailed studies which they carried out in a fairly large series of patients using deep electrodes. These authors found that in the vast majority of cases the deeper zones of the cerebral cortex, from which recordings cannot be made via surface electrodes, were already producing seizure discharges before any such activity could be detected in the superficial regions of the cortex. It therefore seems reasonable to suppose that, in the presence of forced normalisation too, a great deal of pathological electrical activity is in fact taking place in the brain, but in areas of the temporal lobe that we cannot reach with conventional electro-encephalography. In this connection, I would point out that only about one-quarter of the cerebral cortex is actually in direct contact with the vault of the cranium and, as such, accessible to electro-encephalographic recording. In the case of the temporal lobe, the ratio is as low as approximately 1:20, i.e. only about one-twentieth of the surface of the temporal lobe lies directly beneath the calvaria. But we do know something more about conditions governing the transmission of electrical activity from the brain to the scalp: studies on intracerebral and cortical activity in cases of Kojevnikovian epilepsy revealed that here the E.E.G. patterns often showed no abnormalities, despite the fact that a steady stream of spikes was visible in the electrocorticogram and that the clinical picture was one of partial continuous epilepsy. Only occasionally were spikes encountered over Rolando's area. BANCAUD et al. found in such cases that spikes can be seen in the E.E.G. only if and when they appear in relatively synchronised fashion over quite a large region in the electrocorticogram. The reason for this is that the conducting layers in general, and the C.S.F. in particular, distort the pattern of electrical activity in an unpredictable manner; consequently, a fairly extensive area beneath the electrode has to be discharging more or less synchronously before anything becomes visible in the E.E.G. at all. The difference between what the electrocorticogram and the electro-encephalogram reveal is something that I usually try to explain by means of a simile: the relationship between the electrocorticogram and the electro-encephalogram is rather like that existing between a magnificent Babylonian temple and the hillock of rubble to which it becomes reduced after thousands of years of exposure to the elements.

H. REISNER: In the comments he made following Dr. KIELHOLZ's remarks, Dr. BIRKMAYER touched upon a problem about which I too should like to say a few words from the standpoint of a neurologist. The problem I am referring to is that posed by those cases of epilepsy which, as it were, hover between neurology and psychiatry. When I was in charge of the clinic in Graz, I was working both as a neurologist and as a psychiatrist, and in this capacity I was quite often confronted with transient psychoses in epileptic patients; it was nevertheless always the somatic manifestations of the epilepsy, in the form of seizures, that occupied the foreground. But once psychiatry and neurology become separated – as is the case, for example, at our clinic in Vienna – we neurologists no longer encounter any predominantly psychopathological cases, and the psychiatrists no longer see any epileptics in whom seizures are the main feature

---

* BANCAUD, J., TALAIRACH, J., GEIER, S., SCARABIN, J.-M.: E.E.G. et S.E.E.G. dans les tumeurs cérébrales et l'épilepsie (Edifor, Paris 1973)

of the clinical picture. Given this situation, what should we do to avoid such risks as it may entail for the patient? Epilepsy belongs to a sort of no-man's-land between neurology and psychiatry, and there can be few other diseases the treatment of which so obviously calls for knowledge and experience of both these branches of medicine. Now that training in psychiatry and neurology have been separated from each other, one cannot expect every neurologist to have an equally thorough mastery of both branches. It would therefore be highly desirable if, particularly in polyclinics, arrangements could be made for a neurologist to work together with a psychiatrist, or if a consultant could be appointed who – as in the case of my colleague Prof. Pateisky at the out-patient clinic for epileptics in Vienna – is an excellent neurologist and psychiatrist and is thus equally at home in both disciplines. These, I suggest, are the two practical alternatives at present open to us. Either way, there would then be hardly any risk of transient psychotic episodes being overlooked or misinterpreted or, as in my experience has also sometimes happened, of epileptic manifestations being simply ascribed to hysteria. Needless to say, such a partnership between neurology and psychiatry would likewise help to improve the treatment given for epilepsy, because then all the therapeutic possibilities that have been discussed here could be effectively exploited both to combat transient psychoses and to bring the seizures themselves under control.

I should also like to address a remark to Dr. Helmchen. You will remember that, when pentetrazole shock treatment and electroconvulsive therapy were introduced for the management of psychiatric disorders, one of the ideas put forward in this connection was that in cases of schizophrenia the shocks produced would be tantamount to treating the patient by inducing epileptic seizures – a practice which was upheld on the grounds that in schizophrenic psychoses there is no danger of actually provoking genuine epilepsy. This, of course, raises the question as to what schizophrenia really is – a question which we are not here to discuss now. From what Dr. Helmchen has said, however, it would seem that transient epileptic psychoses merely simulate schizophrenic reactions, but do not constitute genuine forms of schizophrenia. Although personally I doubt whether it is true to say that schizophrenia never occurs in association with epilepsy, I would certainly agree that such an association is a very rare occurrence; to this extent it strikes me that the idea I mentioned, dating back to the early days of shock therapy, now once again appears to have some justification.

M. Parsonage: It has been said during this discussion that neurologists rarely, if ever, see psychiatric disorders in patients with epilepsy. This is certainly not true in my own case, because the psychiatric colleagues with whom I work have taught me how to recognise these disorders. I feel that it is a handicap for a neurologist not to be able to do this. In the care of people with epilepsy, neurologists and psychiatrists can indeed collaborate most effectively in the way that Dr. Reisner has suggested, and I believe that a combination of the two disciplines is immeasurably more effective than either alone. In my part of England we set up in 1966 a neuropsychiatric service in which neurologists and psychiatrists can work together and readily communicate with one another – much more easily than they can in many other parts of the country. From the very beginning we realised that this service would be admirably suited for the care of patients with epilepsy, and I am glad to say that our expectations have been fully realised over the years.

H. Helmchen: I'd like to reply first of all to what Dr. Reisner has just said about epilepsy and schizophrenia. The historically conflicting notions concerning an antagonism between epilepsy and schizophrenia are of a semantic nature. There is no proof that, as nosological entities, schizophrenia and epilepsy are mutually exclusive. Though at one time references were frequently made in the literature to the occurrence of epileptic seizures in schizophrenic patients, one hardly ever comes across such reports today. One reason for this may be that nowadays most patients presenting with both syndromes are no longer classified as schizophrenics, but preferably as epileptics with schizoid psychoses. Turning from the nosological to the phenomenological plane, however, we find that observations relating to an antagonism between schizophrenic symptoms and epileptic manifestations in the form of seizures are still by no means rare. TELLENBACH*, for example, has coined the term "alternative psychoses" to describe psychotic symptoms alternating with epileptic seizures. But, as I have also pointed out, this antagonism is only encountered in a portion of those acute reversible psychotic episodes that chiefly occur pre-paroxysmally, and it is hardly ever apparent in the case of chronic psychoses present during intervals between attacks. Incidentally, as was observed by SLATER and BEARD** in 20 out of 69 epileptic patients, psychotic episodes may be a prelude to chronic psychoses. According to FLOR-HENRY***, psychoses running an intermittent course correlate with minimal, and chronic psychoses with maximal, morphological brain lesions.

May I at this point add a comment on Dr. PETSCHE's remarks, which I fully endorse. The cerebral factors responsible for causing schizoid psychoses in the presence of epilepsy apparently include the ratio between morphological and functional lesions, as well as the shifts which this ratio undergoes in the course of time. Quite a number of clues have in fact already been obtained which enable one to specify with at least some degree of accuracy both the site and the nature of the main lesions concerned. Since I have dealt with this topic in detail elsewhere****, I need only give a brief summary here.

Regarding the site of the lesions, it can be said that schizoid psychoses appear to occur particularly often where the lesions are located in the "temporal" region. Though such lesions are a necessary contributing factor, they are certainly not sufficient in themselves to give rise to a psychosis – as confirmed by the fact that many epileptic patients showing evidence of "temporal" foci in the E.E.G. or in the pneumoencephalogram do not develop psychoses. It would often seem that an additional prerequisite for the development of a psychosis is the presence of bilateral lesions. Finally, there are also reasons for supposing that the form in which the psychotic disorder manifests itself may depend on which side of the brain the lesions are located in.

With reference to the nature of the lesions, two main questions arise, namely: what are the factors limiting propagation of the epileptic excitation, and in what respects does limitation of the excitation differ in a psychomotor attack as compared with a psychotic episode? Here, there is evidence to suggest several possible answers. Firstly, the excitation may be limited by the presence of multiple, circumscribed disturbances of cerebral function. In this connection, I would remind you, for example, of the particular frequency with which psychotic episodes tend to occur in patients developing bilateral E.E.G. foci in the course of chronic progressive forms of epilepsy, as well as in those suffering from multifocal cerebral damage associated with residual epilepsy. Secondly, the excitation may be limited by drugs; it is a well-known fact, for instance, that psychotic episodes can be provoked by anti-epileptic agents and eliminated by major tranquillisers, which as a rule lower the seizure threshold. Thirdly, psychic

---

* TELLENBACH, H.: Epilepsie als Anfallsleiden und als Psychose. Über alternative Psychosen paranoider Prägung bei «forcierter Normalisierung» (Landolt) des Elektroencephalogramms Epileptischer. Nervenarzt *36*, 190 (1965)
** SLATER, E., BEARD, A.W.: Schizophrenia-like psychoses of epilepsy. Brit. J. Psychiat. *109*, 95 (1963)
*** FLOR-HENRY, P.: Schizophrenic-like reactions and affective psychoses associated with temporal lobe epilepsy: etiological factors. Amer. J. Psychiat. *126*, 400 (1969)
    FLOR-HENRY, P.: Psychoses and temporal lobe epilepsy. A controlled investigation. Epilepsia (Amst.) *10*, 363 (1969)
**** HELMCHEN, H.: Zerebrale Bedingungskonstellationen psychopathologischer Syndrome bei Epileptikern. In Helmchen, H., Hippius, H. (Editors): Entwicklungstendenzen biologischer Psychiatrie (Thieme, Stuttgart 1975; printing)

stimuli may also have the effect of limiting epileptic excitation. Marked fluctuation is a feature repeatedly observed in E.E.G. tracings recorded from psychotic epileptics. This fluctuation might perhaps be one reason for the pronounced discrepancies between reports on E.E.G. findings obtained in epileptics during acute psychotic episodes. I consider it at all events important to point out here that we have yet to investigate to what extent external psychic stimuli of a momentary nature, such as the fact of being subjected to an examination, may have an influence on the E.E.G. patterns and possibly even restore them to normal, and on the other hand to what extent there may be no point in attempting to make E.E.G. recordings at all except when the patient is passing through a phase of the psychosis in which he is free from anxiety and relatively relaxed.

The so-called psychotropic effect of Tegretol in the treatment of convulsions of cerebral origin in children

by A. RETT*

When one has been using ®Tegretol (carbamazepine) for 15 years in the treatment of children subject to convulsions of cerebral origin, the experience gained during this time must inevitably prompt one to form certain impressions as to the drug's activity. Though of course largely of a subjective nature, such impressions nevertheless affect one's line of action, one's approach to treatment, and one's assessment of the results obtained; they have at all events a decisive influence on the choice of indications, on the dosages employed, and on the way in which the therapeutic response is evaluated. Where, as in our case, the series of patients treated is quite a large one, totalling over 900 children, there may perhaps be "safety in numbers", in the sense that possible sources of errors in judgment become correspondingly narrowed down. Be this as it may, the fact remains that children are particularly difficult patients in whom to assess the anticonvulsive effect of a drug. Assuming that an observation period of at least five years is required before any even approximately valid conclusions can be reached about the therapeutic efficacy of an anticonvulsive agent, the child will during this period have passed through various developmental stages involving physical, emotional, and intellectual modifications to which the anticonvulsive medication needs to be progressively adapted.

Another aspect of which due account has to be taken when assessing the response to treatment is that the epileptic child lives his life "at second hand", as it were. In other words, he is essentially dependent on his environment, e.g. on the mental and emotional attitude of the mother towards his affliction, on the mother's confidence in the treating physician and in the therapy prescribed, on her intelligence and conscientiousness in administering the daily doses of medication and in recording the frequency, type, and severity of his attacks, and above all on the upbringing and education he receives.

It is precisely the abundance of such conditioning factors which often makes it so frustratingly difficult for us to arrive at a verdict on the treatment we have prescribed that can be regarded as reasonably accurate, objective, and reliable.

Bearing in mind all the imponderables which I have merely touched upon here, one is almost tempted to conclude that statistical data relating to a whole series of patients are meaningless and that, in the last analysis, only the study of

* Abteilung für entwicklungsgestörte Kinder, Neurologisches Krankenhaus der Stadt Wien-Rosenhügel und Ludwig-Boltzmann-Institut zur Erforschung kindlicher Hirnschäden, Vienna, Austria.

194

individual cases has any real justification. In the course of our work as clinicians, we nevertheless try to review our results collectively and are even wont to base our future actions on the findings which emerge from such reviews. This, indeed, is the customary – and perhaps necessary – practice, but it is a practice that is bound to some extent to engender scepticism, uncertainty, and mental reservations. I can therefore only hope that the relatively large number of cases we have studied is sufficient to salve our "statistical consciences" and to lend added weight to our observations.

An analysis of the cases in question suggests three conclusions which I propose to present here and which we believe can reasonably be drawn from our experience of these cases. Before submitting our three conclusions for discussion, I should like to emphasise that the very fact that our patients were accepted for treatment at a clinic for developmentally disturbed children implies a certain process of selection and that the special features characteristic of our series of cases would therefore have to be taken into account when attempting to make comparisons with other groups of patients. Finally, due attention would also have to be paid to the paediatrically oriented approach adopted in our clinic, an approach which upon closer analysis would probably be found to differ somewhat from neurological and/or psychiatric schools of thought on methods of examination, diagnosis, assessment, and treatment.

The three conclusions emerging from our experience with Tegretol over the past 15 years are as follows:

1. It is our impression that the response to Tegretol in juvenile grand mal exhibits age-dependent differences, inasmuch as the older the child the better the response elicited by the drug is likely to be.
2. It is a fact which cannot be overlooked that in our series of patients positive results were more frequently recorded in the girls than in the boys; in other words, gynaecotropism seems to be a feature of the therapeutic activity of Tegretol.
3. Among our patients we were unable to obtain evidence of the so-called psychotropic effect of Tegretol, which has been described by many authors and is regarded as having been confirmed in adults.

I propose now to describe the attempts we made to investigate these empirical impressions of ours with a view either to confirming or to disproving them.

Material and methods

From the total of approximately 900 cases treated over a period of 15 years a randomly selected series of 100 patients fulfilling the following criteria was studied:

1. For at least four years they had received regular treatment with Tegretol to the exclusion of all other drugs.

2. The response to this treatment had on the whole been positive, the classification adopted in assessing the response being as follows:

    I Seizures completely abolished

    II Seizure frequency reduced by about 75% as compared with the fre-
quency prior to treatment

    III Seizure frequency reduced by about 50%.

    (It was obviously impossible to assign cases to Groups II and III with ab-
solute accuracy, and in this connection it should also be pointed out that
frequency figures based on observations reported by members of the patient's
family are not necessarily reliable.)

3. Throughout the period of observation, responsibility for treating and following the patients had been entirely in our hands, and the patients concerned
were also suitable for follow-up study.

Results

Given in Figure 1 is a breakdown of the results obtained with Tegretol, classified in terms of the three groups already mentioned; the sex distribution in
each group is indicated at the bottom. In Group I, i.e. the group showing the

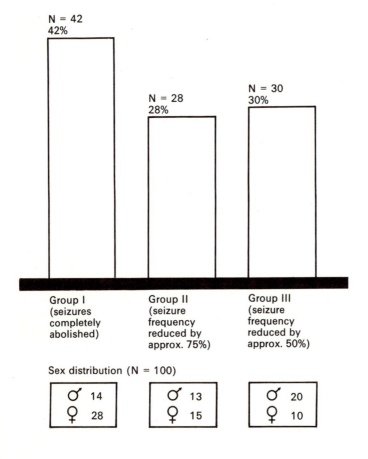

N = 42
42%

N = 28
28%

N = 30
30%

Group I
(seizures
completely
abolished)

Group II
(seizure
frequency
reduced by
approx. 75%)

Group III
(seizure
frequency
reduced by
approx. 50%)

Sex distribution (N = 100)

♂ 14
♀ 28

♂ 13
♀ 15

♂ 20
♀ 10

Fig. 1. Results
obtained with
Tegretol in the 100
patients studied.

best response to treatment, the number of girls is significantly larger than that of the boys. Whereas in Group II the two sexes are evenly balanced, in Group III there is once again a statistically significant difference, the boys outnumbering the girls by 2:1. From these findings it can be concluded that, the better the response to Tegretol, the greater the likelihood that the patients concerned will be of female sex.

Shown in Figures 2–4 is the age and sex distribution of the patients belonging to each of the three groups. The data presented here in graphic form indicate

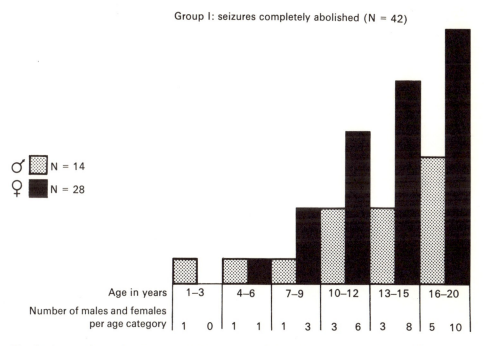

Fig. 2. Age and sex distribution of the patients belonging to Group I, in which treatment with Tegretol completely abolished the seizures.

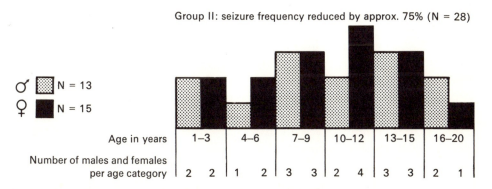

Fig. 3. Age and sex distribution of the patients belonging to Group II, in which treatment with Tegretol reduced the seizure frequency by approximately 75%.

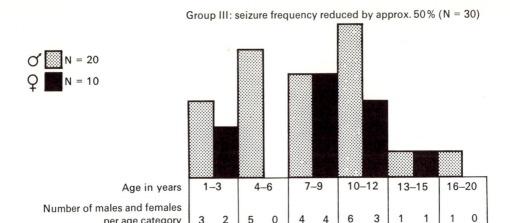

Group III: seizure frequency reduced by approx. 50% (N = 30)

♂ N = 20
♀ N = 10

Age in years	1–3		4–6		7–9		10–12		13–15		16–20	
Number of males and females per age category	3	2	5	0	4	4	6	3	1	1	1	0

Fig. 4. Age and sex distribution of the patients belonging to Group III, in which treatment with Tegretol reduced the seizure frequency by approximately 50%.

the existence of a close correlation between age and sex. In Group I (Figure 2) it is the older patients in general and the girls in particular who preponderate. In Group II (Figure 3) both the age and the sex distribution is relatively even. In Group III (Figure 4) we find more boys than girls, and the bulk of the patients are aged between four and 12 years.

Hormone analyses

In the literature published on Tegretol to date, we have found no confirmation of, or even any allusion to, the gynaecotropism which in our experience appears to characterise the drug's therapeutic effect. Our suspicion that the tendency for Tegretol to produce better results in girls might be due to hormonal factors prompted us to undertake a series of tests along the following lines:

Two groups of patients, designated A and B, were studied. Each group comprised ten girls, aged 14–17 years, who were living under approximately the same conditions. The tests, which took the form of measuring the excretion of total gonadotrophins, follicle-stimulating hormone, and 17-ketosteroids, were performed twice, with an interval of three weeks between one set of analyses and the next. The girls in Group A were receiving treatment with anticonvulsants other than Tegretol. Of the girls in Group B, five were under treatment with Tegretol alone, and five were being given Tegretol in combination with other anticonvulsive drugs.

Neither among girls belonging to the same group nor between each of the two groups and subgroups could we discern any differences whatsoever in the hormone values recorded.

In 1973 we carried out a further series of tests, this time on a double-blind basis. Sixteen girls, whose ages in this instance happened to range from 13 to 16 years, were divided into two groups which were once again designated A and B. Each of the eight patients per group was receiving treatment with Tegretol alone and underwent the same hormone analyses as already described. Whereas in Group A a placebo was temporarily substituted for the Tegretol medication after the first analysis of hormone excretion had been performed, in Group B the treatment with Tegretol was continued unchanged. The hormone determinations were repeated after one or two weeks and again after three or four weeks.

In this study, too, there was no evidence of any shift in the hormone values, either among patients of the same group or in patients of one group as compared with the other.

The gynaecotropism displayed by Tegretol thus remains for us an aspect of the drug's activity for which the only proof we can offer is the higher response rate we have observed in girls as opposed to boys. It is a phenomenon for which we cannot at present furnish any explanation. What it certainly cannot be ascribed to are differences in the dosage or in the mode of administration in girls as compared with boys, since there is no reason to suppose that there were any such differences either in the dosage for the two sexes or in the regularity with which the drug was administered by members of the patients' families or by our hospital staff.

The psychotropic effect of Tegretol

Reports referring to the psychotropic effect of Tegretol, which is now largely acknowledged as having been confirmed, have been published by numerous authors. Most of their observations, however, were confined to non-epileptic patients; moreover, the question as to what is meant by the term "psychotropic effect" – or, rather, what the various authors mean by it – is one to which no generally acceptable answer can be given.

To what degree it is possible to measure such an effect also depends to a great extent on the test procedures employed, and these – selected as they are in the light of each author's personal experience – are by no means in every instance the same. Consequently, with regard at least to the methodology used in testing for evidence of psychotropic activity, assessment of the various results reported involves a considerable element of uncertainty.

Like all other investigators, we too have resorted in our research to those methods which we in the course of the years have found to prove reliable as experimental tools in the field of pharmacopsychology. To study the psychotropic effect of Tegretol, we felt obliged – since this called for long-term investigations – to employ our own standard routine methods, i.e. the same ones as we use for our initial examinations of patients, as well as for all subsequent clinicopsychological check-ups routinely performed once a year.

The epileptic child, considered not only as a paediatric problem but also as a person trying to cope with the mental and emotional situation in which he finds himself, is dependent on a host of ponderable and imponderable factors.

Psychic manifestations of the type frequently met with in this connection are most certainly not conditioned solely by the extent and localisation of organic changes in the brain. The child's original level of intelligence, the amount of care devoted to him by members of the family, and the quality of the remedial training he receives also play their role in addition to such supplementary psychic effects as anticonvulsive drugs may exert. There can be no doubt that the physical and emotional difficulties he encounters during puberty likewise have a decisive influence on the epileptic child's psyche.

Let us now see what light we can shed on the question as to the effect exerted by Tegretol on the psyche of epileptic children. Here, I should perhaps begin by explaining that what, in very broad terms, we understand by a positive psychotropic effect is one characterised by brightening of the sensorium, improved attentiveness and speech, an increase in intellectual performance and powers of concentration, and greater perseverance at work. We have often observed an effect of this kind in cases where a child has been switched fairly rapidly from conventional anticonvulsants to Tegretol. When, on the other hand, a child is given Tegretol as its first and only anticonvulsive therapy, such an effect is either not seen at all or is so minimal that it might equally well be attributable simply to the enhancement of mood that a very good response to the drug's anticonvulsive action might be expected to elicit.

A "psychotropic" effect achieved by switching children from other anticonvulsants to Tegretol is, as I have already mentioned, frequently encountered, and members of the family sometimes wax lyrical in their descriptions of it. In many cases of this kind, we too had the impression that the child's personality had changed for the better, an impression also substantiated by an improvement in such psychomotor tests as the Walther test, threading beads on a string, and climbing stairs; but this response tended to be of rather brief duration, i.e. within about 4–6 weeks the effect had levelled out again.

At this point it should perhaps be added that, in certain cases (amounting to some 2–5% of the children receiving Tegretol as their first drug), Tegretol not only failed to produce any so-called positive psychotropic effect but also gave rise to sedation which, though persisting for no more than a few days, often proved very severe while it lasted.

On the basis of observations such as I have just outlined, it was not possible for us to reach any firm conclusions concerning the psychotropic effect of Tegretol. We therefore decided to undertake a long-term pharmacopsychological investigation, particularly since, as I have explained previously, the test procedures to be employed for this purpose already formed part of the routine clinicopsychological check-ups carried out by us in every case of epilepsy.

Patients studied

The patients investigated, consisting of children and adolescents chosen from among our grand mal cases, were divided into the following three groups:

Group A: ten patients (four girls and six boys aged 13–16 years) who had previously been treated for grand mal with various anticonvulsants, e.g. primidone, mephenytoin, methylphenobarbitone, phenobarbitone, sultiame, ®Apydan (a combined preparation containing phenytoin, phenobarbitone, sodium and ammonium bromide, and caffeine), phenytoin, barbexaclone, etc.

The first psychological examination was performed while these patients were still receiving their previous treatment. After the tests had been completed, they were then transferred over a period of one to three weeks to monotherapy with Tegretol. The second psychological examination was undertaken after the patients had been on Tegretol for not less than 11 months and not longer than 12 months.

Group B: ten patients (four girls and six boys aged 12–16 years) who had been referred to our clinic as suffering from grand mal and who either had never been treated with anticonvulsants at all or had been receiving no anticonvulsive medication for at least six months.

All these ten patients were placed on treatment with Tegretol alone. Since one of them subsequently dropped out, we were able to assess only nine cases in Group B.

Group C: of the ten patients in this group (four girls and six boys aged 13–16 years) three were given primidone alone, two mephenytoin alone, two primidone plus Apydan, one primidone plus phenytoin, one primidone plus a paediatric form of phenytoin, and one primidone plus ®Dintospina (a combination of phenytoin, phenyl-N-methylbarbituric acid, and β-phenylisopropyl-amine).

For the psychological examinations performed, the following tests were employed:

1. Verbal I.Q.
2. Practical I.Q. } Hamburg-Wechsler Intelligence Scale for Children
3. Overall I.Q.
4. Motor function (Walther test)
5. Affectivity
6. Activity
7. Psychic manifestations } Rorschach test
   a) P% (perseveration)
   b) A% (animal responses)

Findings obtained

The findings obtained in each of the three groups are presented in Tables 1–3. From the values recorded in Group A it is apparent that, despite the long interval of 11–12 months elapsing between the first and the second examination, no decisive changes were observed in any of the tests; such tendencies towards a change as we did detect were not statistically significant. In Group B there was a significant improvement in the results of the Walther test, which we regard as being probably the most suitable test of psychomotor function; but this improvement was the only evidence we could find of a possible psycho-tropic effect in response to Tegretol. From Table 3 it can be seen that no

Table 1. Results of psychological examinations performed in Group A (four girls and six boys, all with grand mal seizures) during treatment with various anticonvulsants other than Tegretol (first examination) and during monotherapy with Tegretol (second examination).

	Intelligence			Motor function (Walther test)	Affectivity	Activity	Psychic manifestations	
	V.I.Q.	P.I.Q.	O.I.Q.				P%	A%
First examination	101	100	99	217.40	2.90	10.75	42.50	72.15
Second examination	108	99	104	208.10	1.60	11.45	47.10	70.65
Significance	n.s.	n.s.	n.s.	n.s.	n.s. (trend)	n.s. (trend)	n.s.	n.s.

V.I.Q. = verbal I.Q.; P.I.Q. = practical I.Q.; O.I.Q. = overall I.Q.; P% = perseveration; A% = animal responses; n.s. = not significant; (trend) = trend towards an improvement

Table 2. Results of psychological examinations performed in Group B (four girls and six boys, all with grand mal seizures) prior to (first examination) and during (second examination) monotherapy with Tegretol.

	Intelligence			Motor function (Walther test)	Affectivity	Activity	Psychic manifestations	
	V.I.Q.	P.I.Q.	O.I.Q.				P%	A%
First examination	90.20	79.20	77.95	235.70	2.80	12.45	54.95	69.15
Second examination	85.15	79.75	77.55	209.35	1.60	11.45	47.10	76.65
Significance	n.s.	n.s.	n.s.	P < 0.005	n.s. (trend)	n.s.	n.s. (trend)	n.s. (trend)

Table 3. Results of psychological examinations performed in Group C (four girls and six boys, all with grand mal seizures) prior to (first examination) and during (second examination) treatment with various anticonvulsants other than Tegretol.

	Intelligence			Motor function (Walther test)	Affectivity	Activity	Psychic manifestations	
	V.I.Q.	P.I.Q.	O.I.Q.				P%	A%
First examination	89	103	95	216.60	1.80	13.15	52.25	65.15
Second examination	101	99	100	228.35	2.60	13.00	62.10	69.20
Significance	n.s. (trend)	n.s.	n.s. (trend)	n.s. (trend)	n.s. (trend)	n.s.	n.s. (trend)	n.s.

statistically significant changes were demonstrable in Group C, although the trend towards an improvement in quite a number of the tests is worth noting.

Assessment of findings

Except in the case of motor function (Walther test) in the group of patients treated for the first time with Tegretol alone, our long-term psychological examinations failed to reveal any statistically significant changes in the parameters studied. Various objections can, of course, be raised against the methodology we adopted. The period of 11–12 months separating the two examinations, our choice of tests, and also our method of selecting the patients can be criticised – and I must admit that we ourselves view them with a critical eye. But, until such time as better methods become available, we believe we are justified in attaching some significance to the findings we have thus obtained.

Needless to say, however, we regard these findings merely as affording certain tentative clues, which may be worth considering when planning further investigations. The report I have presented therefore simply provides an empirical review of one aspect of our work on what is undoubtedly an interesting drug. Tegretol is known to exert several different effects on the central nervous system. From the indications that have thus far emerged for this drug, moreover, it is evident that its mechanisms of action are extremely complex; and about the interplay between these mechanisms we know just as little as we do about the "pharmaco-genetic" principles underlying them.

Our results do, it is true, conflict to some extent with the experiences reported by other authors. But the very fact that there are also authors whose empirical findings lend support to our conclusions does at least point to the existence of various unresolved questions which require further study.

Summary

In the light of 15 years' experience with Tegretol in the treatment of epileptic children and adolescents, it is clear that this preparation occupies a position of special importance within the gamut of anticonvulsive drugs currently available. That it exerts an effect on the mechanism involved in the production of seizures is beyond dispute. From results obtained in some 900 patients treated with Tegretol, either alone or in combination with other anticonvulsants, the following conclusions can be drawn:

1. The response rates recorded indicate that Tegretol exhibits gynaecotropism, insofar as girls are more likely to react well to the drug than boys.
2. When the response rates are analysed by reference to the patients' ages at the start of treatment, it can be seen that older children and adolescents derive benefit from the drug more frequently than younger children, and that infants and small children have only a poor chance of responding favourably.

3. We were unable to obtain evidence that in children Tegretol has a direct, primary action on the psyche. Whatever may be meant by the term "psychotropic effect", the fact remains that, with the exception of the psychomotor test, the various tests which we employed in our long-term examinations failed to furnish proof of such an effect in response to Tegretol.

Bearing in mind, however, what a multitude of imponderables is involved in the treatment of children and adolescents subject to convulsions of cerebral origin – imponderables relating not only to the patient, to members of his family, and to his environment, but also to the treating physician and to the drug itself – it must be realised that the observations reported in the present paper should be treated with the same reserve as any comparison between results obtained in different groups of patients invariably calls for.

Discussion

W. Grüter: On the basis of my own experience with ®Tegretol (carbamazepine), Dr. Rett, I should like to take the liberty of propounding a standpoint which conflicts with your interpretation of the drug's psychotropic activity. It must of course be acknowledged that an effect may result purely and simply from the withdrawal of other drugs exerting a sedative action. As long ago as 1966, however, we had already obtained sufficient evidence, both in adults and in children, for us to feel justified in postulating that Tegretol possesses intrinsic psychotropic properties. In the report in which we then published our findings*, we distinguished between two categories of cases: firstly, patients who had previously been receiving no treatment, but who nevertheless showed a marked psychic improvement in response to Tegretol; and, secondly, patients in whom Tegretol exerted no anticonvulsive action but in whom a marked psychotropic effect was registered. Cases to which both these criteria applied were regarded as affording particularly conclusive proof of the drug's psychotropic activity, since they lend strong support to the view that this psychotropic activity is unlikely to be merely a secondary effect resulting from the anticonvulsive action of Tegretol.

Let me now briefly outline my experience with Tegretol by reference to a few figures. The cases treated (Table 1) consisted of 295 patients ranging in age from four to 72 years. One remarkable aspect of the responses recorded is, first of all, the fact that in not a single case did we ever observe an increase in the frequency of attacks, although a large majority of the patients had been receiving other drugs before we transferred them to monotherapy with Tegretol. Secondly, the relatively good response rate in petit mal – which also came as quite a surprise to me at the time – strikes me as being worthy of attention. I suspect that Tegretol is not tried often enough in

Table 1. Results obtained with Tegretol in 295 epileptic patients aged 4–72 years.

Type of attack	N	Reduction in frequency of attacks			
		Complete	> 50%	< 50%	Frequency not reduced, or even increased
Grand mal	158	93 (59%)	50 (31%)	15 (10%)	–
Psychomotor seizures	44	22 (50%)	14 (32%)	8 (18%)	–
Grand mal + psycho-motor seizures	19	12 (63%)	4 (21%)	3 (16%)	–
Grand mal + petit mal	22	4 (18%)	15 (68%)	3 (14%)	–
Petit mal	38	15 (39%)	8 (22%)	15 (39%)	–
Other seizures (cerebro-organic, focal)	14	7 (50%)	7 (50%)	–	–
Total	295	153 (52%)	98 (33%)	44 (15%)	0 (0%)
		(85%)			

* Knauel, H., Grüter, W.: Über psychotrope Wirkungen des Tegretal. Zbl. ges. Neurol. Psychiat. *188*, 18 (1967); abstract of paper

Table 2. Psychotropic and anticonvulsive effect of Tegretol in 160 epileptic patients with psychic disorders.

Type of effect	N	
Both psychotropic and anticonvulsive	86	(54%)
Psychotropic only	13	(8%)
Anticonvulsive only	48	(30%)
Neither psychotropic nor anticonvulsive	13	(8%)
Psychotropic, total	99	(62%)
Anticonvulsive, total	134	(84%)
Psychotropic and/or anticonvulsive, total	147	(92%)
Ineffective	13	(8%)

this form of epilepsy, for the simple reason that from the very beginning petit mal has not featured in the literature as an indication for Tegretol. It seems to me, however, that in refractory cases of petit mal Tegretol is well worth a trial. Thirdly, a failure rate of only about 10% in grand mal suggests to me that Tegretol – purely on the strength of its anticonvulsive activity, and regardless of its psychotropic effect – deserves to rank as one of the very foremost of the so-called basic anti-epileptic drugs. In contrast to what Dr. GROH said in the discussion following the papers by Dr. JANZ and Dr. DREYER, I have not found that Tegretol is liable to aggravate petit mal when employed to treat patients suffering from grand mal plus petit mal. I should perhaps also add that Tegretol proved ineffective in two cases of epileptic psychosis, and that, of ten patients subject to twilight attacks, only six derived benefit from the drug and one actually deteriorated.

Of the total of 295 patients, 160 showed clear evidence of psychic changes. In 54% of these 160 cases, Tegretol produced an anticonvulsive as well as a psychotropic effect; in 8% it exerted only a psychotropic effect, and in 30% only an anticonvulsive effect (Table 2). In other words, it elicited either one or both of these effects in 92% of cases, and failed to achieve any response in only 8%.

Now for a few final words about the nature of the drug's psychotropic activity. Among the 295 patients, there were 43 (approximately 27%) who had received no pretreatment and of whom 29, i.e. 67% or two-thirds, showed a marked psychic improvement. Of the 160 epileptics with psychic changes, 57 were children aged four years or older. Tegretol produced a clear-cut psychic improvement in 40 of them; although 17 of the 57 children had had no pretreatment, 13 of these 17 also responded with a marked psychic improvement.

I regard it as proven beyond doubt that Tegretol has an intrinsic psychotropic effect which is either largely or completely independent of its anticonvulsive activity. The drug's psychotropic effect, moreover, may manifest itself even without any accompanying decrease in the epileptic seizures, although this is admittedly less often observed than an anticonvulsive action associated with no evidence of a psychotropic effect.

D. JANZ: You mentioned in your paper, Dr. RETT, that in your experience girls respond better to carbamazepine than boys. In this connection, I should be interested to know what the average daily doses used in the girls amounted to in mg./kg. body weight as compared with those prescribed for the boys. We have noted that there is a tendency to employ relatively higher dosages of anti-epileptic drugs in women than in men, and I therefore wondered whether this was also the case in your patients.

P. L. MORSELLI: You also said, Dr. RETT, that carbamazepine seemed to elicit a better response in older children. With regard to the age dependence of the therapeutic effect, one factor to be considered is that very important differences in pharmaco-kinetics occur between the ages of three and 17 years. We know today that the elimination rate of some drugs – such as diphenylhydantoin, the benzodiazepines, and phenobarbitone – in children aged between three and six years is about twice or three times faster than in older children. Perhaps this might help to explain the difference in the therapeutic response that you observed with carbamazepine.

H. REMSCHMIDT: In the first question I have for Dr. RETT, I should like to revert to the psychotropic activity of carbamazepine. There is quite a lot of evidence indicating that in adults this drug does indeed produce a psychotropic effect. Since you have come to the conclusion that no such effect is discernible in children, may I point out that in all probability the initial psychopathological status of the patient plays a major role in this connection, and may I therefore also ask whether your decision to resort to carbamazepine was dictated in certain cases by the nature of the patient's psychic manifestations?

Another point I'd like to raise concerns the series of tests you employed, Dr. RETT. From experience – acquired once again in adults – we know that carbamazepine exerts an effect on psychomotor function, drive, and mood, as well as on certain cognitive functions which depend, for example, on the patient's powers of attention and concentration. But intelligence tests such as you used cannot, of course, provide any indication as to whether or not a drug has had an influence on these functions. Curiously enough, and this is something that I find extremely interesting, the test of motor function which you employed did reveal a significant difference in favour of carbamazepine in one of the groups. In my experience, it is differentiated procedures designed for the assessment of psychomotor function that do in fact serve as the best indicators of psychotropic activity. Provided the results yielded by tests of psychomotor function are analysed with sufficient thoroughness, they may even furnish objective evidence of effects exerted on the patient's mood. All in all – as you yourself, Dr. RETT, have already implied in your paper – it would seem that certain difficulties are involved in the use of your battery of tests for the purpose of detecting such psychotropic effects as carbamazepine may produce.

R. KUHN: The boys and girls studied by Dr. RETT showed such a striking difference in their response to carbamazepine that I certainly think this difference warrants serious consideration. We, too, have made observations pointing in the same direction. When recording the case histories of patients treated on an ambulant basis, we make it a practice to mark the record sheets grey for males and yellow for females. In the course of preparing our papers for the present symposium, my wife and I went through these records in order to note down the numbers of successes and failures we had had with carbamazepine in non-epileptic children suffering from behavioural disorders; after we had excluded all the patients whom we had been unable to follow up properly, we were left with 50 case records, almost every one of which bore the yellow marking. In other words, of the children with behavioural disorders whom we had been successfully treating with carbamazepine over a period of years, the vast majority were girls. This is even more surprising when one bears in mind that there are always about a third more boys than girls among the patients seen in child psychiatry. One possible explanation for this finding of ours might be that girls take their drugs more regularly than boys, although Dr. RETT has discounted this possibility in his cases.

One further point: Dr. REMSCHMIDT has just drawn attention to the difficulties and shortcomings which some test procedures entail. Quite apart from the fact that the tests sometimes employed in this connection are inappropriate, I should like to add a general warning that tests can obviously only shed light on the patient's behaviour while the test is actually in progress. One of the snags with juvenile behavioural disorders, for example, is that they tend to manifest themselves, not so much during the situation of a test, but rather within the family circle and in the child's everyday life.

Consequently, clinical differences in the child's behaviour before and after treatment can hardly ever be revealed by tests, the sole exception being – and here I would absolutely agree with Dr. REMSCHMIDT – tests of psychomotor function. Dr. RETT's studies, too, showed that the psychomotor test was the only one to disclose a significant difference.

A. RETT: To begin with, I must emphasise once again that I am of course fully aware that the findings I have reported apply only to the patients we ourselves actually studied, that these findings lend themselves only to evaluation from the paediatric standpoint, and that I certainly would not wish to generalise from them. I also realise that the patients treated in my clinic constitute a special selection of cases, the peculiarities of which likewise have to be taken into account. Another point I wish to stress, Dr. GRÜTER, is that for us, too, Tegretol is a basic drug – so basic, in fact, that in children with grand mal, as well as in those with focal and psychomotor attacks, we make it a rule to start treatment with Tegretol and we employ no other drugs as initial therapy. Only if Tegretol fails to elicit the desired response do we switch to other preparations. I must admit, however, that the percentage of failures, or of cases in which a deterioration even occurs under treatment with Tegretol, is somewhat higher than you have reported among your patients. This, of course, may be due to differences between your cases and ours.

But what of the psychotropic effect of Tegretol? I think, Dr. GRÜTER, that the two of us ought to get together and discuss this, particularly since I as a paediatrician may perhaps see this whole question somewhat differently from you. I also believe that the drug's so-called psychotropic effect should only be assessed on a long-term basis and that what one observes initially may possibly not always be "genuine". Be that as it may, I don't really think there is any fundamental contradiction between your findings and our own.

In reply to the question raised by Dr. JANZ, I should explain that we try where possible to employ the same doses in boys as in girls, the average daily dosage ranging from 10 to 15 mg./kg. But I am sure that a review of the patients treated by us would show that the girls do indeed tend to receive higher doses than the boys. This brings me to Dr. KUHN's comment: given the fact that, at least in my experience, children are enormously dependent on their elders, I don't believe that whether or not they take their Tegretol regularly depends on their sex; I think it depends solely on the intelligence and conscientiousness of the mother.

In answer to Dr. REMSCHMIDT, may I point out that, if you examine the tables I presented in my paper, you will find that practically all the patients had psychopathological symptoms; in other words, in this respect their initial status was a "negative" one. With regard to the test procedures we used, I would emphasise that, precisely because we have spent many years carrying out trials with various anticonvulsants and psychopharmaceuticals, we realised perfectly well that it is psychomotor tests which are of by far the greatest use and that even on a short-term basis they can provide very clear information. In our studies on the effect of Tegretol – in which the Walther test of motor function proved a particularly good one – we carried out daily tests over a period of one to two weeks and were astonished at the wide fluctuations in performance we encountered. Incidentally, in some cases, including ones in which a good anticonvulsive effect was observed, a very marked slowing down of motor function occurred initially, i.e. during the first few days.

Finally, I should like to thank Dr. KUHN most warmly for reporting his own observations in support of the finding that Tegretol seems to exhibit a tendency to gynaecotropism.

Some reflections on the pathophysiology of behaviour

by W. Birkmayer*

Behaviour can be described as a reaction to endogenous or exogenous stimuli and thus as a motor function in the widest sense of the term. Behaviour implies action. And just as any action issues from a particular state, so the term "behaviour" is ineluctably linked with the notion of a "state of being". This state of being, resulting from an inflow of afferent impulses, constitutes together with behaviour, which is an efferent response, a permanent functional circuit like that of affect and emotion. The afferent nature of the forces underlying a person's state of "*affect*", and the element of movement involved in the response which this elicits in the form of "*emotion*", are clearly indicated by the etymology of the two terms.

Specific states of being trigger off specific behavioural responses. The appetite for food, for example, is a subjective sensation which will act as a stimulant leading to an aggressive quest for food, whereas sexual appetite entails a specific mood which will provoke emotional behaviour aimed at the acquisition of a partner. Once these appetites have been satisfied, the individual's behavioural pattern undergoes an appropriate change and his mood reverts to normal; via a feedback mechanism, this in turn has the effect of restoring him to a neutral state of being.

Normal behaviour is always concerned with the attainment of a functional objective and is never an end in itself. Under pathological conditions – such as a psychomotor seizure, for instance – impulses are discharged from the neurones without any concrete objective being achieved. The behaviour of a normal human being, however, invariably subserves the dual instinctual aim of self-preservation and perpetuation of the species. This implies that behaviour must be integrated into the sphere of the instincts and into the depths of the personality, i.e. that it is intimately bound up with the fluid balance existing between the biogenic amines of the brainstem. It is true, of course, that the ethical concepts and character traits contributing towards a person's behaviour are also conditioned by cortical "imprints" dating from his childhood and adolescence. But, in the light of long experience, I would suggest that one should beware of ascribing too much importance to this aspect of human behaviour. Often, in fact, one has the impression that the inculcation of ethical standards of conduct merely serves to camouflage instinctual behaviour. On the other hand, it must be acknowledged that the imposition of moral and intellectual restraints on man's instinctual behaviour does make it possible within certain limits to keep behavioural disorders under control.

---

* Ludwig-Boltzmann-Institut für Neurochemie, Vienna, Austria.

Let us now consider the sphere of the instincts a little more closely. Every living creature is endowed with adaptational energy which helps it to withstand the pressure of selection and which is potentially determined by its genetic code. This adaptational energy manifests itself in the form of kinetic aggressiveness, which enables both man and animals to acquire the territory they need as an essential prerequisite for self-preservation and perpetuation of the species. Whereas FREUD and LORENZ regard aggressiveness as an innate, stereotyped instinct, there are others, including Anglo-Saxon research workers in particular, who account for it in terms of environmental influences.

In his latest book, the psychoanalyst ERICH FROMM[1] has the following to say: "We must distinguish between *two completely different types of aggressiveness* in man. The first type, which man shares with all animals, is a phylogenetically programmed impulse to attack (or to flee) as soon as his vital interests are threatened. This *defensive*, benign aggressiveness serves to ensure survival of the individual and of the species; it is a biologically adapted aggressiveness which peters out once the threat has disappeared. The second type is a 'malignant' aggressiveness marked by *destructiveness and cruelty;* it is specific to man and is virtually absent in most mammals. It is neither phylogenetically programmed nor biologically adapted; it serves no purpose, except to gratify the lust of those who indulge in it."

Frankly, I do not feel that much is to be gained from drawing this distinction between a benign, biologically expedient, instinctual aggressiveness and a cruel, destructive one. When considering an act of destruction, we are still dealing with the instinctual sphere, i.e. with what FREUD referred to as the "death instinct". That man is the only creature who goes so far as to murder his opponent during an act of aggression, is – I would suggest – ascribable to the fact that, in addition to his instincts, man also possesses the ability to reason logically, to anticipate the future, and thus to realise that only by killing his enemy can he effectively eliminate the danger threatening him. Stripped of its semantic overtones, homicide is an instinctual act performed, in order to remove a given threat once and for all, by an individual into whose behavioural code no feedback mechanism incorporating moral restraint has yet been programmed. There can be no doubt, for instance, that a sex murder represents an extreme form of destructive violence and that it is also an instinctual act which, owing to the lack of any cortical inhibition involving logical patterns of thought, is perpetrated in the absence of a feedback mechanism. It is therefore my opinion that the attempt to differentiate between a benign, animal form of aggressiveness and a malignant, human form serves little purpose.

In my view, aggressiveness is synonymous with the kinetic energy which is programmed into the individual's genetic code and which shapes his behaviour in such a way as to afford him the greatest possible chance of survival. The peculiar form of aggressiveness displayed by man, which also encompasses the killing of his enemies, would appear to be biologically expedient inasmuch as man alone is capable of realising that a successfully repelled enemy may well at some time in the future present a renewed threat to his existence.

A feedback control such as that operating in animals, which refrain from biting a rival to death once the latter has assumed a cringing posture, exists only in rudimentary form in man. The cringing of a punch-drunk boxer in the ring does not dampen the aggressiveness either of his opponent or, in particular, of the spectators; on the contrary, not until the loser has been knocked out does the crowd's vicarious aggressiveness subside.

At his present stage of development, man has not yet fully integrated his cortical capacity for intellectual thought into his instinctual animal behaviour. It will probably require several quantum leaps in man's progressive cerebration before he acquires the moral wherewithal to block his aggressiveness.

Let us turn now to another example taken from the instinctual sphere: in the animal world, strutting and posing indulged in by the male undoubtedly serves the biological aim of self-preservation and perpetuation of the species. The rooster ruffling up its feathers, the lion spreading its mane, or the stag displaying its antlers thus contrive to intimidate, and so avoid having to fight, a rival male. This minimises the risk to their own lives insofar as it prevents any conflict from occurring at all. In other words, the biological purpose of such behaviour is to exploit a particular phenotypic image with a view to circumventing a dangerous duel; during the mating season, moreover, the imposing airs assumed by the male afford it a better chance of securing a partner and so help to maintain the species.

But how does this type of instinctual behaviour reveal itself in man? The hollow-chested youth dons a jacket with shoulders so thickly padded that his appearance places him at once in the realm of caricature. The ageing playboy who, though already overtaken by impotence, boasts incessantly of his sexual conquests forfeits all credibility as a result of his vain attempts to impress others. These are but two typical examples of man's strong tendency to exaggerate instinctual patterns of behaviour. His capacity for rationalisation frequently leads him to exceed the bounds of expedient instinctual behaviour, so that he either becomes a mere caricature or ceases to be taken seriously; the whole purpose of instinctual activity is thus defeated. Although instinctual acts also provide the matrix for human behaviour, they often disintegrate under the influence of intellectual cortical functions, and it is precisely this disintegration that results in so many forms of aberrant behaviour in man.

Now for a collective example illustrating the same type of phenomenon: from the cradle to the grave, the modern socialised State goes so far in relieving the individual of the responsibility for taking his own decisions and measures, and in eliminating sources of fear and anxiety, that modern man is now tending to work off his pent-up aggressiveness either in the form of violence directed against the "Establishment" or sadistic ill-treatment of those working under him or of members of his own family or, alternatively, in the form of auto-aggressiveness with all its attendant neurotic or psychosomatic symptoms; whichever of the two guises it assumes, such gratuitous aggressiveness constitutes an utterly nonsensical use of biological energy.

The biological purpose of human behaviour is to enable man to react appropriately to his situation with the aim of protecting or promoting his existence.

Under ideal circumstances this aim can be achieved thanks to the presence of an intact afferent-efferent system, a readily evocable general arousal reaction, and a biochemical equilibrium between the body's transmitter substances.

Although it is possible, on the basis of clinical observations and descriptions, to distinguish between a wide variety of characteristic patterns of pathological behaviour, there are still very few behavioural syndromes which – as in the case, for example, of Parkinson's syndrome or the syndrome of depression – can be related to a deficiency of dopamine, noradrenaline, or serotonin. In many other instances, what emerges as clearly recognisable is some distinctive symptom which, depending on the type of illness in question, stands out as a prominent feature of the resultant behavioural disorder, e.g. the sluggish thought processes and narrowed consciousness of the patient with a cerebral tumour, the poverty of thought and emotion displayed by the schizophrenic, the "stickiness" of the epileptic, the submissive demeanour of the depressive, and the destructive violence of the brain-damaged child. Besides these behavioural disorders involving a causative noxa, there is also the large group comprising psychopathic personality disorders, in which the patient's pathological behaviour is due to faulty programming of his genetic code. The psychopath has an abnormal personality, the abnormalness of which entails suffering both for society and for himself. KURT SCHNEIDER[2] claimed that attempts to classify psychopathic disorders into various types fail to disclose any characteristic differences between these disorders, which very frequently overlap into one another. It is my impression, however, that psychopathic modes of behaviour occur in the form both of plus variants, characterised by excessive activity, and of minus variants in which activity is subnormal. The hyperthymic psychopath who is always on the go, the fanatical psychopath in a state of sustained emotional tension, the self-assertive psychopath full of his own importance, or the explosive psychopath all display one set of features in common, namely, unrestrained activity, aggressiveness, and enhanced drive; and I find it tempting to speculate that these may reflect the uncontrolled release of catecholaminergic transmitters. Psychopaths of the depressive type, on the other hand, including those lacking self-assurance and will-power, as well as irresolute and asthenic psychopaths, would appear to fall into the category of minus variants, characterised by a deficiency of catecholaminergic transmitters in their biochemical code. Purely speculative though this twofold classification may now be, it might eventually prove possible to substantiate it chemically, thereby providing us with a type of target symptom that is amenable to biochemical correction. Meanwhile, the only compensatory means at present available for neutralising plus variants consists in the use of minor and major tranquillisers, and the only method of raising minus variants to a normal level is that based on treatment with the amine precursor L-dopa.

In adults these pathological modes of behaviour are usually refractory to therapy, whereas similar behavioural abnormalities in children and adolescents mostly take the form of transient syndromes. The behavioural aberrations of modern youth have been ascribed to a multitude of factors, the relative importance of which is variously assessed, depending on the *Weltanschauung*, the political persuasions, or even the professional background of the assessor.

As a general rule, it may be said that, when the adaptational capacity imprinted in an individual's genetic code becomes overtaxed, that individual's behaviour will exhibit signs of decompensation. The extent to which his system can cope with biological overtaxation is, of course, also subject to variation. It is obvious, for example, that the changes taking place inside a child during puberty are associated with a decrease in its capacity to adjust itself to conditions outside; and it is precisely for this reason that abnormal modes of behaviour occur more frequently in the puberal stage of development. The abundant supply of information reaching the teenager exerts an accelerating action which almost invariably gives rise to asynchronous development, and the resultant temporal disharmony between his physical, mental, and emotional maturation has the effect of reducing his ability to adapt himself to the demands his environment makes upon him.

In this connection, a special problem is posed by children suffering from organic brain damage, who, owing to their diminished adaptational capacity, find it even harder to cope with the exigencies of life. Further problems arise from a host of other factors. For example, the young child whose mother goes out to work spends much of its time in an affective vacuum, as a result of which it has difficulty in establishing its identity *vis-à-vis* its environment. Where the child is living in a broken home, an even heavier strain is imposed on its adaptational capacity, a strain which is almost bound to lead to behavioural disturbances. In the absence particularly of a paternal image to serve as a guide, the child is deprived of one of the main biological supports which it requires during its development, and this deprival is likewise conducive to behavioural decompensation. Despite such pathogenetic social factors, however, abnormal modes of behaviour in children and adolescents, provided they are not attributable to organic brain damage, usually prove of a transient nature; in other words, by the time the person in question has reached maturity – and I would say that nowadays this does not occur until the age of 25 years – his behaviour will in many cases have reverted to normal.

Since, in my experience, the pathological behavioural patterns that are now so frequently encountered in our society cannot be corrected either by psychotherapy or by social measures, they confront the pharmaceutical industry with a massive challenge to discover and develop drugs capable of rectifying the biochemical balance and thus of restoring normally adapted behaviour.

References

1 Fromm, E.: Anatomie der menschlichen Destruktivität, p. 3 (Deutsche Verlagsanstalt, Stuttgart 1974)
2 Schneider, K.: Klinische Psychopathologie, 9th Ed. (Thieme, Stuttgart 1971)

Discussion

J. Obiols Vié: I should like at this point to say how very happy I am to have been invited to this symposium, particularly since the participants include both psychiatrists and neurologists. Although psychiatry and neurology stem, as it were, from the same trunk, efforts have long been made to separate them; and in some instances these efforts have been successful. Now, however, we are conscious of the need to bring them together again – the main reason for this being that psychiatry is becoming increasingly biologically oriented and therefore increasingly aware of the necessity for re-establishing contact with neurology. Whereas today doctrines such as those of Freud are being challenged, or even to some extent relegated to the background, those of other historical figures – like Griesinger, for example – are acquiring renewed importance and gaining some measure of recognition within the framework of our concepts of pathology. One of the best illustrations of what I mean is provided by the domain of "behavioural disturbances" and "psychopathic personality disorders". Terminologically speaking, these are extremely vague diagnoses applicable to any number of syndromes and raising questions the very imprecision of which is hardly calculated to enhance the prestige of psychiatry. Such developments as the antipsychiatric movement, which have given rise to some concern in certain quarters, would never have occurred had it not been for the lack of precision, clarity, and objectivity that too often characterises our diagnoses.

Since the two terms to which I have been referring are applied to so many different syndromes and disorders, I suggest we have to ask ourselves whether the underlying pathological problem is in fact essentially a psychiatric one, or whether sociological and sociopsychological aspects, etc. are not also involved. There obviously does exist such a thing as behavioural disorders, and in this symposium at which there has been so much discussion of epilepsy I think we also have to decide what we mean by behavioural disorders. One answer I would propose is: all disorders of behaviour – including those occurring in adolescents in particular – that are associated with pathological E.E.G. findings. Here, we have what I believe to be a genuine, objectively verifiable, manifestation. But it would be most desirable if it could also be objectified from the phenomenological and clinical standpoints, and this we have not yet completely succeeded in doing.

With regard to what Dr. Birkmayer has termed the "pathophysiology of behaviour", I feel that this embraces a far wider field, and that it poses problems with which psychiatry has already been confronted in the past but which, on the pathological plane, exceed the scope of psychiatry. So long as the psychiatrist confines himself to studying the pathology of the human organism, his objectives remain clear and precise. But, as soon as he turns to the concept of humanity in general and to the troubles besetting it, he is faced with another aspect, which should preferably be studied by adopting different approaches, i.e. those of the social sciences. I think psychiatry should now aim at deliberately refraining from concerning itself with any problem the nature of which is not absolutely pathological within the strictest meaning of the term. I advocate this so that psychiatry may avoid the risk of providing its enemies with ammunition and that it may more effectively put paid to those movements which are seeking to malign our profession. This task can only be achieved if we make it a practice to study in very concrete fashion the syndromes with which we are dealing and to record our findings objectively.

A. Rett: I trust that Dr. Birkmayer, under whom it has been my privilege to study, will pardon me for taking the liberty of repeating the last paragraph of his paper: "Since, in my experience, the pathological behavioural patterns that are now so frequently encountered in our society cannot be corrected either by psychotherapy or by social measures, they confront the pharmaceutical industry with a massive challenge to discover and develop drugs capable of rectifying the biochemical balance and thus of restoring normally adapted behaviour." Allow me to quote in this connection the example of the child who, having spent hours in front of the television set, complains of headache and cannot get to sleep, and who is then given a sleeping tablet. This is a classic error committed by almost all parents, who fondly imagine that a tablet will achieve what they themselves have failed to attain in their upbringing of the child. I fear one must therefore conclude that, at least where children are concerned, neither psychotherapy – in the broadest sense of the term – nor social or educational measures nor recourse to drugs can alone necessarily provide a solution to the problem. There are many cases in which some form of drug therapy is absolutely essential, but there are also many other cases in which appropriate social or educational measures are quite sufficient in themselves to correct the disturbance in psychosomatic regulatory processes which is responsible for the patient's behavioural disequilibrium.

But, to revert to the example I have quoted, the obvious "social" measure would simply be to switch off the television, and the correct "psychotherapeutic" measure would be to convince the child that sitting too long in front of the television set isn't good for him. A drug should only be used if and when all else has failed; once the decision to resort to medication has been taken, however, the treatment should be carried out purposefully and conscientiously. But to expect a psycho-active agent, alone and unaided, to perform miracles in a child strikes one as being a dangerously facile attitude.

M. PARSONAGE: I have one brief remark to make on Dr. BIRKMAYER's most enjoyable paper. It never ceases to amaze me that, when the psychodynamics of human behaviour are discussed, we always hear about FREUD and that no mention is ever made of the work of CARL GUSTAV JUNG who, in my view, has contributed immensely to our understanding of human behaviour. As this symposium is being held in JUNG's own country, it is all the more fitting that we should remember his work.

P. KIELHOLZ: I should like to offer just a short, but admittedly somewhat critical, comment on your paper, Dr. BIRKMAYER. I personally would avoid referring to plus and minus variants in connection with human behaviour, because this distinction implies a judgment of value, which I don't think we are entitled to make. In a person displaying obsessive-compulsive behaviour, for example, this behaviour may be considered by his employers as quite a positive attribute, whereas the family who has to live with him will in all probability regard it as a minus variant.

W. BIRKMAYER: May I begin by hastening to assure Dr. KIELHOLZ that, when speaking of plus and minus variants, I certainly had no intention of making a judgment of value. I simply borrowed these two terms from the field of neurology, in which, for example, muscle spasm – i.e. a spastic increase in muscle tone – is referred to as a plus variant and areflexia as a minus variant. This type of differentiation is one that I think can quite well also be applied to psychic phenomena. There are some individuals who have too much drive and whose behaviour can therefore be said to constitute a plus variant, and on the other hand there are some individuals who show no initiative and no energy and whose behaviour thus represents a minus variant. But I'd be happy if a psychiatrist could suggest two better terms for me to use.

With regard to Dr. PARSONAGE's comment, I should like to assure him, too, that I share his view that JUNG, with his concept of archetypes, shed more light on the personality structure of man than did FREUD.

Dr. RETT has objected to the last paragraph of my paper – in which I stated that in my experience the pathological behavioural patterns increasingly met with in our society cannot be corrected by psychotherapy or by sociotherapy – on the grounds that what is needed, and what indeed holds out promising prospects, is not more drug treatment, but comprehensive psychological guidance and above all appropriate educational measures. This, of course, is perfectly obvious to me as well. When I referred to "psychotherapy" in this context, I was thinking chiefly of psychoanalysis.

And with psychoanalysis you cannot cure an endogenous depression, nor can you cure an aggressive psychopath or a homosexual – who doesn't even want to be "cured" anyway! As for your example of the child glued to the television set, Dr. RETT, this is clearly not a case of faulty behaviour in the child but, if anything, in the mother. She wants her peace and quiet, and this is why the child is allowed to watch television. Here, then, drug treatment would of course be the wrong solution.

Psychic behavioural disorders have existed throughout the history of man's development. In the Middle Ages, women suffering from such disorders were burnt as witches – at least in Europe. At a later period, persons of this type tended to espouse some political cause or other in an effort to relieve their inner tensions. Nowadays, however, neither religious nor political movements seem to be acting as such a strong pole; hence the large number of behaviourally disturbed individuals now encountered in our society. I am accordingly convinced that FREUD – whom I should perhaps apologise for quoting here – was right when, during the last years of his life, he said something to the effect that "though anxiety should for the moment still be treated by psychoanalysis, the time will come when we shall have drugs to cope with behavioural disturbances". I am, in short, a firm believer in biochemistry.

Drug-induced behavioural disorders in man

by H. Heimann *

Human behaviour is governed by the interplay of many different factors. Psycho-active drugs influence metabolism in certain structures of the brain, but the direct effect they exert on these structures represents only *one* of the factors responsible for changes in behaviour. This factor may be of decisive importance – i.e. when the drug in question has a very strong action, as is the case, for example, with a narcotic – but it may also be qualified by other factors if the drug has a more differentiated and milder action. Under these latter circumstances, the initial status of the psychophysiological systems involved plays just as important a role in the modification of behaviour as does the chemical active substance itself. If a person is given an amphetamine, for instance, when he is in a rested and relaxed state, the effect of the drug can hardly be demonstrated at all by psychological tests, but if he is tired as a result of having spent a sleepless night, or if he is a narcoleptic, the effect of the drug will be readily detectable in these tests.

In recent years psychologists engaged in investigating the effect of psycho-active agents in normal subjects have tended to place the main emphasis on one factor in particular, namely, on the *type of personality*. They have endeavoured by means of questionnaires to assess a person's degree of extraversion or introversion and to examine the influence which these two personality types may have on the effect exerted by sedative and stimulant drugs. According to the English school[1,2], sedative drugs cause introverted subjects to become more extraverted, while stimulants cause extraverted subjects to become more introverted.

A second dimension of the personality that has been determined with the aid of questionnaires is the degree of neuroticism. Attempts have been made, with varying success, to demonstrate that the minor tranquillisers produce differential effects depending on a person's neuroticism score: in response to these drugs subjects with a high neuroticism score, i.e. so-called labile persons, show an improvement both in their performance as assessed in psychological tests, as well as in their state of mind; in subjects with a low neuroticism score, i.e. in those with a stable personality, the same drugs cause a deterioration in performance and in state of mind[6].

However, from a review of the literature and from our own investigations it is clear that this approach to personality research in normal subjects leads to contradictory results. The *personality factor* as determined in studies of psycho-active drugs conducted in normal test-subjects is therefore not of cardinal im-

---

* Universitäts-Nervenklinik, Tübingen, German Federal Republic.

217

portance for the investigation of drug-induced behavioural changes in man. Superimposed on this personality factor are, as I shall try to show, *situational circumstances* which have a more immediate bearing on measurable changes in behaviour occurring in response to psycho-active drugs.

A third factor influencing the effect of psychopharmaceuticals in the mentally ill is the *pathological* condition of the patient prior to treatment. The studies reported to date on personality research in connection with psychopharmacology have for the most part been carried out in students, who from the psychophysiological standpoint could still be regarded as normal, even though their scores on the extraversion/introversion and lability/stability scales may have been at the extreme upper or lower limits.

The difference between extreme limits of the normal range and pathological states may be regarded simply as a quantitative one, i.e. as a mere shift in the balance of psychophysiological systems. This interpretation certainly seems plausible in the case of neurotic and psychosomatic behavioural disturbances, and, judging by the results of recent psychophysiological studies, it also holds good for schizophrenia and depression. It helps to explain why the mentally ill can tolerate much higher doses of a psycho-active drug – irrespective of its type – than can normal subjects. This phenomenon was demonstrated as long ago as the late 1940s when STOLL[11] attempted to use L.S.D. in the treatment of schizophrenics. He found that, as compared with normal subjects, these patients were able to tolerate far higher doses without displaying any L.S.D.-induced psychotic manifestations. Similar findings have been obtained with chlorpromazine and clozapine[3, 5]. In normal subjects single doses of tricyclic antidepressants (e.g. 75 mg. imipramine) cause a considerable diminution in alertness and give rise to autonomic nervous disorders which may even include nausea and vomiting. In severely depressed patients, on the other hand, side effects of this nature are not observed; on the contrary, owing to the antidepressant's sedative properties these patients usually experience a feeling of relief within only a few days of the commencement of treatment, and their susceptibility to the autonomic nervous side effects of the drug is extremely low. A similar situation is encountered even in the case of the benzodiazepines: normal subjects react more sensitively to 5 mg. diazepam than do anxious patients to much higher doses.

The factors I have been describing – i.e. type of personality, situational circumstances, and pathological shifts – can be subsumed into a uniform theoretical system by reference to the *arousal theory*.

Figure 1 illustrates schematically the correlation between the organism's general level of arousal and psychological performance (or state of mind). This correlation, which is based on the results of many psychological tests, is not linear, but has the shape of an inverted U. A shift in the level of arousal, as measured by reference to physiological variables such as pulse, respiration, and cutaneous resistance, leads to an improvement in performance or to optimisation of the subject's state of mind in cases where the shift is from a low to a moderate level of arousal. Once this moderate level of arousal (i.e. the optimal level for a given standard of psychological performance) is exceeded, performance deteriorates again. The level of arousal does not necessarily have to be established on the basis of physiological variables. Numerous studies on the correlation between speed of speech and anxiety, for example, suggest that the relationship between, on the one hand, speed of speech as a psychomotor manifestation of anxiety and, on the other, subjectively experienced anxiety as measured by questionnaires likewise assumes the shape of an inverted U. The values for speed of speech are similar at both low and high degrees of anxiety. This explains why correlation studies may yield either a positive or a negative correlation or, alternatively, a correlation that fails to differ significantly from zero[10].

The effect of psycho-active drugs on the general level of arousal, as postulated in accordance with the theory just described, is plotted against dosage in Figure 1. If the test subject is at an optimal level of arousal for a given psychological performance (B), both stimulant and sedative drugs will impair this performance. On the other hand, if his level of arousal is low (A), a stimulant drug administered in an optimal dosage will improve his performance, whereas in an excessive dosage it will again lead to an impairment.

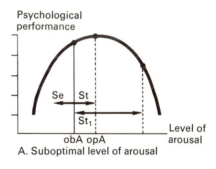

A. Suboptimal level of arousal

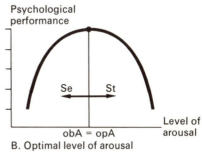

B. Optimal level of arousal

Fig. 1. Relationship between level of arousal and psychological performance, as well as effect exerted by given doses of stimulant and sedative psycho-active drugs on performance. (For details, see text)

opA = optimal level of arousal
obA = observed level of arousal
St   = stimulant drug
Se   = sedative drug
St₁ = stimulant drug given in an overdosage
Se₁ = sedative drug given in an overdosage

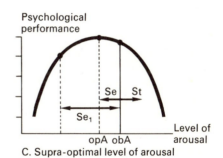

C. Supra-optimal level of arousal

219

In the over-aroused test-subject, the situation is reversed (C). Here, a sedative gives rise to an improvement in performance when administered in the correct dose, and to an impairment when the dose is unduly high. The following general conclusions can thus be drawn:

1. Overdosages are bound to lead to an impairment of performance in cases where the level of arousal is either unduly low or unduly high.
2. The contradictory results obtained in many studies conducted in normal test-subjects are probably attributable to the fact that a random sample invariably consists of subjects whose level of arousal prior to administration of the psycho-active agents differs to a varying extent from the optimum.

If we now attempt to fit extraverted and introverted test-subjects into the pattern provided by the general arousal theory, we find that, when assessed on the basis of their average psychophysiological reactivity, the introverts fall into the high-arousal group and the extraverts into the low-arousal group. Common to all normal test-subjects, however, even to those with extreme types of personality, is their ability to adapt their arousal to whatever level is required in a given set of circumstances, a process which we refer to as *"modulating arousal in accordance with the performance demanded"*. In psychiatric patients the situation is quite different: assessed on the basis of their average psychophysiological reactivity, they too are to be placed at either the upper or lower extremes of the arousal scale; that is to say, patients with anxiety belong to the high-arousal group and those with depression to the low-arousal group. The pathological nature of their reactions, however, is revealed by *their limited ability to modulate arousal*; in other words, these patients are no longer able to modulate their arousal to whatever level is required by the performance demanded of them. Patients suffering from anxiety remain at an unduly high level of arousal and are capable of modulating that arousal to only a very limited extent. Depressive patients remain at a low level of arousal, and their ability to modulate is extremely restricted. In pathological states, therefore, as we have demonstrated in the case of patients suffering from anxiety or depression (HEI-MANN and SCHMOCKER, unpublished findings), the effect of psycho-active agents is chiefly to restore a greater capacity for modulation.

So much for the general arousal theory. Let us now revert to the question of studies conducted with psycho-active drugs in normal subjects. Here, we have to bear in mind that different psychological tests call for different optimal levels of arousal, and that this complicates evaluation of the effects of psycho-active drugs. A simple cognitive test, e.g. watching a radar screen for a long time, requires only a low level of general arousal on the part of the organism, a level that corresponds to a moderate degree of attentiveness directed at a relatively limited perceptual field. In a test of concentration, on the other hand, a higher level of general arousal is needed, and at the same time the subject's attention has to be focused on an extremely limited field; what is called for in this instance is maximally selective attentiveness which shuts the subject off from all interfering stimuli emanating from the rest of his perceptual field. A comparison of the psychophysiological conditions required for these two types of test shows that, as far as the effect of psycho-active agents is concerned, the general arousal theory as outlined in Figure 1 can only apply to very basic areas of behaviour. Due account of the essential conditions governing the performance of a cognitive test, or a test calling for psychomotor concentration, can only be taken by combining the general arousal theory with the concept of attentiveness involving selective perceptual processes.

The complex factors involved in the type of performance demanded by many psychological tests are only influenced in a general way by known psycho-active drugs, with the result that the predictability of measurable changes is limited. The experimental conditions under which such tests are conducted confront the test-subjects with a particular psychophysiological situation. These conditions may be regarded as *external situational factors,* and they can be kept relatively constant in individual tests. In addition, however, consideration has to be given to *internal situational factors,* including especially the test-subjects' *motivation,* which can vary from one day to another even though the external conditions of the test may remain the same. The fact that this motivation cannot be manipulated to the same extent as the external situational factors offers in my opinion an explanation for the varying degree to which performance is impaired in different tests, as we have found in identical subjects given psycho-active drugs under identical conditions.

To illustrate this point, let me refer to an experiment we conducted in 20 subjects in an endeavour to test the sedative effect of a dibenzthiepine derivative in two different dosages. The higher dosage was administered on two different days under the same external conditions, and we found that in the *subjective tests* it yielded on both days results which were consistent and which differed to a statistically significant extent from those obtained with placebo. In the *performance tests,* on the other hand, the results were not consistent. As Figure 2 shows, the *alpha integration values in the electro-encephalogram* followed the same consistent pattern as the findings in the subjective tests, inasmuch as the difference between the effect of placebo and the effect of the higher dosage was statistically significant.

In the light of the general arousal theory, we can assume that the test-subjects' level of arousal was reduced by the sedative. Consequently, the results obtained on the two different days on which the subjects received the sedative could be expected to show positive correlations. To test this hypothesis, we correlated the differences between the base-line values recorded in the morning and the values recorded after ingestion of the drug on the two different days. From Table 1 it can be seen that the results of the psychological and subjective tests failed to display any significant correlations which could be interpreted as evidence in support of the arousal hypothesis.

This means that, although in response to the sedative our test-subjects *as a group* showed a significant decrease in their performance in the various tests and a significant impairment of their state of mind, *it was not the same subjects who reacted in the anticipated manner on both days.* Hence, the individual test-subject will probably display a decrease in performance or an impairment in his state

221

of mind on the days on which he takes the drug, but this prediction will not necessarily hold good for every occasion on which the drug is administered to him.

By contrast, we found that the alpha integration values in the E.E.G. recorded with the eyes open generally showed high correlations (cf. Table 1). In other words, as regards alpha activity, the results obtained in *the group as a whole*

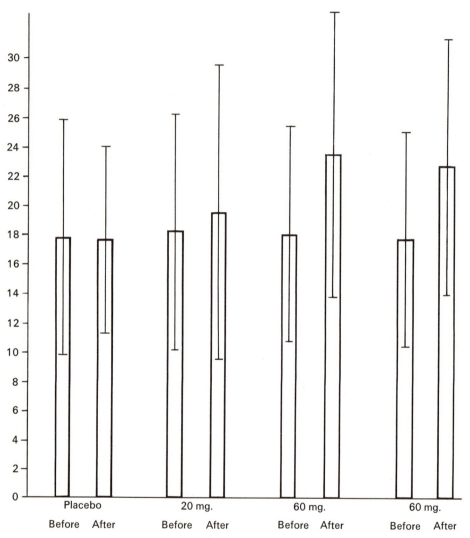

Fig. 2. Mean alpha integration values (± standard deviation) obtained over a period of two minutes in response to placebo and in response to two different dose levels of a sedative (dibenzthiepine). Resting E.E.G. recorded with the subjects' eyes open. Note that alpha activity was significantly and consistently increased following the 60 mg. dose.

60 mg. > placebo   (2α ≤ 0.05)
60 mg. > placebo   (2α ≤ 0.01)
60 mg. > 20 mg.   (2α ≤ 0.01)

(Friedman, as well as Wilcoxon and Wilcox, with difference scores; cf. LIENERT[9])

Table 1. Correlations of difference scores (i.e. result following drug ingestion minus result prior to drug ingestion) obtained with two different doses of a sedative (dibenzthiepine) administered on different days (A, B, and D) in 20 test-subjects. The scores are based on the results of psychological tests and on the alpha integration values recorded in the occipital region over a period of two minutes in E.E.G.s taken with the subjects' eyes open and closed.

	A and D 60 mg. 60 mg.	A and B 60 mg. 20 mg.	D and B 60 mg. 20 mg.
Meili test: time	0.04	0.35	−0.38
Meili test: number of errors	−0.61**	0.75**	−0.58**
Tapping, left arm	−0.03	−0.38	0.03
Tapping, right arm	0.22	−0.45*	−0.12
Minnesota: rate of manipulation	0.29	0.61**	0.38
Lorr Factor 2: "active-energetic"	0.16	−0.27	0.02
Lorr Factor 7: "tired-inert"	−0.07	−0.13	0.03
Polarities list: Subject's estimate of his own worth	−0.12	−0.13	0.26
Polarities list: Familiarity with environment	0.15	−0.11	0.01
Polarities list: Initiative and enterprise	0.16	−0.01	0.23
E.E.G.: Alpha rhythm with eyes open	0.62**	0.64*	0.68**
E.E.G.: Alpha rhythm with eyes closed	0.63**	0.41	0.28

* $2\alpha < 0.05$
** $2\alpha < 0.01$

following treatment with the sedative differed significantly from those recorded following placebo medication; moreover, *those subjects whose alertness was reduced on one of the two days in response to a dose of 60 mg. of the sedative behaved in the same way on the other day when they received 60 mg. and also showed a shift in the anticipated direction even when they received only 20 mg.* Consequently, the alpha integration values in the E.E.G. constitute for this particular sedative and for this particular experimental procedure (E.E.G. recorded with the eyes open) a variable which is not only sensitive but also stable. In this instance, predictability is relatively high even in the case of an individual test-subject.

This example shows that *there is a discrepancy between the effect of psycho-active drugs on physiological parameters – e.g. on alpha rhythm in the E.E.G. – and their effect on variables that can be measured by psychological tests of behaviour.* In a group of subjects the differences recorded in behavioural variables in response to an active drug as compared with placebo are significant only if the random sample is sufficiently large. On the behavioural level, the effect of a psycho-active drug can thus be predicted only on a statistical basis and not by reference to an individual case.

This demonstration of the discrepancy between physiological and psychological variables has, in my opinion, an extremely important bearing not only on the interpretation of results obtained with psycho-active drugs in psychological tests performed in individual patients, but also on the general strategy to be adopted in psychopharmacological research.

223

What conclusions are we to draw, for example, from the results of tests conducted with carbamazepine (®Tegretol) in normal subjects? In our subjective tests carbamazepine produced relaxation and a positive change in state of mind. In this respect, it differed from, for instance, sedatives or minor tranquillisers, the sedative effect of which is as a rule experienced by normal subjects as something unpleasant. At the same time, we even found that, in response to carbamazepine, performance improved to a significant extent in some tests. In the light of these findings one might be tempted to jump to the conclusion that carbamazepine is an ideal minor tranquilliser, since it produces relaxation of a type regarded as positive by the subjects themselves, while also improving psychomotor performance.

In view of the results we had previously obtained with the sedative, however, one objection which could be raised to such a conclusion is that in our tests with carbamazepine we were just particularly fortunate; it could be argued that the values obtained with carbamazepine, as compared with those recorded in response to placebo, showed a shift towards an optimal level of arousal chiefly because the base-line values prior to administration of the drug were such that a positive shift was bound to occur. Since the trial plan did not allow for the use of more than one effective dose level or for a repetition of this dose, we were unable to check the consistency of the beneficial response recorded.

The findings obtained in the psychophysiological study with the sedative were quite in accordance with our assumption that *situational factors, including motivation in particular, on the various days of the test have a greater influence on the effect of a psycho-active agent than does type of personality.* Hence, if we wish to use measurable behavioural variables in order to obtain meaningful results in psychopharmacological studies – results, that is, which will enable us to predict the response to psycho-active agents – we cannot base the selection of our random sample solely on individual values recorded in personality tests, nor can we confine ourselves simply to measuring variables before and after administration of the drug in question. On the contrary, our entire approach to the methodology of such investigations will have to be changed.

The cross-section technique usually adopted hitherto – i.e. the determination of individual values for certain variables at a particular time in a fairly large number of subjects and a single repetition of these measurements after treatment with a drug – does not provide a reliable means of detecting drug-induced changes in behaviour. Only systematic repetition of the measurements in longitudinal studies of as many behavioural and physiological variables as possible in a small number of carefully selected test-subjects will enable us to take account of the internal situational factor of motivation, which cannot be allowed for in cross-sectional studies. In this connection, it must not be forgotten that systematic changes in the external situation, e.g. noise conditions or other situational factors influencing arousal, may reduce the importance of motivation. By adopting such an approach we would be reverting to the method for measuring psychological processes which was impressively described as long ago as 1892 by KRAEPELIN[7] in his monograph entitled "On the influence exerted by several drugs on simple psychological processes". Here, KRAEPELIN drew a comparison between the transience and inconstancy of psychological processes and the movements of a buoy on the surface of the water. Just as the buoy is anchored to the bottom of the sea, so are psychological processes anchored to the subject's "psychophysical constitution", with the result that changes in these processes are subject to certain limitations. Single observations of the position of the buoy, just like single measurements of psychological processes, will therefore fail to reveal any typical, recognisable pattern of change, but repeated observations or measurements must eventually succeed in "providing an accurate picture of the connection between different manifestations".

Summary

Drug-induced behavioural disorders in man are governed not only by the psycho-active properties of the substance in question and by the influence it exerts on metabolism in certain structures of the brain, but also by the following factors: type of personality, situational circumstances, and pathological shifts in the pretreatment status of psychophysiological systems. The arousal theory makes it possible to subsume these various factors into a uniform theoretical system. At the same time, it enables one, firstly, to make predictions about the effect which given doses of stimulant or sedative drugs will exert on the recipient's state of mind and on his performance in psychological tests, and, secondly, to differentiate between the reactivity of normal test-subjects and that of psychiatric patients. Psychiatric patients are unable to modulate their level of arousal in accordance with the performance demanded of them, whereas mentally normal subjects, even if their average psychophysiological reactivity is unduly high or unduly low, are still capable of adapting their arousal to whatever level is required in a given set of circumstances. By itself, however, this theory cannot take adequate account of the conditions governing the performance of psychological tests. These conditions can, in fact, only be properly allowed for by combining the arousal theory with the concept of attentiveness directed at selective perceptual processes. Situational circumstances can be divided into external factors, i.e. factors connected with the psychological tests themselves, and internal factors, i.e. the motivation of the test-subject. The results obtained in a trial in which a sedative was administered to normal test-subjects revealed that, on the behavioural plane, there was a discrepancy between physiological and psychological variables. The effects of psycho-active drugs on behaviour can be quantitatively predicted only on a statistical basis and not by reference to a single drug administration. Their effects on the E.E.G., on the other hand, can be predicted with a relatively high degree of accuracy even for the individual case. This discrepancy between effects on a psychological variable and effects on a physiological variable is due to internal situational factors – i.e. motivation – which exert a greater influence than either type of personality or external situational factors. The

225

influence of motivation must be borne in mind when considering the results obtained in a study on the effect of carbamazepine in normal test-subjects; what is more, it should logically lead to a change in the general strategy adopted in psychopharmacological research.

References

1 EYSENCK, H.J.: Drug and personality: I. Theory and methodology. J. ment. Sci. *103*, 119 (1957)
2 GRAY, J.A.: The psychophysiological nature of introversion/extraversion: modification of Eysenck's theory. In Nebylistyn, V.D., Gray, J.A. (Editors): Biological bases of individual behaviour, p. 182 (Academic Press, New York 1972)
3 HEIMANN, H.: Wirkungsvergleich von Psychopharmaka am menschlichen Verhalten. Beitr. gerichtl. Med. *28*, 155 (1971)
4 HEIMANN, H., SCHMOCKER, A.M.: Zur Korrelation frequenzanalytischer und psychologischer Messwerte. In Schenk, G.K. (Editor): Die Quantifizierung des Elektroencephalogramms, Beitr. Symp. Arbeitsgem. Methodik Elektroenceph., Jongny sur Vevey 1973, p. 631 (AEG-Telefunken, Constance 1974)
5 HEIMANN, H., WITT, P.N.: Die Wirkung einer einmaligen Largactilgabe bei Gesunden. Mschr. Psychiat. Neurol. *129*, 104 (1955)
6 JANKE, W., DEBUS, G.: Experimental studies on antianxiety agents with normal subjects: methodological considerations and review of the main effects. In Efron, D.H. (Editor): Psychopharmacology. A review of progress 1957–1967, Proc. VIth Ann. Meet. Amer. Coll. Neuropsychopharmacol., San Juan, Puerto Rico 1967. U.S. publ. Hlth Serv. Publ. No. 1836: 205 (1968)
7 KRAEPELIN, E.: Über die Beeinflussung einfacher psychischer Vorgänge durch einige Arzneimittel (Fischer, Jena 1892)
8 LEGEWIE, H.: Persönlichkeitstheorie und Psychopharmaka. Kritische Untersuchung zu Eysencks Drogenpostulat (Hain, Meisenheim am Glan 1968)
9 LIENERT, G.A.: Verteilungsfreie Methoden in der Biostatistik, 2nd Ed., Vol. I (Hain, Meisenheim am Glan 1973)
10 MURRAY, D.C.: Talk, silence, and anxiety. Psychol. Bull. *75*, 244 (1971)
11 STOLL, W.A.: Lysergsäure-diäthylamid, ein Phantastikum aus der Mutterkorngruppe. Schweiz. Arch. Neurol. Psychiat. *60*, 279 (1947)

Discussion

W. BIRKMAYER: Many thanks indeed for your paper, Dr. HEIMANN. It seems to me that the line of research which Dr. HEIMANN is pursuing may well help to reintegrate the complex field of psychopharmacology into the overall framework of the natural sciences. Expressions such as "it is my impression that", "it might be supposed that", or "I am inclined to believe that" will have to disappear from the reports we write. Such exact and, above all, such reproducible investigations as Dr. HEIMANN has presented here – and not for the first time either – provide one way in which to arrive at a critically calculated mean when confronted with discrepancies in individual response rates ranging between such crass extremes as 10 and 90%.

H. REMSCHMIDT: I, too, found Dr. HEIMANN's paper extremely interesting, and I believe that it also has important implications with regard to the planning of clinical trials. The varying effects which some psycho-active drugs have been found to exert, e.g. their ability either to activate or to inhibit certain functions, can be satisfactorily explained by reference to Dr. HEIMANN's model and by taking account of all the factors he has mentioned. We have been faced with similar problems in the course of our own studies. When investigating a major tranquilliser, for example, we found that it tremendously accelerated psychomotor performance in simple tests, but that it impaired psychomotor performance in such complex tests as those involving multiple choices. Phenomena of this kind become readily understandable if, when drawing up the plan of a trial, one pays due attention to the factors Dr. HEIMANN has referred to. There is also another factor to be borne in mind, which I regard as very important, but which is generally overlooked in clinical trials. This factor is the subjective effect of psychopharmaceuticals, which can and should be taken into account and for which relatively accurate allowances can be made. It is a factor which – assuming a placebo is being used for purposes of comparison – may well have a major bearing on the assessment of a psycho-active drug's activity.

R. DREYER: I should like to ask Dr. HEIMANN whether the improvement which carbamazepine (®Tegretol) produces, and which cannot be achieved with sedatives or minor tranquillisers, is not simply a placebo effect attributable to the fact that the patient is to some extent anticipating a favourable response. If this were so, would one be justified in inferring that the drug has a psychotropic effect?

R. KUHN: I have a couple of questions for Dr. HEIMANN. When you refer in your Figure 1 to an "optimal level of arousal", is this an optimum based on empirical observation of a given patient, or is it a theoretical optimum arrived at in consideration of the fact that both an activating and an inhibiting drug may exert a negative effect? Incidentally, Dr. HEIMANN, I should like to add that I, too, found your paper most interesting, because the very elegantly presented findings contained in it shed light on a number of puzzling problems which we encounter again and again in connection with drug therapy.
The second question I'd like to put to you concerns the modulation of arousal. What exactly do you mean by modulation in this context? I ask this because I believe that, when tackling the problem of drive, it is also absolutely essential to consider the role played by what might be termed higher cerebral functions, and that it is of fundamental importance to determine these superordinate controlling functions as accurately as possible.

H. HEIMANN: The observations reported by Dr. REMSCHMIDT tally closely with findings which we have obtained both in healthy subjects as well as in patients, in whom some tests revealed an improvement in response to psycho-active drugs and others a deterioration. This phenomenon, as I have tried to show, is bound up with the fact that a certain optimal level of arousal is required for the performance of a given task; precisely where that level lies depends on the type of task concerned.

In reply to Dr. DREYER, I should mention that the studies in question were carried out, not in patients, but in 20 healthy subjects. The doses of carbamazepine given amounted to 200 mg. on one day and 400 mg. on another. The subjects received a placebo on two days, and carbamazepine – in the doses I have just mentioned – on the other two days. The battery of tests employed to assess performance and state of mind indicated that carbamazepine exerted quite a clear-cut psychotropic action, as confirmed by the significant differences in comparison with the placebo. This psychotropic action is particularly interesting inasmuch as the tranquillising effect experienced subjectively in response to carbamazepine was, curiously enough, actually accompanied by a certain degree of stimulation. This is a finding which, in our experience, clearly distinguishes carbamazepine not only from diazepam and other minor tranquillisers, but also from major tranquillisers and antidepressants. Carbamazepine is, in fact, the only tricyclic compound which, in our experience to date, produces an improvement in performance (namely, in a test of digital dexterity) in healthy subjects.

To answer the first of Dr. KUHN's two questions, the figure of mine to which he referred was meant as a diagrammatic representation. I nevertheless believe that it is possible to establish a correlation between a subject's psychological performance in a given test and the optimal level of drug-induced arousal, and that this can be done, for example, by measuring his performance under various conditions of arousal. Our own experience suggests that performance can be tested, for instance, under noisy as compared with quiet conditions, because noise is conducive to arousal. The only problem arising in this connection is that of deciding by reference to which physiological variables one should determine the level of arousal. What I have called the "optimal level of arousal" is thus not simply a theoretical optimum inferred from the fact that stimulating or sedating drugs are always also liable to impair performance, but an optimum which – though its determination in a given case admittedly entails considerable time and effort – is nonetheless objectively measurable. Incidentally, I should perhaps add that the whole concept I have presented is based on the results of psychological studies which also included tests performed without psycho-active drugs; it is a concept deduced from a wealth of data elaborated by psychologists. Here, when the general level of arousal was correlated with psychological performance, the same non-linear correlation in the shape of an inverted U was found time and again.

Now for the question Dr. KUHN raised concerning modulation of the arousal level – a notion I have derived from psychophysiological studies on healthy subjects, as well as on depressives and patients suffering from anxiety states. It is clearly apparent to us that the depressive is incapable of adequately modulating his level of arousal, which remains confined within very narrow limits. On the other hand, a healthy individual – even if he has a personality type bordering on the pathological, i.e. if he displays a high degree of neuroticism or of extraversion or introversion – is able to modulate over the whole arousal scale as soon as he is called upon to perform a certain task. This, by the way, has been confirmed by the results of DÜKER tests conducted with sedatives*, in which the so-called reactive increase in tension also constitutes a motivational element. The healthy volunteers felt sedated under the influence of a sedative, but still worked better and more quickly than in response to a placebo, because they were capable of compensating the sedative effect. This is something which depressives, for example, cannot do, or at least not to the same extent. The findings obtained in these Düker tests support your contention, Dr. KUHN, inasmuch as they suggest that higher psychic functions have a very important bearing on measurable changes in behaviour elicited by psycho-active drugs. Moreover, there is every reason to suppose that the functional processes in question are not exclusively

---

* DÜKER, H.: Über reaktive Anspannungssteigerung. Z. exp. angew. Psychol. *10*, 46 (1973)

confined to the brainstem, but that the cerebral cortex is probably also involved on quite a large scale.

W. Birkmayer: Thank you very much, Dr. Heimann. I should like to emphasise once again how fascinating I find the research work you are doing. I am convinced that studies of this kind provide the modern psychiatrist with ways and means of arriving at exact facts and data.

Finally, just one last remark. Already 20 years ago, the Nobel prizewinner Ulrich von Euler devised a method for detecting plasma noradrenaline levels in micro-gramme amounts. Meanwhile, thanks to more modern techniques, it has now become possible to perform determinations expressed in picogrammes, i.e. in thousandths of a nanogramme. The methods employed by Dr. Heimann strike me as leading in a similar direction and will therefore, I am sure, contribute to a better scientific understanding of the effects exerted by psycho-active drugs.

Behavioural disorders in children and the possibilities offered by drugs in their treatment

by G. Nissen*

Whereas in the U.S.A. in particular a typological differentiation is made between "behavioural disorders" and "character disorders", in German-speaking countries virtually *all* the psychopathological syndromes encountered in children are classified as "behavioural disorders" *(Verhaltensstörungen)*. To give this term such a wide connotation may serve a useful purpose if it helps one to arrive at a rough, preliminary definition of these syndromes. The expression "difficulties in schooling and upbringing", formerly employed for the same purpose and defining the sociological setting in which psychic disorders of a fairly subtle type are most likely to be observed, has now largely been replaced by "behavioural disorders" as a descriptive diagnosis. This diagnosis, however, sheds no more light on questions of pathogenesis than do expressions such as "acute abdomen", "gait disorders", or "retention of urine"; like these latter descriptions, "behavioural disorders", too, is a term which is of little significance, especially as regards choice of treatment and prognosis, until it has been supplemented by a nosological diagnosis.

The behaviour of a child at a particular age or stage of development is assessed by reference to traditional standards and average values which, in turn, are liable to vary from one epoch to another and from one culture to another. Since in the last ten years or so behavioural disorders have aroused the interest not only of child psychiatrists, whose task it is to diagnose and treat them, but also of educationalists who have been endeavouring for obvious reasons to obtain statistics on their prevalence, of sociologists who include them in their studies of social conditions, and of psychotherapists who draw a sharp distinction between such disorders and the neuroses, the resultant confusion of terminology is worthy of the tower of Babel.

Let me illustrate this by quoting a few examples. The German Educational Council[1] states: "A person is adjudged to be suffering from a behavioural disorder if, as a result of organic damage – especially of cerebral origin – or of an unfavourable upbringing, he is disturbed in his psychosocial behaviour, reacts inappropriately in social situations, and cannot cope with even minor conflicts." From the sociological standpoint[18], abnormal behaviour is defined as "an affront to the expectations of a large majority of the members of a society"; furthermore, a behavioural disorder is deemed to be present "if a person's behaviour elicits negative reactions from third parties". As can be seen, these two sociological definitions are based on the concept of standards and average values.

---

230   * Städtische Klinik für Kinder- und Jugendpsychiatrie Wiesengrund, Berlin.

At the First World Congress of Psychiatry, the Commission on Nomenclature of the Child Psychiatry Section[20] recommended that the term "behavioural disorders", or "behaviour disturbances", be used to denote maladjustment to family life, maladjustment to school, and social maladjustment. It is this connotation which will be adopted in the present paper because, though not satisfactory for various reasons (especially from the nosographic point of view), it does form a useful *point de départ* for a discussion of the theme in question.

Whereas the expression "difficulties in schooling and upbringing" delineates the field of study concerned without implying any value judgments, the term "behavioural disorders" focuses attention on the child himself, who, in cases where the disturbance in question is a behavioural disorder in the narrower sense of the term, usually suffers less from his abnormal conduct than do the people around him. This approach, however, entails the risk of overlooking the causal connection between induced or reactive behavioural disorders in children and faulty attitudes on the part of their parents. In the last analysis, it may mean that treatment is directed only at the symptoms of the disorders, symptoms which the parents, by their very attitude, provoke and sustain in the child. Drug therapy, if administered indiscriminately and without obeying certain rules, may make this vicious circle even more difficult to break. It may, indeed, simply serve to confirm the parents' view that the child is either at fault or ill, and it may harden their already negative attitude to the child's upbringing. At worst, the elimination of symptoms by means of drugs may promote a pathological personality development against which the child might perhaps have successfully defended himself by displaying even more pronounced symptoms. Although I am deliberately emphasising this scepticism towards the use of drugs in children, a scepticism which is particularly widespread in the German Federal Republic, I feel that for various reasons it is nowadays no longer so unreservedly justified.

Viewed from the nosological standpoint, the concept of "behavioural disorders" loses its phenomenological unity as soon as an attempt is made to break it down in terms of aetiology and pathogenesis. One often runs into difficulty with such attempts, because behavioural disorders due to varying causes seldom display a specific symptomatology. As a rule, these disorders take the form of psychic anomalies which, stemming as they do from a plurality of causes connected with the child's environment, psychological development, and cerebral function, call for differentiated and graduated treatment. It is a pity that STERN[25] did not succeed in his endeavour to persuade teachers, social workers, educational advisory centres, etc. to make use of the concept of "character disorders" in addition to that of "behavioural disorders". Even if the introduction of this concept of character disorders had failed to give rise to an informative discussion on the causes of abnormal modes of behaviour – as it has finally failed to do even in the U.S.A. – it might at least have encouraged us in German-speaking countries to carry out a long-overdue analysis of the reasons for minimising and denying the importance of the role played by genetic, organic cerebral, and endocrine factors in the pathogenesis of abnormal behaviour patterns in children (Figure 1).

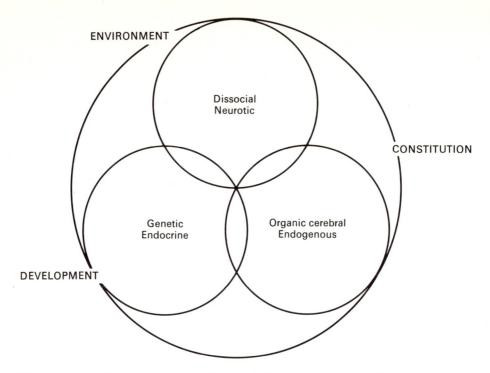

ENVIRONMENT

Dissocial
Neurotic

CONSTITUTION

Genetic
Endocrine

Organic cerebral
Endogenous

DEVELOPMENT

Fig. 1. Causes of behavioural disorders in children. Behavioural disorders of varying aetiology seldom display symptoms centred on one particular set of causes. They usually involve psychic anomalies which are determined directly or indirectly by a variety of different factors – factors relating to the child's psychological development, to his reactions to his environment, and to organic cerebral processes – and which call for differentiated and graduated therapy.

For the somatic and psychic development of a human being genetic codes are just as necessary as environmental influences; it is these genetic codes, in fact, which, interacting with the individual's constitution, are responsible for the way in which man reacts to his environment. Human geneticists today are convinced proponents of the environment theory, because they know that it is often only in an unfavourable environment that an hereditary predisposition becomes manifest; in a favourable environment, on the other hand, the predisposition may remain permanently latent.

Psychoanalysts with a critical turn of mind, such as HARTMANN[6], acknowledge that the existence of "autonomous ego cores" imposes biological limits on the extent to which environment can affect the individual, and that these ego cores may even perhaps play a decisive role in governing neurotic developments[23]. The neuropsychologists are convinced that there is a psychophysical correspondence between all psychic and somatic processes and even that all central nervous processes are subject to determinism[22]; this does not, however, lead automatically to a belief in fatalism, because the stimulus-producing setting in which we live is essential for our existence.

A descriptive and nosological classification of behavioural disorders in children may be of secondary importance for teachers and sociologists, because it is only to a limited extent that educational measures can be specifically directed at the cause of the disorder, and because the major problem confronting the sociologist is not to detect the underlying cause, but to consider the consequences for society. Doctors, on the other hand, should endeavour, as advocated by the Swedish psychiatrist Essen-Möller[2], to arrive at a multifactorial diagnosis by taking into account not only the clinical picture, but also the child's personality structure, the onset and course of the behavioural disorder, and its primary and secondary causes. Only in this way can one avoid the danger of administering polypragmatic therapy instead of the polycentric treatment that is required.

In the "Diagnostic and Statistical Manual (D.S.M. – II)" of the American Psychiatric Association[4], behavioural disorders are classified as being less severe than well-defined psychopathological syndromes such as neuroses, psychoses, and personality disturbances. If we were to try to fit these behavioural disorders – i.e. behavioural disorders in the narrower sense of the term – into the system of classification normally employed by us, we would designate them as *syndromes due to disturbances in psychological development* ("childhood deficiencies"), and as *frustration-induced disturbances* (emotional frustration syndromes), which, though ranking nosologically between the "psychic reactions" and "dissocial developments", cannot always be clearly distinguished from them. As regards their aetiology, prognosis, and sociological implications, these four groups of disorder are characterised by the following three features: 1. The child's environment is invariably involved in the development of the behavioural disorder; 2. The child himself usually feels less troubled by the behavioural disorder than do the people around him; and 3. The prognosis is relatively favourable if measures designed to correct the child's environment, as well as psychotherapy, can be instituted in good time.

As can be seen from Figure 2, behavioural disorders in the narrower sense of the term therefore include not only emotional frustration syndromes and disturbances in psychological development, but also – albeit in attenuated form – chronic psychic reactions and simple dissocial developments. Structured neuroses, psychoses, psychosyndromes of organic cerebral origin, and personality disorders would *not* be covered by this concept, because they are clinical pictures with a special aetiology and prognosis. Figure 2 shows that, for the purposes of description, all psychopathological syndromes can be regarded as behavioural disorders; but only those syndromes represented by the four shaded segments can be designated as behavioural disorders in the narrower sense of the term.

Concerning the *prevalence* of behavioural disorders in general, there is a large measure of agreement among teachers, psychologists, and doctors, most of whom put the figure in schoolchildren at between 25 and 30%[3, 5, 26, 28].

Using criteria of assessment which, from the methodological point of view, were fairly strict, Scholz[24] found "very severe behavioural anomalies" in 1–1.5% of schoolchildren, whereas Kluge[10] reported that 3.3% of the school-

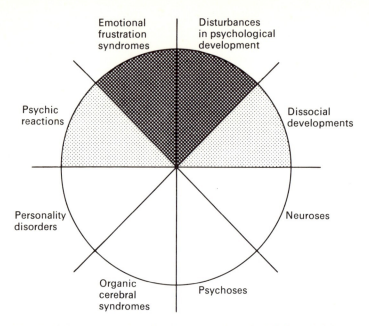

Fig. 2. Behavioural disorders in general and childhood behavioural disorders in the narrower sense of the term. From a descriptive standpoint, all psychic disturbances in children and in adults can in principle be regarded as behavioural disorders. Behavioural disorders in the narrower sense of the term comprise, in children, syndromes due to disturbances in psychological development ("childhood deficiencies") or to frustration (or deprivation), which are to be classified nosologically between the psychic reactions and dissocial developments.

children he studied displayed "obviously abnormal behavioural patterns". These two differing figures clearly reveal how necessary it is to define the borderline between mild and severe behavioural disorders; in the absence of such a definition no exact data can be obtained on the incidence of the two categories.

The methods of *treatment* available for use in behavioural disorders comprise: environmental therapy, remedial training, psychomotor treatment, psychotherapy, behaviour therapy, and drugs. The choice of a suitable approach to treatment is dependent upon numerous conditioning factors, of which it is impossible to give a complete list here. They include, however, the following: age of the child and his stage of development, parents' skill – or lack of skill – in bringing up the child and their readiness to seek and accept advice, nature of the symptoms, and availability of a suitable therapist.

The basic rule of therapy is that psychogenic behavioural disorders should as far as possible be corrected by psychotherapy, and that abnormalities which are predominantly of constitutional or organic cerebral origin should be treated by a combination of remedial training and drugs. This rule does not exclude the possibility that psychogenic disorders may be favourably influenced by drugs or that psychosyndromes of organic cerebral origin may respond to

234

psychotherapy. Moreover, it should be borne in mind not only that behavioural disorders in children usually have very complex causes, but also that the various members of the child's family are apt to attach, often without realising it, widely differing degrees of importance to these disorders.

The success of treatment for a behavioural disorder depends very largely on the readiness both of the child and of all the persons with whom he is in regular contact to play their part in the treatment and also to accept that the aim of therapy is to achieve a cure. This precondition can by no means be taken for granted, because we know that the majority of these children come from a discordant environment, in which they act to some extent as symptom-carriers for their parents. In such instances, the parents cannot automatically be regarded from the outset as useful assistants to the therapist. At the start, and in many cases for a long time afterwards, they themselves require the doctor's attention, and his most difficult task may well be to recognise those facets of the parents' personalities that are still sound and can be put to good account in the treatment of the child.

In small children and young schoolchildren, causal treatment for the behavioural disorder represents the most rational approach. That is to say, the wrong mental attitude of one or both parents towards the child should be corrected by means of psychotherapy or psycho-active drugs, thus creating the necessary preconditions for improving or eliminating the child's behavioural disorder. The older the child, the more he himself becomes the focal point of therapy. But even in the case of adolescents, the parents, just like the marriage partners of adult patients, should not be left out of account in the treatment programme. Anxious, obsessive-compulsive, or depressive mothers or fathers may induce symptoms of anxiety, obsession, compulsion, or depression in their children not merely during certain phases of early childhood but at all ages, and may thereby help to perpetuate a disturbed personality structure.

The question as to whether psychotherapy should in principle be given priority in the presence of psychogenic disorders or diseases no longer gives rise to much discussion. The problem which worries most child psychiatrists nowadays and causes them insuperable difficulties is that of ensuring that at least those children who obviously *must* have psychotherapy do actually receive it. The present dearth of specialists in this field will certainly not be remedied in the foreseeable future, and, in view of the lengthy period of training psychotherapists require and of the fact that one psychotherapist can treat only a small number of patients, it probably never will be. Nor can this unfavourable situation be decisively improved by resorting to short courses of psychotherapy or to group-therapy. In their daily work psychotherapists who deal with children, as well as child psychiatrists who use psychoanalysis and also attach importance to remedial training, are liable to be particularly troubled by their consciences when they perceive the need for a unilateral method of treatment but are unable to satisfy that need owing to lack of time or of qualified assistants. This conflict of conscience on the part of the therapist, who realises that he cannot devote his energies solely to a small privileged group of children requiring optimal care, may give rise to the paradoxical situation in which a large number of children suffering from behavioural disorders and neuroses, who could be relieved of their symptoms simply by recourse to drugs, receive no treatment at all because the therapist considers a course of psychoanalysis or of remedial training to be more appropriate but lacks the resources to carry it out. In the majority of his cases, therefore, the child psychiatrist is faced not with the choice of whether to employ either psychotherapy or drugs, but with the need to seek a compromise between the two. Moreover, in certain clinical pictures, such as enuresis, for example, this compromise approach has indeed proved superior to unilateral methods.

In the psychiatric treatment of children on an ambulatory basis a rough differentiation of behavioural disorders into various types – such as is customary in the nomenclature used for neuroses and psychopathies and such as is, in fact, also to be found in the International Classification of Diseases (308) – has shown itself to be most useful as a means of facilitating a decision to use certain forms of treatment.

This differentiation takes account of practical requirements and meets the parents' desire to see that treatment is focused chiefly on the cardinal symptoms of the child's behavioural disorders. On the other hand, since the advent of the psycho-active drugs, typologies which may almost be regarded as classic today – such as the one which HOMBURGER[8], following in the footsteps of KURT SCHNEIDER, introduced into the psychopathology of childhood diseases – have been undergoing a renaissance, although they no longer feature the old aetiological concept.

HOMBURGER[8] described nine types of abnormal personality in children, STUTTE[27] 12, LUTZ[12] eight, and JENKINS[9] six. The reason why I should like here to restrict the number of types to three is not that new fundamental information has become available on the subject. On the contrary, such a restriction is dictated solely by pragmatic considerations – i.e. it is based on achievable therapeutic results. The first and foremost aim of treatment is to give the anxious child a certain measure of self-assurance, the apathetic child more spontaneity, and the hyperkinetic child more balance, and thus to facilitate their integration into society. Inasmuch as the elimination of symptoms by the use of drugs cannot change a human being's personality structure, it is to be regarded as falling under the heading of "prosthetic medicine". This designation may sound disparaging, but it is of course applicable to symptomatic methods of treatment in virtually all branches of medicine and not only in psychiatry.

On pragmatic grounds, then, behavioural disorders in children can be divided into the following three broad categories, each of which displays its own characteristic symptoms:

1. The *anxious child*. Children in this category have unmotivated bouts of weeping, screaming, or sadness. Their sleeping-waking rhythm is often disturbed, and pavor states accompanied by severe anxious excitation, sweating, and mild disorientation are fairly common. These timid and sensitive children often

withdraw into day-dreams, have little contact with others, or behave in a mutistic fashion. They often have speech impairments, wet or dirty their beds, or refuse to attend kindergarten or school. Owing to their lack of self-confidence and their feeling of inferiority, they cannot tolerate separation from the persons with whom they have their closest relationships.

2. The *child displaying inhibition of drive* and apparent or actual reluctance to participate in everyday life. These children are unenterprising, withdrawn, and shy. They are largely incapable of asserting themselves, sometimes show signs of dysphoria and depression, and tend to develop psychosomatic symptoms. They are backward in playing and learning, give up too early, and are apt to find themselves always relegated to "the end of the line". In cases where a child suffering from lack of drive is of below-average intelligence or displays weakness in certain fields of performance, his basic attitude of resignation is made even worse by his constant failures.

3. The *hyperkinetic child*. Children belonging to this category exhibit psychomotor restlessness, lack of concentration, and an inability to regard objects or people dispassionately. They seldom maintain firm contacts for long, and they are impulsive. They are persistently obstinate and defiant, they tend to be hetero-aggressive or auto-aggressive, and they often develop dissocial attitudes. In schoolchildren, the predominant features are disturbances of concentration, distractability and general disinhibition, as well as a tendency to destructive acts and explosive reactions.

For various reasons it is particularly difficult to evaluate the *effectiveness of psycho-active drugs in children*, and this is also a field that has not yet been adequately studied. As children belonging to different age groups, and thus at different stages of development, display a plurality of symptoms of differing origin, it is not easy to form homogeneous series in which to assess the effect of a drug. Moreover, so many different psycho-active drugs are available on the market that the individual investigator can reach a reliable verdict only on those drugs with whose use, properties, and side effects he is himself familiar.

Consequently, drugs can often be tested only in very small groups of children displaying the same symptomatology, with the result that it is not always possible to make a sound assessment of them. Comparative studies are difficult to perform, not only because insufficient knowledge is available on the pharmacodynamic effects of drugs in children, but also because of the types of drug involved and the way in which they are administered; drug therapy in children, in fact, does not call simply for a good doctor-patient relationship, but also requires that due account be taken of a much more complicated set of relationships involving the doctor and the child, the doctor and the parents, and the doctor, the child, and the child's family. The aim is to ensure not only that the patient takes the drug regularly, but that all members of his family accept the approach to therapy proposed by the doctor and do not expect the drug he has prescribed to exert effects which it cannot or must not exert. A child's fear of being abandoned by his mother may be neutralised for a time by chemical means, but it should not be eliminated altogether, because this

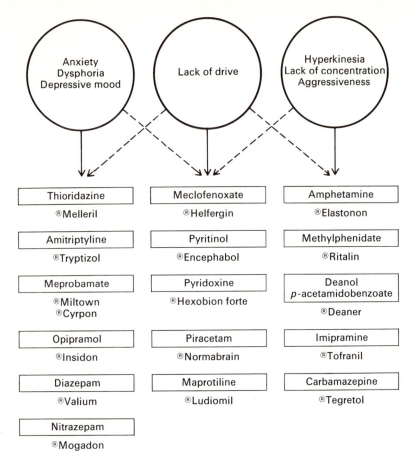

Anxiety Dysphoria Depressive mood	Lack of drive	Hyperkinesia Lack of concentration Aggressiveness

Thioridazine	Meclofenoxate	Amphetamine
®Melleril	®Helfergin	®Elastonon

Amitriptyline	Pyritinol	Methylphenidate
®Tryptizol	®Encephabol	®Ritalin

Meprobamate	Pyridoxine	Deanol p-acetamidobenzoate
®Miltown ®Cyrpon	®Hexobion forte	®Deaner

Opipramol	Piracetam	Imipramine
®Insidon	®Normabrain	®Tofranil

Diazepam	Maprotiline	Carbamazepine
®Valium	®Ludiomil	®Tegretol

Nitrazepam
®Mogadon

Fig. 3. Cardinal symptoms encountered in behavioural disorders in children, and drugs indicated in their treatment. In this figure the disorders have deliberately been grouped according to their symptomatology and not according to nosological criteria. As the interrupted lines indicate, drugs listed as being effective against one group of symptoms may also prove beneficial in other groups. Some of the preparations have consequently been listed, not under their main indications, but under groups of symptoms which appear to constitute additional indications for them in children.

might in turn rid the mother of possible guilt feelings, the presence of which could help to resolve the conflict between mother and child.

Before the physician prescribes drug therapy, he must first decide what type of behavioural disorder the child is suffering from. Instead of presenting a mere summary review of the drugs available for use in this connection, I therefore now propose – by analogy with the outline given in Figure 3 – to discuss briefly the indications for the various categories of psycho-active drug by reference to the cardinal symptoms encountered in behavioural disorders of childhood.

In anxious children showing acute symptoms (constant paroxysms of weeping and screaming, initial or delayed insomnia and nightmares, fear of separation leading to difficulties in social adaptation, refusal to attend kindergarten or school, circumscribed phobias, or bouts of anxiety), thioridazine (®Melleril) and maprotiline (®Ludiomil) have proved very useful – also thanks to their virtually complete absence of side effects. In cases where generalised synchronous potentials are found in the E.E.G. and where the patient's symptoms become acute at night, we commonly resort to the benzodiazepines (®Valium, ®Mogadon) or to carbamazepine (®Tegretol), all of which possess anticonvulsive properties in addition. On the other hand, we employ meprobamate less often now than we used to.

In children displaying lack of drive (both retarded children and those with organic cerebral damage), drugs are unable to produce effects on individual symptoms, such as lack of concentration or inattentiveness. Treatment with "neurostimulants", which supply the nerve cells with nutrient substances and energy carriers, is therefore based not on target symptoms but on the principle of stimulating without exciting and tranquillising without depressing[19]. It has been demonstrated in animal experiments that, for example, meclofenoxate (®Helfergin) and pyritinol (®Encephabol) are indeed capable of improving brain metabolism (e.g. glucose metabolism). Both drugs may serve to step up the child's response to teaching, but in children with brain damage they occasionally give rise to diffuse states of restlessness. The administration of piracetam (®Normabrain) or of vitamin B_6 (in the form of ®Hexobion forte) still has its indications, especially in cases where meclofenoxate or pyritinol are contra-indicated because of their tendency to lower the convulsion threshold.

For the treatment of hyperkinetic children, methylphenidate (®Ritalin) and amphetamine (®Elastonon) have been used to good effect for many years, particularly in the U.S.A. The improvement rates achieved with methylphenidate reportedly amount to 80%[14] or 70–90%[13, 15], those with amphetamine to approximately 70%[14], and those with deanol p-acetamidobenzoate (®Deaner) to 47%. Good responses have also been elicited with imipramine and carbamazepine in a high percentage of cases. In hyperkinetic children it is advisable to combine drug therapy with remedial training designed to impose a certain discipline on both body and mind (e.g. handball, table-tennis, piano-playing).

In the last two years we have employed methylphenidate in combined treatment programmes of this type in more than 100 hyperkinetic children and have obtained clear-cut, and in some cases dramatic, improvements in about 60% of them. We prefer to administer the drug in small doses, giving the children 10–20 mg. methylphenidate in the morning and only in rare instances a further 10 mg. at midday. In small children we do not use drugs. In the case of schoolchildren, methylphenidate is discontinued during holidays or during intercurrent illnesses. Where a good response has been achieved, methylphenidate is replaced after 3–4 months – at the latest after six months – by deanol p-acetamidobenzoate, imipramine, or carbamazepine. Only if the improvement in behaviour fails to persist under this medication is treatment with methylphenidate resumed. In some children it has been possible after a period of treatment lasting six to eight months to stop all drugs for some

239

considerable time, because the improvement in behaviour following the discontinuation of drugs, though not so pronounced as during treatment, was nevertheless still quite appreciable. In our experience, hyperkinetic syndromes definitely known to be of organic cerebral origin respond more often and more markedly to psycho-active drugs than those in which an organic cause has not been established.

The therapeutic armamentarium of the child psychiatrist, too, has thus been enriched by the advent of the psycho-active drugs, though not to the same extent as that of the psychiatrist called upon to treat psychoses in adults. Successful treatment for children with behavioural disorders depends not only on a thorough knowledge of the indications, dosages, psychodynamic properties, and side effects of a number of selected drugs, but also on a series of practical and psychological factors, of which special account has to be taken in children and also in adolescents.

Many parents become worried and alarmed when they read the list of indications in the package leaflet for a drug. They sometimes jump to the conclusion that the doctor has not told them the whole truth about their child's behavioural disorder, or they are afraid that the drug's possible side effects may impair the child's learning ability and performance. Adolescents are apt to think that the doctor is trying with the aid of drugs to force them to accept their parents' educational demands. The parents frequently administer inadequate doses of the drugs prescribed, or else they discontinue the medication prematurely, while adolescents may either try to avoid taking their drugs or even refuse to take them at all; for obvious reasons, the doctor is often not informed about this. Hence, whenever drugs are prescribed, the parents and also, to an appropriate extent, the schoolchild or adolescent himself must first be enlightened as to the aim of the treatment and as to the action and possible side effects of the drug concerned.

A judiciously selected psycho-active drug administered in a suitable dosage not only exerts a beneficial influence on the child's behaviour, but also indirectly alters the attitude of the parents towards the child. A placebo effect must also be allowed for, because children are more easily influenced than adults and because the mere fact of having to take drugs regularly over a certain space of time for a disorder hitherto regarded simply as a difficulty in schooling or upbringing can also modify the child's habitual reactions. In cases where a child has been successfully treated with psycho-active drugs, his parents' attitude towards him generally improves, because the disappearance of the symptoms facilitates the child's social adaptation and makes him more accessible to teaching. Some children who have responded well to drug treatment, however, are exposed to an additional danger, inasmuch as their parents may for ever afterwards regard them as sick children. This is yet another reason why drug therapy directed at the symptoms of a disorder should only be embarked upon after the child's past history and family history have been examined with particular care.

From the medical point of view, the value of combining psychotherapy and drugs is indisputable in all cases where it benefits the child. But such combined measures, though usually desirable, are not always to be recommended. If a child has a disturbing tic, for example, the use of a drug may well eliminate the tic, but it may also thereby block the one and only path leading to a deeper exploration of the parent-child relationship. As regards psycho-active drugs themselves, no final verdict on a particular preparation can be reached until its pharmacodynamic effects have been carefully distinguished from its psychodynamic properties. The essential preconditions for the testing of drugs in this way are that the concept of what is and what is not a behavioural disorder should be defined as accurately as possible in both descriptive and nosological terms, and that due account should be taken not only of criteria relating to the child's age, stage of development, or sex, but also of the results of neurological and neurophysiological examinations. Long-term observations of behavioural patterns in children, carried out with the object of evaluating the effects of psycho-active drugs, are apt to be unreliable, because a child's psychological development and biological maturation do not proceed at a uniform pace, and because familial and sociological factors involved in the behavioural disorder often cannot be accurately assessed.

References

1 DEUTSCHER BILDUNGSRAT: Empfehlung zur Pädagogischen Förderung Behinderter und von Behinderung bedrohter Kinder und Jugendlicher (Third draft; No. 3.4.9)
2 ESSEN-MÖLLER, E.: On classification of mental disorders. Acta psychiat. scand. *37*, 119 (1961)
3 FALK, W.: Versuch einer Analyse der Schulreife aufgrund ärztlicher Untersuchungsergebnisse eines Hamburger Einschulungsjahrganges. Gesundheitsfürsorge *8*, 187 and 199 (1959)
4 FREEDMAN, A. M., KAPLAN, H. I., SADOCK, B. J.: Modern synopsis of comprehensive textbook of psychiatry, p. 613 (Williams & Wilkins, Baltimore 1972)
5 HARNACK, G.-A. VON: Nervöse Verhaltensstörungen beim Schulkind (Thieme, Stuttgart 1958)
6 HARTMANN, H.: Ich-Psychologie. Studien zur psychoanalytischen Theorie (Klett, Stuttgart 1972)
7 HELWIG, H.: Psychopharmaka im Kindesalter. Mschr. Kinderheilk. *121*, 114 (1973)
8 HOMBURGER, A.: Psychopathologie des Kindesalters (Springer, Berlin 1926)
9 JENKINS, R. L.: The runaway reaction. Amer. J. Psychiat. *128*, 168 (1971)
10 KLUGE, K. J.: Verhaltensauffälligkeiten in Grundschulen. Heilpäd. Forsch. *5*, 1:1 (1973)
11 KNOBEL, M.: Psychopharmacology for the hyperkinetic child. Arch. gen. Psychiat. *6*, 198 (1962)
12 LUTZ, J.: Kinderpsychiatrie, 2nd Ed. (Rotapfel, Zurich/Stuttgart 1964)
13 LYTTON, G. J., KNOBEL, M.: Diagnosis and treatment of behavior disorders in children. Dis. nerv. Syst. *20, 334* (1959)
14 MILLICHAP, J. G.: Drugs in management of minimal brain dysfunction. Ann. N.Y. Acad. Sci. *205*, 321 (1973)
15 NICHAMIN, S. J., COMLY, H. M.: The hyperkinetic or lethargic child with cerebral dysfunction. Mich. Med. *63*, 790 (1964)
16 NISSEN, G.: Moderne Behandlungsmethoden in der Kinder- und Jugendpsychiatrie. Prax. Kinderpsychol. *19*, 161 (1970)

17 Nissen, G.: Zur Behandlung von Verhaltensstörungen bei Kindern. Ther. d. Gegenw. *113*, 387 (1974)

18 Opp, K.-D.: Abweichendes Verhalten und Gesellschaftsstruktur. Soziologische Texte, Vol. 101 (Luchterhand, Darmstadt/Neuwied 1974)

19 Rett, A.: Kritische Betrachtungen zur Verwendung von Psychopharmaka bei Kindern. Wien. med. Wschr. *116*, 726 (1966)

20 Sanctis, C. de, et al.: Minutes of the meetings of the Commission of Nomenclature. In Ey, H., Marty, P., Lang, J.L. (Editors): Ier Congr. mond. Psychiat., Paris 1950; VII Psychiat. infant., p. 133 (Hermann, Paris 1952)

21 Satterfield, J.H., Lesser, L.I., Saul, R.E., Cantwell, D.P.: EEG aspects in the diagnosis and treatment of minimal brain dysfunction, Ann. N.Y. Acad. Sci. *205*, 274 (1973)

22 Schaefer, H., Novak, P.: Anthropologie und Biophysik. In Gadamer, H.-G., Vogler, P. (Editors): Neue Anthropologie, Vol. I: Biologische Anthropologie, Part I, p. 22 (Thieme, Stuttgart 1972)

23 Schepank, H.: Erb- und Umweltfaktoren bei Neurosen. Tiefenpsychologische Untersuchungen an 50 Zwillingspaaren (Springer, Berlin/Heidelberg/New York 1974)

24 Scholz, D.: Ergebnisse der Einschulungsuntersuchungen 1969 in Berlin (West). Senator für Gesundheit und Umweltschutz, III C (Offprint 1972)

25 Stern, E.: Über Verhaltens- und Charakterstörungen bei Kindern und Jugendlichen (Rascher, Zurich 1953)

26 Steuber, H.: Zur Häufigkeit von Verhaltensstörungen im Grundschulalter. Prax. Kinderpsychol. *22*, 246 (1973)

27 Stutte, H.: Kinderpsychiatrie und Jugendpsychiatrie. In Gruhle, H.W., et al. (Editors): Psychiatrie der Gegenwart, Vol. II, p. 952 (Springer, Berlin/Göttingen/Heidelberg 1960)

28 Thalmann, H.-C.: Verhaltensstörungen bei Kindern im Grundschulalter (Klett, Stuttgart 1971)

29 Tramer, M.: Lehrbuch der allgemeinen Kinderpsychiatrie, 4th Ed. (Schwabe, Basle/Stuttgart 1964)

30 Zeh, W.: Bemerkungen zu einem Klassifikationsvorschlag der psychischen Störungen von Erik Essen-Möller, Lund. Nervenarzt *33*, 404 (1962)

The use of carbamazepine in the treatment of behavioural disorders in children

by R. M. PUENTE *

In a previous paper[2] we discussed the problem posed by the high proportion of children in Mexican primary schools who have to repeat one or more years' schooling; in the period 1967–1969 this proportion amounted to roughly one-fifth (22%) of the school population. Subsequently, in an investigation carried out among 12,458 pupils from 13 primary schools (5,695 girls and 6,763 boys), it was discovered that 8.14% of these children were suffering from cerebral damage.

The question of behavioural disorders in children has aroused considerable interest in Mexico, and, when we came across publications referring to the use of carbamazepine (®Tegretol) in the management of the typical symptoms of these behavioural disorders, we decided to give this drug a trial.

Experience in Mexico with carbamazepine in the treatment of behavioural disorders is based on studies conducted in altogether 83 children; in one series of 56 cases, the studies were carried out under open conditions[1,3], whereas in a second series of 27 children we ourselves tested carbamazepine against placebo in a double-blind trial. The findings obtained in both series will be briefly described.

Open non-comparative study

RUÍZ CASTAÑO[3], as well as KRASOVSKY et al.[1], studied a total of 72 children (55 boys and 17 girls) whose ages ranged from three to 12 years (average: 7.9 years) and who were suffering from behavioural disorders of varying origin. This group did not include any patients displaying a manifest neurological disease.

The most common symptoms were as follows: inattentiveness, disobedience, anxiety, aggressiveness, impulsiveness, low frustration tolerance, perseveration, hyperkinesia, backwardness in learning, unpredictable behaviour, destructiveness, lack of interest, irritability, sleep disturbances, emotional instability, and nail-biting. Other less frequent symptoms comprised: enuresis, night terrors, extreme passivity, and tics.

The children were given carbamazepine orally in an initial dosage of 50 mg. three times daily, which was gradually raised by increments of 50–100 mg. every three or four days. The optimal dose was found to be 300 mg. daily,

* Hospital Psiquiátrico "Fray Bernardino Alvarez" y Escuela Superior de Medicina del Instituto Politécnico Nacional, Mexico City, Mexico.

the maximum being 600 mg. In some cases, as little as 100 mg. daily proved sufficient. Throughout the period of treatment the children did not receive any other drug acting on the central nervous system. Carbamazepine was administered for periods ranging from nine to 23 weeks (average: 12 weeks), 17 cases being treated for the maximum period of 23 weeks.

The results were evaluated in two ways. Firstly, using a severity scale graded 0–4, the symptoms were assessed prior to treatment and also, depending on the response and on the cooperativeness of the patients and their relatives, every one or two weeks during treatment. The initial and final severity of each symptom was compared by reference to the arithmetical means of the scores recorded. If by the end of treatment the overall score had decreased by 90–100%, the response was considered to be excellent; a decrease of 70–89% was regarded as good, one of 40–69% as unsatisfactory, and one of 39% or less as nil. The second method of evaluation consisted of psychological tests (psychometric, projective, and perceptional-motor tests), which were carried out before and after treatment in 38 cases.

The results presented here refer to only 56 out of the total of 72 cases, because 16 of the children dropped out of the trial and could therefore not be fully evaluated. The responses elicited in the case of each symptom are indicated in Table 1.

Table 1. Effect exerted by carbamazepine on the symptoms in 56 children with behavioural disorders (open study).

Symptoms	Response				
	Excellent	Good	Unsatis-factory	Nil	Totals
Inattentiveness	20	18	17	0	55
Disobedience	16	18	11	4	49
Anxiety	19	15	13	0	47
Aggressiveness	14	18	14	0	46
Impulsiveness	14	13	18	0	45
Low frustration tolerance	10	14	15	3	42
Perseveration	13	15	12	1	41
Hyperkinesia	11	13	14	1	39
Backwardness in learning	6	11	17	5	39
Unpredictable behaviour	6	15	12	1	34
Destructiveness	8	11	12	0	31
Lack of interest	5	12	6	1	24
Irritability	3	8	11	0	22
Sleep disturbances	7	9	1	0	17
Emotional instability	7	4	4	1	16
Nail-biting	2	6	2	3	13
Enuresis	6	2	1	0	9
Night terrors	3	3	0	0	6
Extreme passivity	3	1	1	1	6
Tics	2	0	0	0	2

Indicated in the last column is the number of cases (out of the 56 evaluated) in which the relevant symptom was present.

In the children in whom psychological tests were performed, it was noted that some of the disturbances in visual perception and motor function revealed by the Bender *Gestalt* test had disappeared following the treatment. Significant improvements were likewise observed in the children's interpersonal relationships, in their adaptation to their environment, in their mental approach to problems, in their ability to coordinate their ideas, and in their vocabulary; the children also became less anxious and less obviously in need of affection.

Double-blind comparative study

We ourselves carried out a double-blind, comparative, within-patient study with carbamazepine and placebo in 30 children, and were able to evaluate the findings in 27 of them[2]. The children, all displaying cerebral damage or dysfunction, were aged from five to 13 years (average: 8.7 years); 12 were boys and 15 girls. Determination of their intelligence quotients with the aid of a battery of psychological tests showed that 11 of the children were mentally defective (in six the deficiency was slight and in five severe); in 14 cases the I.Q. proved to be normal, and in two it was not ascertained. Each child was subjected to a clinical and psychiatric examination, as well as to psychological tests (psychometric, projective, and perceptional-motor tests) and to educational tests. All these examinations and tests were performed before and after treatment, and the psychological tests were also repeated halfway through the trial. The children's symptoms were assessed once a week.

In 88–100% of the cases the following symptoms were encountered: inattentiveness, backwardness in learning, reluctance to participate in group tasks, low frustration tolerance, emotional instability, and unpredictable behaviour. Symptoms such as hyperkinesia, impulsiveness, destructiveness, speech disorders, hetero-aggressiveness and auto-aggressiveness, pathological disobedience, and lack of interest were observed in 81–85% of the children. Perseveration, anxiety, and extreme passivity were present in 51–77%, and nail-biting, night terrors, enuresis, and sleep disturbances in 18–40%.

The 27 patients were divided into two groups of 13 and 14, respectively. The first group was given carbamazepine for four weeks, and then, following a drug-free interval of one week, placebo for four weeks. In the second group, placebo was administered for the first four weeks, followed, after a drug-free interval of one week, by carbamazepine for four weeks. The dosage of carbamazepine employed was 300 mg. daily (100 mg. t.i.d.) for the first two weeks, followed by 200 mg. daily (100 mg. b.i.d.) for the last two.

The final evaluation of the results was made by calculating the percentage reduction in each patient's symptoms by reference to a severity scale graded 0–4. Patients whose symptoms were reduced by 41% or more were classified as "improved", and those with a reduction in symptoms of 40% or less as "not improved".

The results obtained are summarised in Table 2. In the group that received carbamazepine first, nine of the 13 patients improved in response to carbam-

Table 2. Symptomatic effect of carbamazepine in 27 children with behavioural disorders (double-blind study).

Final assessment	Sequence of treatment			
	Carbamazepine followed by placebo		Placebo followed by carbamazepine	
No. of cases improved	9	1	4	8
No. of cases not improved	4	12	10	6
Totals	13		14	

azepine and only one in response to placebo. In the other group, only four patients improved on placebo, as against eight on carbamazepine.

In the patients given carbamazepine first, the W.I.S.C. (Wechsler Intelligence Scale for Children) and Goodenough tests revealed an improvement of 15–30% in attentiveness, comprehension, retention, memory, abstraction, concentration, and observation; in response to placebo, the improvement in the same patients was 0–12%. In the group that was given placebo first, the degree of improvement recorded in the same tests ranged from 2 to 10%, and increased to 20–30% in response to carbamazepine.

In the Bender *Gestalt* test, the group receiving carbamazepine first showed better integration of the *Gestalt*, fewer mistakes in direction and visual perception, as well as a decrease in perseveration, during the period of treatment with the active drug; these improvements tended to disappear again following medication with placebo. In the other group, we observed better integration of the *Gestalt* and a decrease in rotation during the placebo period, and these improvements were maintained during treatment with carbamazepine. A placebo response is not surprising in this type of patient.

Tolerability

As the patients' ages and the doses of carbamazepine employed were similar in each of these Mexican studies, there is no need to analyse the trials separately in respect of drug tolerability. Of the total number of 83 children, 26 developed side effects, but these did not necessitate discontinuation of the treatment. They comprised: transient drowsiness in 16 cases, nausea and malaise in three, malaise and vomiting in one, urticaria in three, epigastric pain in two, and headache in one.

Conclusions

The importance of the problem of behavioural disorders in children requires no emphasising, especially as this is a problem which is not confined to particular countries or regions, but is of universal magnitude.

We have used carbamazepine to treat far more children than those reported on in this paper, but, for technical reasons, we have not been able to collect the data on the total number treated. When reviewing the studies conducted with carbamazepine in Mexico, we found that in altogether 83 children the case records were complete enough to be properly evaluated.

While being fully aware of the fact that an overall treatment programme based on a multidisciplinary approach is called for in the case of these patients, we consider ourselves justified in resorting to carbamazepine in order to control the symptoms associated with behavioural disorders.

The drug produces a clear-cut symptomatic improvement, as demonstrated for virtually all presenting symptoms in an open study. Our own double-blind trial, in which carbamazepine was compared with placebo, showed that the drug leads to a considerable reduction in the signs and symptoms of children with behavioural disorders, thereby improving their performance at school, their family relationships, and their adaptation to their environment and to society in general; at the same time, the drug makes the children more accessible to psychological, psychiatric, and psycho-educational methods of treatment.

References

1 Krasovsky Z., J., Villanueva, R., Hernández, O.: La carbamazepina en el tratamiento sintomático de los trastornos de conducta infantil. Münch. med. Wschr. (Ed. mex.) *114*, 619 (1972)
2 Puente, R. M., Barriga, F., Morales, M. T.: Estudio doble-ciego con carbamazepina en un grupo de escolares con daño cerebral. Comunicación preliminar. Medicina (Méx.) *53*, 97 (1973)
3 Ruíz Castaño, G.: Uso de carbamazepina en niños con trastornos de la conducta. Pren. méd. mex. *37*, 215 (1972)

Discussion

W. BIRKMAYER: In the comprehensive review which Dr. NISSEN gave us in his paper, he strongly emphasised the importance of environmental factors, and I am sure we all agree with him on this point. But I should nevertheless like to draw attention once again to the monograph published by SCHEPANK, a colleague of Dr. NISSEN's in Berlin. This study, to which Dr. NISSEN also referred, deals with neuroses in twins, in whom it was found that only 50% of the neuroses were attributable to unfavourable environmental circumstances, the other 50% being of hereditary origin. FREUD, incidentally, arrived at the same percentages. But, since – thank goodness – we are not able to tinker with the genetic code, all we can hope to do is to change the environment.

P. KIELHOLZ: I should like to thank Dr. NISSEN not only for his critical appraisal of psychopharmacotherapy in children, but also for having stressed the value of environmental therapy – although, of course, we all know that it is adults, rather than children, who prove the most difficult to educate. I do not quite agree with Dr. NISSEN, however, when it comes to the indications for antidepressants. Together with Dr. KUHN and with colleagues from the Bechterew Institute in Leningrad, we have shown in our clinic that depressive children, like depressive adults, also have to be treated by reference to the target symptoms of anxiety, retardation, and sadness, and that, instead of prescribing any arbitrarily selected antidepressant, one has to employ a drug whose activity pattern is appropriate to the child's target symptoms. I should be interested to know whether Dr. NISSEN would agree with this.

A. RETT: Speaking as a paediatrician, I feel I cannot thank Dr. NISSEN enough for the clarity with which he has exposed many of the problems confronting us. But there is one thing I wish to emphasise: behavioural disorders of the kind that have just been described here are no longer simply a problem for the family or for the school, but have now come to assume tremendous significance as a sociopolitical issue. The judgments of value implied by such epithets as "lazy, stupid, vicious, timid, naughty", etc., which many teachers employ, are simply no longer tolerable in this day and age. What we have to do is: firstly, to analyse these judgments, which all too often entail such dramatic consequences as transference of the child from one school to another, or even to a special home, thereby radically affecting the child's future and the lives of other members of the family; secondly, to discover and interpret the causes responsible for the behavioural disorders, and to inform teachers and parents accordingly; and, thirdly and lastly, also to institute appropriate treatment. In this connection, Dr. NISSEN has drawn attention to the frustrating discrepancy between, on the one hand, progress achieved in the diagnostic field and, on the other, the meagre scope of the psychotherapeutic possibilities open to us. Isn't it true to say that in most instances the only therapist we can hope to find is an informed and understanding teacher who is convinced of the need for analyses of the kind I have in mind? But where *are* these teachers who are ready and willing to cooperate wholeheartedly with us? It may be all very well and good to conclude that we simply have to work with drugs because we can't alter the child's educational and social milieu, but this is not a satisfactory solution, especially when one bears in mind how often drug treatment is downright sabotaged by teachers! Just a word or two more about how drugs should be employed: it is impossible to predict precisely what effect either a stimulant or a sedative will produce in a given case, nor can one lay down any rules of thumb regarding the dosage to be employed; consequently, one has to discover by trial and error which drug is the best one for each individual child and adapt the dosage to the fluctuations occurring in its behaviour. It is obvious that, here once again, success can be achieved only if the family, the teacher, the kindergarten mistress, or whoever is responsible for the child's education, cooperate with the treating physician.

Now for a brief comment on so-called paradoxical therapy with methylphenidate (®Ritalin) or amphetamines in hyperkinetic children. Among our patients, too, we have sometimes obtained spectacular results with this "paradoxical" treatment. But I disapprove of the practice, which seems to be quite a common one in the United States, of administering such drugs as an aid to differential diagnosis and of concluding that a child who responds well to the medication must *post hoc propter hoc* be suffering from a hyperkinetic syndrome. I say this because similar dramatic responses can also be attained with psycho-active agents possessing other activity patterns; it's all a matter of finding out which drug "works" in a particular case.

To sum up, I would say: drug treatment – yes, but if possible never without at the same time ensuring that the child also receives comprehensive care and guidance; drug treatment – yes, but only under proper control.

R. KUHN: I would certainly endorse the comments of the last two speakers. As regards the final part of Dr. NISSEN's paper, may I suggest that – for the purpose of adapting the treatment as closely as possible to the individual requirements of each case – it might be preferable to begin by analysing the behavioural disorders nosologically and only afterwards to attempt a descriptive analysis, because the nosological method involves far fewer ambiguities than the descriptive approach.

Another point I'd like to mention is one that has often occurred to me in connection with the way in which the relationship between the environment and the child now tends to be viewed in modern child psychiatry. We hear so much nowadays about the attitudes adopted by the parents, the teachers, or other persons involved in the child's upbringing, and about the repercussions which these have on the child. But little if any thought seems to be given to the repercussions of the child's behaviour on the parents. Very often, in fact, abnormal behavioural patterns encountered in parents are no more and no less than reactions to impossible behaviour on the part of their children. I therefore feel that one should begin by examining the dichotomy underlying this whole problem and that one should first try to determine where the primary cause is located. If we take a look at all the members of the family, we may well discover that two, three, four, or even more children are absolutely normal in their behaviour and that only one child stands out like a sore thumb. The reactions of the parents and of others responsible for this child's upbringing and education may be found to encroach on the pathological, and we as psychiatrists must then provide treatment for them too, because they have been so severely tormented by the child that they are utterly at the end of their tether. Such, to put it bluntly, are some of the sobering aspects of child psychiatry.

I. GAMSTORP: I, too, have a few comments to make on Dr. NISSEN's paper. Firstly, he referred to the many children who display the hyperkinetic syndrome and are seen by child psychiatrists in particular. In my experience, a large proportion of these schoolchildren will already have shown movement disorders at a younger age and still do when they start school. They are clumsy children who exhibit obvious neurological signs if you examine them in a paediatric neurological way, as opposed to the manner in which an adult would be examined neurologically. They have slow clumsy movements and lots of crude movements – a sign that their ability to move is immature. This creates many problems for them in school. We try to find these children at an early age, i.e. when they are three or four years old, and we start them on physiotherapy. Physiotherapy not only produces at least some improvement in the child's movements, but also makes the parents realise that something is organically wrong with the child; this realisation that the child cannot be blamed for the disorders lessens the feelings of guilt on the part of both the child and the parents. Moreover, physiotherapy gives the child a little more confidence when he starts school. I should be interested, Dr. NISSEN, to hear your views on this subject.

Secondly, amphetamine and methylphenidate are two drugs that have virtually disappeared from my country. We are not allowed to use them, except in individual cases for which we require special permission from the authorities. However, I cannot say that we miss them. The reason why they were forbidden in Sweden is that they were misused. Instead of giving them to their children, parents sold them, and they appeared on the black market for misusers. I wonder whether this problem has also been encountered in the German Federal Republic.

My final comment concerns the high incidence of behavioural disorders in school-children. You, Dr. NISSEN, quoted a figure of between 25 and 30%, and I have seen similar figures mentioned in many other studies from Stockholm and elsewhere. To me this always suggests that there must be something wrong either with our limits for normality or with the school, but certainly not with the child. I feel that measures could perhaps be taken to improve the schools, and that then we should have less need for drugs.

G. NISSEN: I should like to assure Dr. KIELHOLZ that I do, of course, entirely agree with what he said about the selection of antidepressant drugs for use in children. Classifications based on differential typology are, I would say, necessary not only in the case of depressive children but also for the treatment of all behavioural disorders. What I presented in Figure 3 of my paper was only a crude and simplified outline of the indications for the drugs listed; it is based primarily on phenomenological criteria and most certainly needs to be supplemented from the differential-typological angle. One major problem encountered in children with behavioural disorders lies precisely in the fact that usually the symptoms are not yet fully developed; instead, they tend to be rudimentary and to appear in varying combinations. This only goes to show once again how necessary it is to find more accurate ways and means of distinguishing behavioural disorders not only from abnormal psychic reactions but also from neuroses and psychopathic personality disorders.

I fully concur with Dr. RETT's comments. We don't stick to any rigid dosage schedule either; on the contrary, we always find ourselves obliged to adopt an individualised approach. The decision as to when a particular drug is indicated, however, is one that we reach largely on the basis of experience, which – since the circumstances of the case may often be difficult to elucidate – does not always prove a reliable guide. Every now and again we encounter massive side effects in response to quite small doses of major tranquillisers, for example, whereas we find that in other children these drugs produce no side effects, even when taken in considerable overdosages. Until three years ago I never treated hyperkinetic children with methylphenidate or amphetamines, despite the fact that I was of course already familiar with the American literature on their use. Then, one day a woman from Berlin, who happened to be a qualified pharmacist and who had been staying together with her child in the U.S.A., returned home to Berlin and brought the child along to my surgery. The child had been treated in the United States with amphetamines, and the mother told me about the dramatic transformation this medication had produced. I carried on treating the child in the same way and became convinced myself of the value of the amphetamines. Later on, I began using these drugs in cooperation with parents who were very critical, most of them being either school or university teachers themselves. I took great care to warn them of the possible side effects, although, according to the experience of American child psychiatrists, these appeared to be relatively rare. In many of the cases concerned, I once again observed some astonishingly good responses. An essential prerequisite for the success of this treatment too, however, is that the therapist should genuinely believe in the possibility of its exerting a beneficial effect – a belief which helps to motivate both the child and the parents. Incidentally, studies in the U.S.A. have shown that the improvement rate tends to increase in proportion to the number of neurological symptoms present.

In reply to Dr. GAMSTORP's remarks, I should like to say that in children drug treatment must be regarded, not as the first, but rather as the last resort. We must nevertheless beware of the arrogant attitude adopted by some psychoanalysts, who would preferably do nothing for a child that does not fall within the category of psycho-therapy. We are dealing after all, not with just a few children, but with hundreds of them, for whom we simply cannot provide the requisite psychotherapeutic facilities. Herein lies the cardinal advantage of drug treatment. In the case of our hyperkinetic children, we often find a history of pathological data relating to the mother's pregnancy or to the birth itself. Moreover, these children also tend to suffer from disturbances affecting fine motor functions, as reflected particularly in poor handwriting, they also have difficulty in distinguishing forms and shapes, and they exhibit neuropathological signs. We try to treat such cases by endeavouring to improve the child's psychomotor functions. Each country, of course, has its own schools of thought on this approach to treatment. We have been tackling the problem along the lines adopted in the studies undertaken in Hamm by HÜNNEKENS and KIPHARD*, but, in addition to the methods employed by these investigators, we are becoming increasingly aware of the great importance of the FROSTIG programme**, which has now also been translated into German.

With regard to the amphetamines, Dr. GAMSTORP, restrictions have also been imposed on their prescription in my country, although the doctor is still free to decide whether or not he wishes to prescribe them. In view of these difficulties, we are very pleased that there are now a number of other drugs – as listed in Figure 3 of my paper – which can be employed in lieu of the amphetamines or methylphenidate. Imipramine (®Tofranil) in particular has yielded excellent results in some cases, and the same applies to carbamazepine (®Tegretol) and to deanol p-acetamidobenzoate, a recently introduced drug with which, however, I must admit that I have lately encountered a few side effects.

I should like to thank Dr. BIRKMAYER for his reference to the fact that there is quite a large measure of agreement on various aetiological aspects. The genetically de-termined contribution to the pathogenesis of behavioural disorders is something that we must try to establish individually in each child, particularly as I am sure that constitutional factors often do play a preponderant role. But, as you have already pointed out, Dr. BIRKMAYER, since these factors cannot be altered, we can only hope to change the child's environment – and unfortunately this is not possible either in every case. Here once again, then, we may have to fall back upon drugs, employed of course together with environmental therapy and remedial training.

Finally, I should particularly like to thank Dr. KUHN for his critical comments. His preference for a nosological rather than a descriptive analysis of behavioural disorders is one that I do, in fact, entirely share. It is true that the outline I presented in my paper was phenomenologically oriented, but the reason for this was that I wanted to provide a simple practical guide to the use of certain drugs. The fact of the matter is that in many cases we have no idea either of the pathogenetic constellation or of the cause of such behavioural disorders, nor can we always contrive to elucidate them under the conditions of ambulant practice.

You also referred, Dr. KUHN, to the role of the parents and to the suffering which the child's behaviour may cause them. In this connection, I should add that we also make it a practice to note the extent to which the abnormal behaviour of disturbed or mentally impaired children has induced a morbid atmosphere in their environment. We know, for example, what alienating effects a screaming, fretful, or grizzling infant may provoke in the family, and that the mother's reactions to such a strain are liable in turn to prove pathogenic, inasmuch as they may lead to secondary neuroticism in the child. Such complicated interreactions are sometimes very difficult indeed to sort out! One case that springs to my mind in this connection was that of a child suffering

---

* HÜNNEKENS, H., KIPHARD, E.: Übung der Motorik als therapeutische Methode bei entwicklungsrückständigen Kindern. Jb. Jugendpsychiat. *2*, 177 (1960)
** FROSTIG, M.: Movement education: theory and practice (Follet Educational Cor-poration 1970)

from mild brain damage who kept the whole family on tenterhooks; the mother told me that she had six normal children and only this one "cuckoo's egg", which fate had, as it were, foisted upon her and which didn't really belong to the family. It is precisely children of this kind, however, who, because of their behaviour and the reactions it evokes, run an added risk of developing neuroses.

The psychotropic effect of carbamazepine in non-epileptic patients, with particular reference to problems posed by clinical studies in children with behavioural disorders

by H. Remschmidt[*]

1. Introduction

Despite the clinical experience acquired so far with carbamazepine (®Tegretol) in the management of behavioural disorders in non-epileptic patients, and although several systematically conducted trials have been undertaken with the drug in such patients, its use in this indication may still be regarded as constituting a new departure in psycho-active pharmacotherapy. I cannot therefore offer any definitive answers to the questions that arise in this connection, nor do I intend to report on purely empirical observations of my own. My task, as I see it, is simply to outline various considerations which might perhaps help to shed further light on this indication for carbamazepine. To begin with, however, let me first dwell for a moment on another aspect of the drug's use to which I have devoted particular attention – namely, to its effect on the personality changes encountered in epileptic children.

Several authors have come to the conclusion, on the basis of well-documented studies, that carbamazepine exerts a beneficial influence on epileptic personality changes[3, 5, 7], inasmuch as it:

1. Activates *psychomotor function*;
2. Improves certain *psychopathological symptoms* belonging to the "core" syndrome of epileptic personality changes, such as sluggishness of thought, "stickiness", instability of mood, dysphoria, automatism, and stereotypy[10, 11];
3. Improves *social behaviour* (the patients become better adapted to life at home and at work, they take more interest in their surroundings, they indulge in more outward-going activities, and they show more initiative).

Some of these effects are regarded as being indicative of the drug's "psychotropic" action. While the majority of authors acknowledge that carbamazepine does in fact possess psychotropic properties, some (e.g. Rett[15]) doubt whether these properties can be demonstrated in children. This, however, is a matter which time does not permit me to go into in detail here. Let me merely point out that, since epilepsy is invariably associated with the types of disorder mentioned above, the possibility of there being a connection between anti-convulsive and psychotropic activity cannot be rejected out of hand.

Several of the symptoms I have listed as showing a fairly reliable response to carbamazepine are also encountered in non-epileptic children suffering from

---

* Klinik für Kinder- und Jugendpsychiatrie der Universität, Marburg-Lahn, German Federal Republic.

behavioural disorders. In the present paper the term "behavioural disorders" is employed in a very broad sense to denote all disturbances in adaptation which, whether accompanied or unaccompanied by organic disease, are reflected in changes in *psychomotor function* and *social behaviour*, as well as in certain *psychopathological phenomena* such as instability of mood, inability to concentrate, aggressiveness, or loss of drive.

These disorders are being widely discussed nowadays under the headings of "minimal brain dysfunction" (M.B.D.), "hyperkinetic syndrome", "learning disabilities", and "behavioural disturbances marked by aggressiveness". Although it would appear a logical step to treat behavioural disorders with a drug capable of influencing target symptoms of this kind, there are several fundamental considerations which have to be borne in mind in this connection and to which I should like to draw attention here.

2. Some fundamental considerations

First of all, findings obtained in epileptics cannot be applied to non-epileptics for the following reasons:

1. In my opinion, it is not yet clear whether, and, if so, in what way an *anticonvulsive* effect is connected with a *psychotropic* effect (cf. LEDER[5]). If such a connection did exist, it would of course have repercussions on the mode of action of carbamazepine in non-epileptic patients as well.

2. There is evidence that carbamazepine exerts a strikingly good effect in cases of epilepsy characterised by certain distinctive psychopathological syndromes. This raises the question as to the patient's "initial psychopathological status" and the extent to which the latter might be responsible for considerable variations in the therapeutic efficacy of carbamazepine.

3. The response to carbamazepine is particularly favourable in the presence of non-specific E.E.G. abnormalities.

These considerations suggest that in non-epileptic patients carbamazepine offers especially good prospects in cases where psychic disorders are associated with – but not necessarily caused solely by – disturbances of organic cerebral origin. The drug's mode of action in patients with no organic cerebral disease could, in principle, be completely different; but, so far as I am aware, no meaningful studies have yet been carried out in this field. The problem thus arises as to whether there is any justification for using the drug in entirely disparate behavioural disorders, irrespective of their aetiology. To my way of thinking, this use is justified under certain conditions, among which I would mention:

1. Provided no other, more causal method of treatment is available, which is known to yield good responses in a certain percentage of cases.

2. Provided the disorder in question is chronic and is considered by the physician in charge of the case to require treatment.

3. Provided the drug employed causes few side effects.

4. Provided careful attention is paid to the patient's family setting and occupational environment, in order to make sure that these do not contain any sources of conflict responsible for maintaining the symptoms. In some cases, the presence of such conflicts may even be a contra-indication for drug therapy.

3. Results obtained with carbamazepine in non-epileptic children with behavioural disorders

At a recent meeting in Basle, at which child psychiatrists, paediatricians, clinical psychologists, and pharmacologists exchanged their views and experiences on this subject, the conclusion was reached that beneficial clinical results can be achieved with carbamazepine in the following target syndromes, more or less irrespective of their origin: hyperactivity and hypo-activity, hyperkinesia and hypokinesia, lack of concentration, behavioural disturbances marked by aggressiveness, and mood disorders of a dysphoric type.

According to the literature available to me, 28 clinical trials have so far been carried out with carbamazepine in altogether more than 800 children and adolescents displaying very heterogeneous patterns of disturbed behaviour. The quality of the methods employed in these trials varied, but the results can be summarised as follows:

1. The seven double-blind trials conducted to date in children exhibiting various behavioural disorders (with and without pathological E.E.G. findings) have yielded widely differing results. In three of them (GROH et al.[1]; PUENTE[8]; PUENTE et al.[9]) the superiority of carbamazepine over placebo was found to be statistically significant as regards enhancement of drive, promotion of purposeful activity, improvement in mood, and social adaptation. In two other investigations [KIVALO et al.[4]; SCHIFINO et al. (unpublished findings, 1969)], in which carbamazepine was likewise compared with placebo, there was a tendency for the former to exert a better overall effect on the behavioural disorders. Finally, in the remaining two double-blind studies [BETTSCHART et al. (unpublished findings, 1969); NISSEN et al.[6]] no difference could be found between carbamazepine and placebo.

2. In the 21 non-comparative studies, of which only 17 could be evaluated, carbamazepine was reported to have exerted a positive effect on the target symptoms of *hyperkinesia* (in nine out of the 17 studies) and *aggressiveness* (in five out of the 17).

In ten of these 17 studies the investigators point out that carbamazepine elicits particularly good responses in the presence of non-specific pathological E.E.G. findings. This might be interpreted as evidence of a correlation between anticonvulsive and psychotropic properties (a more detailed discussion of this question is to be found in the paper by LEDER[5]).

3. None of the known studies conducted in non-epileptic children with behavioural disorders makes any reference to a subjective improvement such as

has been reported in adult epileptics treated with carbamazepine (cf. LEDER[5]). While the assessment of subjective improvement admittedly poses methodological problems, these problems are not insoluble.

4. Thirteen of the 28 studies carried out in non-epileptic children and adolescents contain detailed information on *side effects* (relating to altogether 413 patients). Side effects were in fact reported in 26% of the patients and necessitated withdrawal of the drug in 2.7%. The commonest side effect was tiredness (17.4% of cases), followed by skin reactions (4.4%), dizziness, and nausea.

4. Conclusions

The results obtained to date show that carbamazepine brings about certain changes in behaviour and in state of mind in both epileptics and non-epileptics.

As regards its effect on *behaviour*, there is, I feel, some objective evidence that the drug exerts an influence on psychomotor function, drive, and mood. Concerning its effect on the patient's *state of mind*, it seems that in response to treatment with carbamazepine the patients become less plaintive, show less of a tendency towards hypochondriasis, and experience a diminution in anxiety and tension, while at the same time their mood brightens, their drive becomes enhanced, and their initiative increases. State of mind and behaviour must always be considered in relation to the social setting in which the patient lives. Changes in the patient himself invariably also evoke alterations in his environment – and it is often virtually impossible to separate these alterations from the effects of the drug as such. This also makes clinical trials extremely difficult.

From the data that have been reviewed in this paper the following conclusions can be drawn:

1. It is essential to find satisfactorily measurable variables which would make it possible to obtain reliable objective evidence of the effects of carbamazepine on behaviour *and* on the patient's state of mind. For this purpose, close attention should be paid to tests of *psychomotor function,* the possibilities of which are far from having been exhausted and which can serve as subtle indicators of changes in many different dimensions, such as drive, arousal, and mood. On the other hand, if tests of motor performance are included in a plan of clinical trials, the extent to which the results are affected by carbamazepine may vary widely depending on the complexity and difficulty of the tests and also on the patient's initial psychopathological status. This is a problem we have highlighted in a study with thioridazine, in which we found that the drug exerted a clear-cut positive effect on simple motor performances (e.g. in tapping tests), but was not superior to placebo in complex multiple-choice tests[13]. Another methodological difficulty connected with the use of psychomotor variables is that of creating a situation approximately commensurate

with the type of behaviour it is desired to record. Only if this problem is satis-factorily solved can meaningful data be obtained.

2. Even in the case of children, it is absolutely essential, in my opinion, to take account also of *changes in the patient's state of mind*. These changes can be objectively assessed in a *direct* manner by resorting to appropriate interrogation, and also *indirectly* by asking the patient's relatives about his behaviour. Indirect information of this kind, however, should be treated with caution. In a study on parent-child relationships in families in which there was an epileptic child, we found that the ability of the parents to assess the behaviour of their children depended to a large extent on the type of personality displayed by the parents themselves; this applied in particular to extreme abnormalities of behaviour, such as violence, destructiveness, and fits of rage[12].

3. Also indispensable is the need to provide the child's parents or relatives with extremely detailed advice and to explain to them exactly what *role* car-bamazepine should play in the *overall treatment schedule*. In this connection, due account must be taken of the well-known possibility that the drug will be regarded by the parents as affording them an *alibi* which absolves them from the obligation to modify their own behaviour.

4. Finally, there is also a question of *ethics* to be borne in mind. If drugs are used to treat all forms of abnormal behaviour irrespective of aetiology, there is a risk that they will mask the real underlying cause and possibly do more harm than good. Obviously, this is not a risk that should be taken if the aetiology is known. On the other hand, the physician is often confronted with complex and chronic disorders of adaptation, the cause of which is usually unknown or which are due to so many different factors that it is difficult to obtain a clear-cut picture. In such cases, there seems to be good reason for administering a drug which is claimed to bring about an improvement in certain well-defined patterns of abnormal behaviour and to produce no serious side effects. Whether or not carbamazepine fully justifies this claim is a question which, despite the experience reported in this paper, can only be answered after further detailed studies have been carried out.

References

1 Groh, C., Rosenmayr, F., Birbaumer, N.: Psychotrope Wirkung von Carbam-azepin bei nicht-epileptischen Kindern. Med. Mschr. *25*, 329 (1971)

2 Ketz, E.: Vorläufiger Bericht über Behandlungsergebnisse mit dem neuen Anti-epileptikum G 32883. Joint meeting of the German, Swiss, and Austrian E.E.G. Societies, Zurich 1963

3 Ketz, E.: Tegretol – ein neues Antiepileptikum. Praxis *53*, 264 (1964)

4 Kivalo, E., Seppäläinen, A.-M., Lydecken, K.: Om behandling med carbam-azepin (Tegretol) av orotillstånd uppträdande i samband med svåra fall av hjärnskador och utvecklingsrubbningar [The treatment of the agitated and most severe cases of cerebral injury and cerebral palsy with carbamazepine (Tegretol)]. Nord. psykiat. T. *22*, 44 (1968)

5 Leder, A.: Tegretal: Zum Problem der psychotropen Wirkung. Nervenarzt *41*, 59 (1970)

6 Nissen, G., Spilimbergo, A., Flach, D.: Tegretal bei kindlichen Verhaltensstörungen. Polycopied manuscript (ciba-geigy, Basle)

7 Pakesch, E.: Untersuchungen über ein neuartiges Antiepileptikum. Wien. med. Wschr. *113*, 794 (1963)

8 Puente, R.M.: The use of carbamazepine in the treatment of behavioural disorders in children. In Birkmayer, W. (Editor): Epileptic seizures – behaviour – pain, Int. Symp., St. Moritz 1975, p. 243 (Huber, Berne/Stuttgart/Vienna 1975)

9 Puente, R.M., Barriga, F., Morales, M.T.: Estudio doble-ciego con carbamazepina en un grupo de escolares con daño cerebral. Comunicación preliminar. Medicina (Méx.) *53*, 97 (1973)

10 Remschmidt, H.: Experimentelle Untersuchungen zur sogenannten epileptischen Wesensänderung. Fortschr. Neurol. Psychiat. *38*, 524 (1970)

11 Remschmidt, H.: Testpsychologische und experimentelle Untersuchungen zur Psychopathologie der Epilepsien. In Penin, H. (Editor): Psychische Störungen bei Epilepsie. Psychosen, Verstimmungen, Persönlichkeitsveränderungen, XIVth Ann. Meet. Dtsch. Sekt. Int. Liga Epilepsie, Bonn 1972, p. 135 (Schattauer, Stuttgart/New York 1973)

12 Remschmidt, K., Keil, S., Niebergall, G., Merschmann, W.: Untersuchungen zur Eltern-Kind-Beziehung in Familien mit einem epileptischen Kind. In preparation

13 Remschmidt, H., Mewe, F., Mewe, G., Dauner, I., Merschmann, W.: Der Einfluss von Thioridazin (Melleril) auf Psychomotorik, Konzentrationsverhalten und Reaktionsvermögen bei verhaltensgestörten Kindern. In preparation

14 Rett, A.: Zur Beurteilung der Wirkung von Anticonvulsiva im Kindesalter – ein klinisches und entwicklungsphysiologisches Problem. Neue öst. Z. Kinderheilk. *7*, 178 (1963)

15 Rett, A.: Zur Frage der sogenannten psychotropen Wirksamkeit des Tegretol in der Behandlung der kindlichen Epilepsie. In Pateisky, K., Lechner, H. (Editors): Sozialmedizinische und therapeutische Aspekte der psychischen Veränderungen bei Epilepsie, Wiener Symp., 1968, p. 103 (Basle 1970)

The psychotropic effect of Tegretol in non-epileptic children, with particular reference to the drug's indications

by C. Groh*

Before discussing the psychotropic effect of ®Tegretol (carbamazepine) in non-epileptic children, I think it would be advisable to consider the reasons justifying the drug's use in this type of patient.

In the very first publications on Tegretol attention was already drawn to the beneficial influence which this preparation had been found to exert on behavioural disorders and personality changes in epileptic patients. Subsequently, however, this so-called psychotropic activity – which is considered to constitute a distinctive advantage of Tegretol as compared with other antiepileptic agents, but which often tends to be described in more general terms such as "a brightening effect on epileptic personality changes", "an ability to make patients more active and communicative", or "a capacity to improve sociability" – has not gone unchallenged, doubts having been cast both on the quality of the effect as such and on its existence as an intrinsic feature of the drug's pharmacological profile. Hence the double-blind clinical studies which have been performed on children in particular in an attempt to furnish objective evidence of the psychotropic effect of Tegretol and to confirm that it is indeed distinct from the drug's other properties.

The greater the importance attached to the role played by somatic factors in the pathogenesis of behavioural disorders in children, including especially factors connected with minimal brain dysfunction, the more convincing a case one can make out in favour of the view that for the treatment of such syndromes what is required are not only psychotherapy and remedial training – which still remain essential elements of any holistic approach to child psychiatry – but also drugs for use in support of these methods.

The observation that behavioural disorders in children are not infrequently associated with abnormal electro-encephalographic findings and that in such cases treatment with anticonvulsants may prove effective should, of course, not prompt one to jump to a diagnosis of "latent epilepsy" or "masked epilepsy"; but it nevertheless does provide a strong argument for the use of a special, psychotropically acting, anticonvulsant in the management of behavioural abnormalities. What is more, a number of reports on open studies have in fact already been published from which it is apparent that children suffering from behavioural disturbances of varying symptomatology and aetiology may in some cases show a marked improvement in response to Tegretol.

* Allgemeines Krankenhaus der Stadt Wien, Universitäts-Kinderklinik, Vienna, Austria.

Difficulties arise, however, when one attempts to make a summary evaluation of the results contained in the relevant publications[4]. What one expects to obtain from a review of the literature are, above all, answers to the following two questions:

Firstly, can the so-called psychotropic effect of Tegretol be demonstrated objectively?

Secondly, what form does this effect take, and on which target symptoms or syndromes is Tegretol most likely to exert a favourable influence? In other words, what are the indications for Tegretol in non-epileptic children?

Regarding the first of the two questions, in view of the results obtained in open studies it seems probable that Tegretol does have an intrinsic psychotropic effect. Moreover, although the number of controlled trials is relatively small and only some of them have been statistically evaluated, their findings, too, point in the same direction.

We ourselves have also carried out a study designed to shed light on both of these questions[2]. It consisted of a double-blind crossover trial involving 20 non-epileptic children who were aged 8–14 years and who, though of normal intelligence, displayed various disturbed patterns of behaviour. As shown in Tables 1 and 2, the response to Tegretol as compared with placebo proved to be statistically significant, even though the placebo also appears at first sight to have been by no means ineffective. Although we attempted in addition to pinpoint the main features of the drug's effect by reference to certain target symptoms (Table 3), we found it impossible to draw up a spectrum of indications for Tegretol, and this for two reasons: firstly, the number of cases treated was not large enough and, secondly and more especially, our expectations concerning the therapeutic response – coloured as they were by our previous experience with Tegretol in epileptic children – led to a certain bias in our selection of the patients to be admitted to the trial.

With regard to the second of the two questions mentioned above, on the strength of the experience we had acquired with Tegretol in the 20 non-epileptic children already referred to, we continued employing the drug as treatment for behavioural disorders in children seen during the day-to-day course of work in our out-patients' department. By using Tegretol in a larger number of patients over a longer observation period, we hoped to obtain a deeper insight into those effects of the drug that are specifically relevant to child psychiatry. Comparisons between the respective data contained in the literature are difficult to make, because of lack of uniformity in the nomenclature used, because the nosological classifications adopted often differ very considerably, and because the patients have been selected on the basis of widely varying criteria. The symptoms most frequently alleged to respond well to Tegretol are hyperkinesia and aggressiveness. In this connection, however, it must be pointed out that individual symptoms may be interpretable in a variety of ways and attributable to a variety of radically differing causes. During childhood in particular, aggressiveness for example may result from excessive, uncontrolled activity, which the child cannot keep in check because he still lacks the requisite powers of self-criticism and deliberation; alternatively, what

Table 1. Overall results obtained with Tegretol versus placebo in a double-blind crossover trial involving 20 non-epileptic children with behavioural disorders. The difference in the response to Tegretol as compared with placebo was found to be highly significant in the chi-square test (P < 0.01).

Medication	Total number of cases	Response			
		Marked improvement	Moderate improvement	No change	Deterioration
Tegretol	20	10	6	3	1
Placebo	20	1	6	12	1

Table 2. Results obtained in the same 20 cases as shown in Table 1, analysed by reference to the sequence in which Tegretol and placebo were administered. Note that the sequence of administration has an influence on the response elicited by placebo: in the case of placebo, the chi-square test revealed a significant difference in the responses (P < 0.05), depending on whether placebo was given in the first (I) or in the second (II) period of treatment; in the case of Tegretol, by contrast, the sequence of administration did not significantly affect the response.

Medication	Treatment period	Number of cases per treatment period	Response			
			Marked improvement	Moderate improvement	No change	Deterioration
Tegretol	I	10	6	1	2	1
	II	10	4	5	1	–
Placebo	I	10	1	5	4	–
	II	10	–	1	8	1

Table 3. Results obtained in the same 20 children as shown in Tables 1 and 2, analysed by reference to target symptoms. These results suggest that the psychotropic activity of Tegretol takes the form chiefly of an increase in drive and a brightening of mood. The drug exerted only a moderate effect on psychovegetative symptoms.

Target symptoms	Number of cases	Medication	Response			
			Marked improvement	Moderate improvement	No change	Deterioration
Impaired drive	7	Tegretol	4	2	1	–
		Placebo	1	2	3	1
Dysphoric mood changes	6	Tegretol	3	1	1	1
		Placebo	–	–	6	–
Anxiety and neurotic symptoms	4	Tegretol	3	–	1	–
		Placebo	–	3	1	–
Psychovegetative syndrome	3	Tegretol	–	3	–	–
		Placebo	–	1	2	–

may well be even more likely is that such aggressiveness is actually a sign of weakness – as when a listless and apathetic child feels himself, and indeed allows himself to be, driven into a corner by his schoolmates and finally becomes violent because he can see no other way of escape. A similar reaction can sometimes also be observed in the children of oversolicitous parents who, when faced with the "harsh realities" of an environment that is new to them, may likewise exhibit symptoms of aggressiveness.

For these reasons, we felt it would be preferable, not to judge the success or failure of psychopharmacotherapy by reference to individual symptoms, but to endeavour to take closer account of clinical reality by basing our evaluation on the results obtained in various psychopathological syndromes. It is by no means always easy, however, to assign a case to a particular syndrome, especially in children. Depending on the child's age and phase of development, the symptomatology is liable to change, and syndromes may appear to dissolve, as it were, or to blend into other syndromes.

It must also be borne in mind that a behavioural disorder can manifest itself only in and through the environment. Even a serious form of personality change may sometimes not only be tolerated by the child's environment, but may be coped with so skilfully by teachers and parents that, despite its continuing existence, the child manages to adapt himself satisfactorily. Conversely, other cases occur in which symptoms of a critical developmental stage that are merely somewhat more pronounced than usual already become regarded as pathological by the child's elders, whose intolerant and unfeeling reactions may possibly aggravate the symptoms and result in their neurotic fixation; examples in point include protracted or intensified phases of defiance, prolonged infantile erethism, puberal crises, and also symptoms of disharmonic maturation (problems of acceleration, partial infantilism).

Hence, the type of "syndromal diagnosis" which we attempt to employ must inevitably be of a provisional nature, because it can often only take account of a cross-section through the various psychopathological symptom-complexes concerned. From the therapeutic standpoint, however, this approach has nevertheless proved practicable.

Let us now see whether, on the basis of such syndromal diagnoses, it is possible to discern any special indications for Tegretol.

When we reviewed the cases treated in our out-patients' department we found a total of 62 non-epileptic children with behavioural disorders who had been treated with Tegretol and kept under adequate observation for a sufficiently long time (at least six months) to enable us to pronounce judgment on their response. Whereas the 35 children who exhibited no change under the treatment had shown various patterns of disturbed behaviour, of the remaining 27 who did undergo an improvement 19 had had a psychopathological syndrome characterised by the following symptomatology: they were emotionally labile, moody or irritable, and quite often evinced paranoid responses to their experiences, as a result of which they tended to react violently at the slightest provocation; all their reactions were unpredictable; signs of anxiety were sometimes present, but more frequent – particularly among the younger children – were motor restlessness and agitation. In cases where the latter two symptoms are a prominent feature of the syndrome, the patient's behaviour bears a close resemblance to that of hyperkinetic-erethistic children. On the other hand – notably in older children, i.e. in those aged over ten years and especially over 12 years – one tends to encounter diminished drive rather than restlessness; such children appear listless and devoid of any interests, they seem incapable of making any effort at school in particular, and are therefore accused by parents and teachers of being lazy.

Among the many and varied symptoms just outlined, the one that strikes us as being of cardinal significance is the emotional lability or moodiness, from which the other behavioural anomalies apparently stem. We would therefore apply to such patterns of behaviour the term "dysphoric or dysthymic syndrome", which – as in the case of depression occurring in adults – can be subdivided into an agitated and a retarded form. It may perhaps also be possible to draw a parallel between the age dependence of these two facets and the age distribution of the "erethistic-hyperkinetic" and "enechetic" syndrome in epileptic children as reported by FREUDENBERG[1] and MATTHES[3].

Another question worthy of interest in this connection is whether the aetiology of the behavioural disorder has any bearing on the indication for treatment with Tegretol. Do patients, for example, in whom examination discloses clinical, psychological, or E.E.G. evidence suggestive of an organic lesion stand a better chance of responding favourably to Tegretol?

Findings reported in the literature indicate that this may perhaps be the case, inasmuch as the successful responses recorded chiefly involve patients with abnormal E.E.G. patterns (although it must be added that negative confirmation – i.e. absence of response in the presence of a normal E.E.G. – is often lacking). In our own double-blind trial, too, only one of the 20 children had a normal E.E.G., despite the fact that they were all selected for the study on the basis of purely clinical criteria and without prior knowledge of their electro-encephalograms. Unfortunately, we are not in possession of adequate data on all the children whom we afterwards treated routinely in our out-patients' department; consequently, we cannot yet answer the question as to the possible influence of the aetiology on the response to treatment, although we certainly regard this as a point deserving of further discussion.

References

1 FREUDENBERG, D.: Leistungs- und Verhaltensstörungen bei kindlichen Epilepsien. Bibl. psychiat. neurol. (Basle) No. 135: 51 (1968)
2 GROH, C., ROSENMAYR, F., BIRBAUMER, N.: Psychotrope Wirkung von Carbamazepin bei nicht-epileptischen Kindern. Med. Mschr. *25*, 329 (1971)
3 MATTHES, A.: Psychische Veränderungen bei kindlichen Epilepsien. Nervenarzt *32*, 2 (1961)
4 REMSCHMIDT, H.: The psychotropic effect of carbamazepine in non-epileptic patients, with particular reference to problems posed by clinical studies in children with behavioural disorders. In Birkmayer, W. (Editor): Epileptic seizures – behaviour – pain, Int. Symp., St. Moritz 1975, p. 253 (Huber, Berne/Stuttgart/Vienna 1975)

Behavioural disorders in non-epileptic children and their treatment with carbamazepine

by V. Kuhn-Gebhart*

At a joint Swiss-Austrian meeting on the subject of electro-encephalography which took place in Vaduz in the autumn of 1966 R. Kuhn and I presented a paper on the problems involved in administering anti-epileptic treatment to apparently non-epileptic children with behavioural disorders. In the course of this paper we described the results of personal observations which at that time extended back over a period of about ten years. On the same occasion, we also mentioned a paper which Anastasopoulos[1] had delivered at the IVth World Congress of Psychiatry held in Madrid a short while previously, as well as personal communications made at this congress by de Oliveira Bastos. The paper presented by Anastasopoulos from Greece, and the observations reported by de Oliveira Bastos from Brazil, fully corroborated our own views on this topic. Most of the results described by these two authors were obtained with carbamazepine (®Tegretol), whereas we ourselves had initially used phenobarbitone and hydantoins and did not start employing carbamazepine until later. At the Vaduz meeting we referred to "surprising positive and unexpected negative results". As our communication was never published, we should like to repeat here some of our findings:

1. In a large series of children with behavioural disorders, some of whom had been followed up for many years, we had found that a considerable number of these patients showed a marked or very marked improvement in response to anti-epileptic treatment, even though their case histories contained not the slightest evidence of epilepsy and even though, with very few exceptions, epilepsy did not manifest itself subsequently.

2. The E.E.G. patterns in these cases are sometimes a little underdeveloped; more commonly, though, they reveal signs of considerable irregularity with a pronounced tendency to theta and delta activity. Hyperventilation often activates the E.E.G., giving rise to synchronous phases of slow activity which are occasionally accompanied by rather sharp waves, but which display no real epilepsy potentials. The E.E.G. patterns may improve along with a clinical improvement, but frequently they do not.

Broadly speaking, the more abnormal the E.E.G. findings, the greater the likelihood that anti-epileptic treatment will prove successful; conversely, the more normal the E.E.G. findings, the greater the likelihood that psycho-active drugs in the narrower sense of the term, including in particular antidepressants of the iminodibenzyl group or phenothiazines, will yield good results.

---

* Kantonale Psychiatrische Klinik, Münsterlingen, Switzerland.

3. In many cases these children with behavioural disturbances have a family history of mental illness, which may take the form of epilepsy, but is more often associated with depression, suicide, schizophrenia, or psychopathic personality disorders.

4. While some of the children display varying degrees of mental deficiency, many of them are of normal or even above-normal intelligence.

5. The clinical pictures they present are extremely varied and sometimes feature apparently contradictory elements. Difficulties in schooling and upbringing are the principal outward characteristics. Frequently encountered in these children are various forms of hyperkinesia marked, for example, by general restlessness, nervousness, hyperactivity, tics, excitability and irritability, quarrelsomeness and aggressiveness, and a tendency to indulge in loud and noisy behaviour. There are also cases – though not so many – in which the clinical picture is dominated by apathy, aloofness, indifference, sluggishness, and loss of drive. As far as mood is concerned, the patients may be shy, anxious, inhibited or even depressive, or else they may be overoptimistic, incapable of realising the abnormality of their behaviour, completely fearless, boastful, and bragging. Genuine mood disorders often play a major role in the clinical picture; in some instances, they may have already persisted for many years, while in others they are phasic or episodic and exhibit a variety of different overtones. Asocial acts – involving truancy, running away from home, lying, stealing, or unrestrained sexuality – are sometimes met with. Nocturnal and diurnal enuresis and encopresis may also be encountered. Sleep patterns are sometimes completely normal, and sometimes marked by restlessness. Occasionally, the predominating symptoms are anxiety and autonomic nervous disturbances such as headache, migraine, abdominal pain, sweating, and tachycardia.

6. The response which these children show to anti-epileptic treatment varies. A general improvement in behaviour may occur in some cases, while in others only certain symptoms are eliminated and the rest persist unchanged. Where a positive response is achieved, it usually sets in within a few days or, at the most, a few weeks. As withdrawal of medication is apt to be followed by a prompt relapse, the drugs must generally be continued for quite a long time.

7. Long-term treatment of this kind can for the most part only be carried out on an ambulatory basis, which means that the physician can never be sure whether the drugs are being taken regularly; moreover, he cannot know whether the child is also being exposed to other factors, such as psychic conflicts in particular, which may interfere with the effect of treatment. Hence, positive results are of relatively greater significance than negative ones.

8. These observations of ours raise a number of questions of general interest: a) Is the effect of a drug in children with behavioural disturbances perhaps no more than a placebo effect? Is the beneficial response achieved with a drug possibly attributable simply to a coincidental spontaneous improvement in the child's condition? Does the mere fact of examining the child and talking to him exert a positive psychological influence which outweighs the effect of whatever drug may be prescribed? When analysing the results obtained in

our patients, we have borne all these critical objections in mind, and we have come to the conclusion that it is extremely unlikely that a successful response would have been achieved in such a high percentage of cases if the drugs used had not exerted a genuine therapeutic effect.

b) Another pertinent question is whether those children whose behavioural disturbances respond to anti-epileptic therapy might not in fact be epileptics whose epilepsy has just not been detected, either because at the time of examination seizures are absent, very infrequent, or occur only at night, or else because the illness takes the form of epileptic equivalents which are not recognised as such. This is certainly a possible explanation in cases where a history of clear-cut epilepsy is found among the patient's close relatives, or where the patient himself displays isolated symptoms of a suspicious nature. It is conceivable that a few of our patients may have had undetected epilepsy, but definitely not the majority of them, because we deliberately excluded from our series all children with a past history of epileptic manifestations.

c) A further point to consider is whether a favourable response to anti-epileptic drugs might not be partly due to the latter's "non-specific" effects, e.g. to their sedative or hypnotic properties. This interpretation may well appear plausible in some cases, particularly in those where the clinical picture prior to treatment is marked by hyperactivity, restless sleep, and anxious excitation. On the other hand, we can point to cases in which all attempts to achieve a sedative effect failed until anti-epileptic drugs were given.

d) The possibility that carbamazepine exerts a distinctive effect on behavioural disorders in children cannot be rejected out of hand, especially since the drug has also been observed to exert a beneficial influence on psychic disturbances in adult epileptics. It can, however, be argued that the same applies to phenobarbitone, hydantoins, and combinations of these two groups of drugs. Nonetheless, we have encountered cases in which the classic drugs failed to elicit a response until they were supplemented by carbamazepine – a finding which suggests that carbamazepine possesses some additional therapeutic property.

e) It is still extremely difficult to explain why modes of behaviour, such as lying and stealing, which are subsumed under the heading of "deficiencies of character and upbringing", should disappear in response to drugs. The same is true of abnormal sexual behaviour and of aggressiveness resulting therefrom. Likewise hard to account for is the fact that one and the same drug should produce a "sedative" effect in one case and a "stimulant" effect in another. In this connection, it should be pointed out that children with behavioural disorders who have a family history of endogenous depression or manic-depressive psychosis often show a dramatic response to antidepressants, especially if their E.E.G. patterns are normal. There also seem to be cases – not only among children but among adults as well – in which an optimal response can only be achieved by combining an anti-epileptic drug with an antidepressant.

In the light of our experience to date, we have the impression that the more the picture is dominated by external signs of neglect, faulty upbringing, and unfavourable social factors, the less likelihood there is of attaining successful results with drugs. Conversely, many of the children in whom we have achieved good responses come from orderly homes. This is, of course, not really surprising, because in cases where the child's family circumstances are unsatisfactory the physician's instructions are often carried out only in desultory fashion, if at all. Furthermore, these children are exposed to damaging external influences which are so strong that any attempt to improve their psychic condition is virtually doomed from the start. Finally, quite a number of these children have a particularly unfavourable family history – and not only in respect of cyclic diseases or epilepsy.

That cyclic diseases and epilepsy, on the one hand, and neglect and faulty upbringing, on the other, may give rise to very similar behavioural disorders, which respond sometimes to a drug and sometimes to educational measures or psychotherapy, merely confirms that there are only a limited number of ways in which a child's organism or psyche is capable of reacting.

So much for the conclusions we had reached eight years ago. Since then we have employed anti-epileptic drugs – occasionally a hydantoin preparation, but usually carbamazepine, which is probably the most effective – to treat many additional cases of a similar nature. In children displaying marked hyperactivity, we sometimes add methylphenidate (®Ritalin) to the regimen in order to reinforce the effect of carbamazepine. In a few instances, it has not been possible to continue treatment with carbamazepine for an adequate length of time owing to the appearance of drug rash. On the whole, however, the results achieved have fully confirmed our previous findings. It should perhaps be added that in many cases we have noticed that a small dose of only 50 mg. carbamazepine once or twice daily yields the best responses.

To obtain some idea of the success rate in our patients, we analysed the results recorded in the last 50 children treated over a sufficiently long period (for as many as eight years in one instance). Of these 50 patients, 30 showed a very good or good response, ten a clear-cut improvement, and the remaining ten no change, except for one child whose condition actually deteriorated.

To sum up, our experience has shown that behavioural disorders in children often respond well to anti-epileptic treatment. These findings of ours indicate once again how little justification there is today for rejecting the principle of treating such disorders with psycho-active drugs and for ascribing their pathogenesis solely to social, educational, and psychogenic factors. On the other hand, it must be admitted that psychotherapeutic guidance and social measures frequently have a decisive role to play in the management of these disorders, inasmuch as they provide the indispensable framework within which drug therapy is able to exert its full effect.

Reference

1 ANASTASOPOULOS, G.: Hysterische Manifestationen bei griechischen Kindern. In López Ibor, J. J. (Editor): Proc. IVth World Congr. Psychiat., Madrid 1966, Part III, p. 1612; Int. Congr. Ser. No. 150 (Excerpta Medica Foundation, Amsterdam etc. 1968)

The psychotropic effect of carbamazepine in non-epileptic adults, with particular reference to the drug's possible mechanism of action

by R. Kuhn*

Certain epileptologists hold the view that anti-epileptic drugs should be administered only in cases of confirmed epilepsy. For decades, however, phenobarbitone has played an important part in the treatment of non-epileptic autonomic nervous syndromes, cerebral circulatory disorders, subjective symptoms occurring as a sequel to brain injuries, and abnormal behavioural patterns. In these indications it is also frequently combined with other substances, as exemplified by such preparations as ®Bellergal and ®Priscophen.

Anti-epileptic drugs subsequently introduced were likewise tested for evidence of psychotropic activity, and attempts made to enhance this activity by modifying their formulation, one example in point being that of ®Atrium. In the case of carbamazepine (®Tegretol), although initial data on the type and degree of the drug's psychotropic properties were somewhat conflicting, the fact that in epileptic patients it does indeed exhibit such properties now appears to be undisputed. Epileptic personality changes characterised by retardation, "stickiness", unrestrained emotional outbursts and other poorly controlled reactions, as well as susceptibility to mood disorders and twilight states, often respond very well to carbamazepine. Depression in epileptic patients – which, owing to the epileptogenic effect of antidepressants, proves very difficult or even impossible to treat with such drugs – usually also shows a spectacular improvement under the influence of carbamazepine.

Pöldinger[5] reported that he had failed to observe any psychotropic effect in non-epileptic adults treated with carbamazepine. Later, however, at a joint Swiss-Austrian meeting on electro-encephalography held in Vaduz we ourselves (cf. Kuhn-Gebhart[4]) gave an account of the positive results we had obtained with anti-epileptic drugs in non-epileptic children. It is probably true to say that any psychopathological symptom encountered in epileptic patients is also liable to occur in persons who have never suffered from seizures and whose E.E.G. recordings are devoid of seizure potentials. Occasionally, evidence of epilepsy may be found in the family histories of such persons, but this is not generally the case. These individuals, to whom the term "epileptoid" is sometimes applied, frequently belong to the depressive, cyclothymic, or hysterical category or show a tendency towards obsessive-compulsive symptoms, and in many cases psychogenic reactions also appear to play a role of considerable importance. In patients of this kind one is therefore tempted to initiate treatment with antidepressants or major tranquillisers or to resort to psychotherapy. In cases where such measures yield little or no response, it has now

* Kantonale Psychiatrische Klinik, Münsterlingen, Switzerland.

for many years been our practice to switch to anti-epileptic medication; for this purpose we have lately been employing carbamazepine, which we have found to be the most effective choice and which frequently produces excellent results.

The prospects of a favourable response are best in those cases in which the pattern of the symptoms is suggestive of some underlying cerebro-organic cause or in which the E.E.G. tracings deviate from normal.

In addition to this very heterogeneous group of abnormal subjects and patients as described above, another new and well-circumscribed indication for carbamazepine has recently emerged. There has of late been an increasing number of reports referring to the problem of habituation to the benzodiazepines. These preparations are often prescribed in circumstances in which they are neither indicated nor therapeutically effective, e.g. in the presence of unrecognised depression. Now, as we all know, it is very difficult to withdraw benzodiazepines in cases where the patient has become habituated to them. The doctor who transfers such patients to an antidepressant repeatedly hears bitter complaints, coupled frequently with the reproach that the new drug he has prescribed causes severe excitation and insomnia. These, however, are not due to the antidepressant as such, but are withdrawal symptoms resulting from discontinuation of the benzodiazepine medication, which often in fact prove so troublesome as to make it impossible to change to a more suitable drug regimen. It was a verbal report from Sweden, referring to the use of carbamazepine in these benzodiazepine-dependent patients in a dosage of $\frac{1}{2}-1$ tablet three times daily, which prompted us to give the drug a trial in such cases. Our own experience to date suggests that this is a highly rewarding indication for carbamazepine. It also seems reasonable to expect that withdrawal symptoms attributable to other substances, as well as so-called "flashback" manifestations, might likewise respond favourably; although we have so far employed carbamazepine to treat only a few cases of this type, the results have been sufficiently encouraging to justify further attempts along these lines. In the presence of severe emotional excitation and mental unrest we have also successfully combined carbamazepine with low doses of a beta-blocker, and, in patients showing psychotic symptoms, with a major tranquilliser or an antidepressant.

In this connection, it is interesting to note that carbamazepine has also been recommended for the treatment of delirium tremens[1]. (Here, incidentally, it would have the advantage of not increasing the risk of road accidents in the case of patients – motorists or pedestrians – who consume alcohol in the course of their treatment, because "carbamazepine does not potentiate the effect exerted by alcohol on the degree or accuracy of perception".[6])

How are these psychotropic effects of carbamazepine to be accounted for? The first explanation which springs to mind is the fact that its chemical structure is akin to that of the iminodibenzyl compounds. This structural affinity may play some role, but – since there are also other anti-epileptic drugs displaying similar psychotropic effects – it can hardly be regarded as the decisive factor.

269

In our opinion it is the influence exerted by carbamazepine on motor function that deserves primary consideration in this connection. Hysterical and obsessive-compulsive phenomena, certain mood disorders (especially those of a depressive or irritable type), and various behavioural disturbances are associated with motor manifestations which differ in their form, intensity, course, and duration from normal patterns of movement, but which usually attract little if any attention. Many of these motor phenomena appear to be similar to the "catastrophe" type of reaction as described by KURT GOLDSTEIN[3]. Anti-epileptic drugs have a pronounced influence on motor function, inasmuch as they are capable of inhibiting the uncontrolled propagation of excitatory impulses which underlies both epileptic seizures as well as the motor manifestations of catastrophe reactions.

In many respects the action of anti-epileptic drugs on motor function is the reverse of that produced by antidepressants, which have the effect of imparting greater freedom of expression and action to the retarded depressive. But this retardation observed in depressive patients is not simply the opposite of excitation. The two extremes cannot be interpreted merely in terms of a deficiency or an excess of drive, because in both instances the production of movement itself is abnormal – which, incidentally, explains why retardation and excitation may also occur in a wide variety of combinations with each other. Perhaps this is one of the reasons why, especially in the presence of disorders associated with hypokinesia, it often proves necessary to administer carbamazepine in combination with an antidepressive drug – for which purpose maprotiline (®Ludiomil) is particularly suitable. The effect exerted by carbamazepine on withdrawal symptoms may possibly likewise be explainable along these same lines.

Bearing in mind how closely motor function is linked with mood and intellect, it would not seem unreasonable to suppose that positive changes in psychic functions might be achieved via an influence exerted in the motor sphere. Suppositions of this kind are, of course, purely hypothetical and, as such, by no means preclude other possible explanations which time does not permit me to consider here.

Finally, psychotropic drugs almost invariably serve to alleviate repercussions resulting from organic disturbances of cerebral function and thus to improve the patient's performance. This is just as true of anti-epileptic agents as it is of all psychopharmaceuticals. Impairment of cerebral function inevitably also renders the sufferer more susceptible to the effects of situational changes without and instinctual forces within, the most obvious initial signs of such enhanced susceptibility taking the form of reactive phenomena. Although KURT GOLDSTEIN[2] already drew attention to this some 50 years ago in an impressive paper entitled "Similarities in the functional causality of symptoms encountered in organic and psychic diseases", it is an aspect that has perhaps not yet received sufficient attention in psychopathology and psychiatry. The experience that has meanwhile been acquired in the realm of psychopharmacology suggests at all events that it is high time for us to reflect anew upon these long-known facts.

References

1 BRUNE, F.: Anhebung der Krampfschwelle als therapeutisches Prinzip bei der Behandlung von Alkohol-Delirien. Nervenarzt *37*, 415 (1966)
2 GOLDSTEIN, K.: Über die gleichartige funktionelle Bedingtheit der Symptome bei organischen und psychischen Krankheiten; im besonderen über den funktionellen Mechanismus der Zwangsvorgänge. Mschr. Psychiat. Neurol. *57*, 191 (1925)
3 GOLDSTEIN, K.: The organism (American Book Comp., New York 1939)
4 KUHN-GEBHART, V.: Behavioural disorders in non-epileptic children and their treatment with carbamazepine. In Birkmayer, W. (Editor): Epileptic seizures – behaviour – pain, Int. Symp., St. Moritz 1975, p. 264 (Huber, Berne/Stuttgart/Vienna 1975)
5 PÖLDINGER, W.: Klinische Erfahrungen mit dem Iminostilbenderivat G 32883. Zbl. ges. Neurol. Psychiat. *184*, 17 (1965/66); abstract of paper
6 SCHWEITZER, H.: Die visuelle Wahrnehmung bei Gabe von Carbamazepin in Kombination mit Alkohol. Blutalkohol *7*, 371 (1970)

Discussion

W. Birkmayer: I should like to thank the four previous speakers for their presentations and also to say how pleased I was that Dr. Kuhn referred in his paper to Goldstein, whose work has unfortunately now been largely forgotten. The book on the structure of the organism which Goldstein wrote after he had emigrated to Amsterdam is a mine of sound and thought-provoking information, and I consider it well worth studying. The discussion is now open.

W. Grüter: As regards the effectiveness of ®Tegretol (carbamazepine) in the management of behavioural disorders in non-epileptics, may I briefly describe my own experiences with the drug in such cases. At the neurological clinic and Hephata institutions in Treysa my colleague Dr. Knauel and I used Tegretol to treat 42 non-epileptic patients with behavioural disorders which had failed to show a satisfactory response to conventional drugs. These patients could be divided into two groups. The first group consisted of 28 mental defectives who had sustained organic cerebral damage in early childhood and who displayed periodic or permanent moodiness and irritability, marked by a tendency to outbreaks of violence. E.E.G. recordings revealed typical seizure patterns in 14 of these 28 patients and non-specific changes in a further six. The other group comprised 14 mentally normal children and adolescents who were being looked after in our remedial training department. These patients, too, exhibited irritability and periodic moodiness. The E.E.G. tracings disclosed typical seizure patterns in two of them and non-specific changes in four.
The results we obtained were, briefly, as follows: the behavioural disorders showed a good or satisfactory response to treatment with Tegretol in 12 of the 28 mental defectives (42%) and in ten of the 14 mentally normal children and adolescents (71%). This difference in the success rates suggests perhaps that mental defectives – even though, as in our series, their E.E.G. tracings more often reveal typical seizure patterns – are likely to derive less benefit.

R. Dreyer: We have heard at this symposium a great deal about the psychotropic activity of carbamazepine. In view of its eminently good psychotropic effect, isn't there a risk that, like so many other psycho-active drugs, it may lead to habituation after a certain time?

P. Schmidlin: I should like to ask Dr. Kuhn a question. How many cases of habituation to benzodiazepines have you personally encountered to date? Were the patients suffering from genuine withdrawal symptoms as described and defined according to internationally accepted conventions? Or was it perhaps simply that the patients' condition deteriorated again after the medication had been withdrawn and that the symptoms were thus not genuine withdrawal symptoms at all? Were you really able to eliminate the symptoms you have described by administering Tegretol alone?

P. Kielholz: I, too, have a brief question for Dr. Kuhn. He mentioned in his paper that he had also given carbamazepine in combination with ®Ludiomil (maprotiline), and this was news to me. We have employed this same combination to treat depressive mood disorders in epileptic patients, and I should therefore be interested to know what dosages he used.

G. Nissen: I think that this is perhaps an appropriate juncture at which to draw attention once again to the fact that – particularly with regard to epileptic mood disorders and episodic behavioural disturbances in children – differences of opinion exist between, on the one hand, psychiatrists and child psychiatrists and, on the other, epileptologists and paediatricians who are more or less neurologically oriented. From discussions at E.E.G. congresses, I know, for example, that there are also leading German paediatricians who advise against treatment for behavioural disturbances in children exhibiting abnormal E.E.G. findings, whereas such treatment is expressly recommended by psychiatrists and child psychiatrists. I fancy there are various reasons for this disparity of views. One explanation may be that epileptic children are mainly dealt with by paediatricians and neurologists, whereas children with behavioural disorders are chiefly referred to child psychiatrists or to child guidance centres. It has also struck me that psychiatrists and child psychiatrists tend to be particularly on the look-out for psychopathological abnormalities, even in children with manifest epilepsy, whereas paediatricians often appear to attach less importance to these aspects.

With reference to the psychotropic effect of carbamazepine, I should like to recall at this point that we obtained negative findings when we carried out a double-blind study in a non-selected group – although I hasten to add that we remain convinced of the drug's psychotropic activity. I also still have the impression, which seems to be borne out by what Dr. Kuhn has said, that behavioural disorders which are definitely due to organic causes respond better to carbamazepine than those of non-organic origin. In this connection, however, I consider it essential that the child psychiatrist should see the patient's E.E.G. records and judge them for himself. It is certainly not a good thing for the child psychiatrist to have to rely on an assessment of the E.E.G. made by a neurologist or psychiatrist who is in the habit of treating adults only. A child psychiatrist who is able to confine himself to the evaluation of E.E.G. tracings recorded in children runs far less risk of ascribing undue significance to the E.E.G. findings, which in children not only vary depending on the patient's age and developmental status but are also liable to be distorted by numerous other influences; while accepting relatively wide tolerance limits and borderline areas, he will nevertheless still be able to detect a number of manifestly "abnormal" findings which call for diagnostic clarification.

Incidentally, in this connection I should perhaps emphasise that we never institute treatment in a child solely on the basis of pathological E.E.G. findings, but only where such findings are accompanied by a periodic behavioural disorder and where, in addition, the case history reveals either that the pregnancy or the birth itself had entailed complications, that the child had previously suffered from isolated seizures, or that its statomotor or speech development had been retarded during infancy. That such children with behavioural disorders can derive benefit from anti-epileptic treatment is so self-evident as to require no further discussion – as I am sure anyone can confirm who has himself witnessed the dramatic disappearance of a behavioural disorder in a child receiving anti-epileptic medication. I remember, for example, the case of a child that had been adopted by a parson's wife who afterwards came from Western Germany to Berlin. This child, which was suffering from a severe behavioural disorder, was referred to a neurologist, who, because the disorder was associated with pathological E.E.G. findings, instituted anticonvulsive therapy. Under this treatment, the child's behaviour already showed an enormous improvement in the space of only one week. The mother, who was a very well-informed and critical woman, was able to give a precise description of the changes that the child underwent in response to the medication, and also of the renewed deterioration which set in when an attempt was made to withdraw the treatment.

R. Kuhn: In reply to Dr. Dreyer's query about the possibility of habituation to carbamazepine, I can assure him that this drug produces no habituation or addiction; the same, by the way, applies to all the antidepressants as well. So far as I am aware, not a single case of habituation or addiction has been reported, and I myself have never yet met a case either. Why this should be so, however, is very curious.

Now let me answer Dr. Schmidlin's question. Although we only recently began tackling the problem of withdrawal symptoms following discontinuation of treatment with benzodiazepines, we have already had six cases which responded favourably to carbamazepine. We have also treated two patients with symptoms resulting from the withdrawal of other drugs, and both of them likewise responded well to carbamazepine. That the patients who had been taking benzodiazepines really were suffering from withdrawal symptoms seems most probable in the light of the clinical picture, the symptoms of which were not identical with those present prior to treatment with the benzodiazepines. The symptoms had originally been largely of the mild depressive type, whereas after withdrawal of the benzodiazepines they took the form almost entirely of excitation states.

Regarding the question Dr. KIELHOLZ raised, I'm afraid I can't quote any hard-and-fast dosage schedules for combined treatment with carbamazepine and maprotiline. I can state, however, that we make it a practice only to add small doses of maprotiline to the carbamazepine, i.e. doses of 10 mg. one to three times daily; we do not raise this dosage until and unless it proves necessary. Generally, we find we can manage with small doses of maprotiline, particularly since carbamazepine itself also has an antidepressive effect. The reason why we prefer to use maprotiline for this purpose, rather than imipramine (®Tofranil) or clomipramine (®Anafranil), is that maprotiline exerts a marked additional sedative effect.

Dr. NISSEN mentioned the negative findings he had obtained in a double-blind study with carbamazepine. The literature contains repeated reports of negative results of this kind in double-blind studies with antidepressants and other psycho-active drugs. A great deal evidently depends on the way in which the study is planned and the patients selected.

As for Dr. NISSEN's plea that child psychiatrists should assess the E.E.G. findings themselves, here I am one hundred percent in agreement with him. Anyone who merely relies upon the verdict of an E.E.G. specialist, however excellently the latter's findings may be formulated, is hardly likely ever to derive from the E.E.G. records any information of much relevance to the assessment of childhood behavioural disorders. It is, in fact, of cardinal importance that the E.E.G. findings should be interpreted in relation to the overall clinical picture, and this applies both to child psychiatry as well as to adult psychiatry.

Lastly, a brief comment on Dr. NISSEN's final remarks. I also completely agree with him that one should never initiate treatment purely and simply on the basis of E.E.G. findings. A neurosurgeon doesn't perform a craniotomy solely on this basis either! It is always the conclusions emerging from the sum total of all the findings that should determine what treatment, if any, is indicated.

W. BIRKMAYER: Thank you very much, Dr. KUHN. I propose that we now leave this boundless topic of behaviour and turn to the third theme of our symposium, i.e. to the problem of pain. Dr. MUMENTHALER has prepared an extensive paper on this subject, which I have already had the pleasure of perusing in Vienna and which will be published *in extenso* in the proceedings of this symposium. I now call upon him to present an abridged version of it.

The pathophysiology of pain

by M. MUMENTHALER *

Tactus simplex, est sensus, quo tactiles quorumvis corporum terrestrium qualitates, ut calor, frigiditas, humiditas, siccitas, laevitas, asperitas, gravitas, levitas, dolor, titillatio, aliaeque similes, ex diverso nervorum, pertotum corpus dispersorum, motu, mediante cute, sentiuntur.

The sense of touch is that by which the tactile qualities of all earthly bodies, such as warmth and cold, humidity and dryness, softness and hardness, heaviness and lightness, pain and titillation, and the like thereof are felt through the skin in response to divers stimuli acting upon nerves distributed throughout the body.

HENRICI REGII: *Fundamenta physices, p. 226*
(Amstelodami 1646)

* Neurologische Universitätsklinik, Berne, Switzerland.

1. Introductory remarks

Pain is a problem confronting all who practise medicine, including especially not only neurophysiologists, neurologists, and neurosurgeons, but also psychiatrists. During the past ten years in particular, both the multifarious nature of this problem and the new therapeutic possibilities opened up by developments in the fields of surgery and medicine have prompted numerous research studies and publications on pain, as well as several international symposia [14, 58, 62, 102].

That, despite all these activities, a great many questions relating to pain still remain unanswered, becomes only too obvious when one begins to examine the voluminous literature on the subject. As I hope to demonstrate in the following paper, however, the work accomplished in recent years has nevertheless made certain valuable additions to our knowledge which, in turn, have also paved the way to new advances in the realm of treatment.

In spite of the obvious drawbacks involved in selecting a clinician, rather than a neurophysiologist, to review the complex pathophysiology of pain, the choice of a clinician for this task may perhaps also have its advantages, inasmuch as he can attempt to explain the fundamental aspects of those phenomena that the clinician actually encounters at the patient's bedside and to answer various questions which have an immediate bearing on the practical approach to treatment.

2. Scope of the following review

On the basis of recent literature, the pathophysiology of the end-organs subserving the sensation of pain will be discussed, together with the mechanism of pain apperception and the specificity of these end-organs. References will also be made to the latest findings concerning the afferent pain pathways in the periphery and their specificity, as well as to the encoding of differing afferent impulses, to regulatory mechanisms operating in the input control centre located in the posterior horns of the spinal cord, to the conduction of pain impulses through the spinal cord to the brainstem and thalamus, and, finally, to the supraspinal control of pain sensation and to the representation of pain in the cerebral cortex. Those pathological forms of pain that are of foremost clinical importance will also be described and their pathophysiology discussed. Tempting though it might have been to dwell upon some of the philosophical aspects of the role of pain in human existence, this temptation has been resisted.

3. The functional organisation of pain

3.1. Pain receptors in the periphery

It has long been known that the skin contains structures of varying histology referred to as sensory end-organs. In 1837, JOHANNES MÜLLER [88] advanced his theory according to which certain receptors are specific for certain physical sensations; and it has since been confirmed that there are indeed various specific functions which can be assigned to the different endings of sensory nerve fibres present in the skin, as well as in other peripheral organs. The existence of such specific correlations has been demonstrated, for example, in the case of the corpuscles subserving touch, the group of lamellated Vater-Pacini corpuscles in the skin (and their analogues in the viscera)[52], the Herbst corpuscles in birds, and the "innominate-type" corpuscles to be found in certain animals[100]. Recent investigations have shown, however, that the specificity of some sensory nerve endings is relative rather than absolute, insofar as it applies only within certain limits. In the nasal skin of the cat, for instance, application of a specific low-temperature stimulus has resulted in the identification of a cold spot, stimulation of which leads to a discharge in an afferent axon of the infraorbital nerve. Electron-microscopic examination of the tissues in question revealed a uniform anatomical substrate in the form, not of a Krause corpuscle, but of a free, ramified nerve ending with an axon belonging to the A-delta type of fibre, the terminal portion of which was devoid of a myelin sheath[47]. A similarly high degree of specificity was at one time claimed for the Meissner and Merkel corpuscles as touch receptors, for the Krause bulbs as cold receptors, and for the Ruffini bodies as receptors for the modality of warmth. More recent studies on the correlations between neurophysiology and histology, however, have disclosed that such claims require to be modified to some extent and have also served to emphasise just how complex the functioning of these peripheral receptors is.

The mechanoreceptors in the skin, such as the Vater-Pacini corpuscles, contain three main components: a mechanical portion, which registers and modulates the stimulus; a transducer, which transforms the mechanical energy into an initial form of electrical energy (the receptor potential); and a portion which initiates within the receptor the impulse that then travels through the axon[106]. The receptor potential is subject to temporal and spatial summation: if the end-organ is mechanically stimulated over a fairly long period, prolonged depolarisation occurs, followed by hyperpolarisation.

Already in 1906, SHERRINGTON[113] drew attention to the fact that a sensation of pain can be elicited by stimuli of widely differing types, e.g. mechanical, thermal, or electrical. He pointed out that "excitants of skin pain have all a certain character in common, namely this, that they become adequate as excitants of pain when they are of such intensity as threatens damage to the skin".

This raises first of all the question as to whether, under certain circumstances, receptors specifically concerned with some other sensory modality may perhaps also function as pain receptors[25]. By recording the impulses passing through single nerve fibres it has been demonstrated that, when individual specific cutaneous receptors are exposed to stimulation ranging from mild to noxious, the afferent signals which they emit do not as such enable any distinction to be drawn between stimuli of damaging as opposed to innocuous intensity[96] (Figure 1).

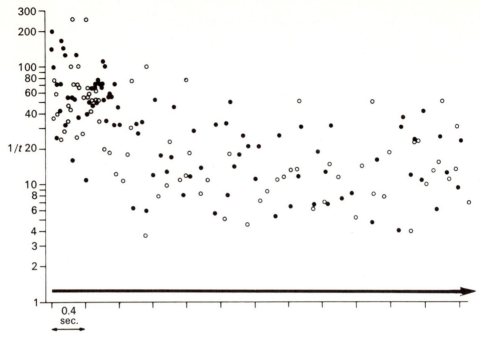

Fig. 1. Instantaneous frequency (**1/t**) of discharge evoked in afferent nerve fibres from a receptor in primate glabrous skin in response to firm but innocuous pressure (filled circles) and to noxious pressure (open circles). (Reproduced from PERL[96] by kind permission of the author and of The Journal of Physiology)

The thermoreceptors in the skin are known to have a very low stimulus threshold for those stimuli which they are specifically designed to appreciate, i.e. for thermal stimuli, whereas they respond only weakly to mechanical stimulation. Strong noxious mechanical stimuli inactivate these thermoreceptors, rendering them unresponsive to subsequent thermal or mechanical stimulation. On the other hand, there are quite a number of mechanoreceptors which, when the skin is subjected to a dynamically constant degree of displacement, vary in their response depending on whether the instrument causing the displacement is blunt or pointed. Sensory units of this kind discharge at a higher frequency when the instrument employed to stimulate the skin has a sharp point; but discharges of the same type and frequency can also be elicited from these units by means of a blunt instrument, provided the latter is made to produce a stimulus of a certain rate or in a certain direction (Figure 2). Thermoreceptors, in turn, may show the same discharge frequency in response both to a harmless increase in temperature as well as to heat of around 45–47 °C., which is strong enough to damage the skin[48]. This confirms that a mechanoreceptor, or a thermoreceptor displaying only a low specific stimulus threshold, is not capable alone of distinguishing between an adequate stimulus and a harmful stimulus. Consequently, the very nature of these receptors is such that alone they cannot serve as nociceptors, i.e. as specific warning devices and differentiated appreciators of painful stimuli.

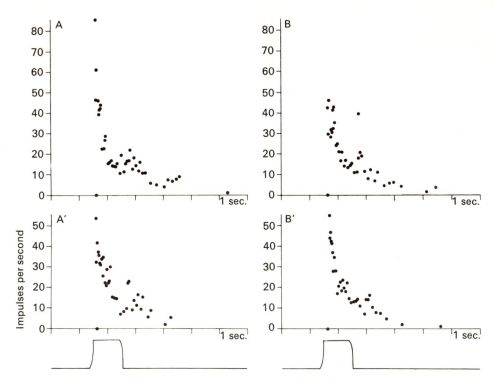

Fig. 2. Responses evoked in an afferent axon from a C mechanoreceptor by innocuous (A and B) and noxious (A′ and B′) mechanical stimuli. The stimulus time and form are shown in the lowermost traces; velocity and displacement were identical for all tests. A (A′) and B (B′) were the first and third of a series at 100-second intervals. For A and B a blunt probe was used, and for A′ and B′ a needle contacting the centre of the same area of skin. (Reproduced from BESSOU et al.[16] by kind permission of the authors and of The Journal of Neurophysiology)

On the basis of studies undertaken by VON FREY[40] and his school, it was at first believed that warmth and cold, as well as pressure and touch, are registered by specific nerve endings enveloped in a sheath, whereas the receptors serving specifically to appreciate pain are free nerve endings. It was later discovered, however, that the role of the free nerve endings involves more than simply registering pain. Reference has already been made to the finding that in the cat's nose free nerve endings also act as specific thermoreceptors for cold[47]. In order to make a closer analysis of the cutaneous receptors, it was therefore necessary to begin by investigating their function, for which purpose receptors with a high stimulus threshold were studied[96]. When the afferent discharges from such high-threshold receptors were recorded in experimental animals, no discharge could be detected in response to over 100 grammes of pressure with a blunt instrument, whereas discharges already occurred at a pressure of 100 grammes with a pointed instrument. Pinching with serrated forceps elicited particularly intensive discharges[96] (Figure 3). Experiments of this type have confirmed that cats and monkeys possess sensory units fulfilling a specific nociceptive function[24,25]. Among these nociceptive sensory units are some which

279

A

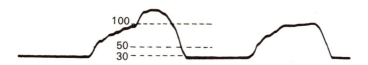

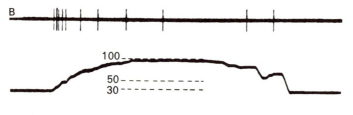
B

Fig. 3. Upper traces in A and B: responses of a mechanical nociceptor with a myelinated afferent fibre to graded mechanical stimuli. Lower traces in A and B: output of calibrated probe in grammes. A = blunt tip of 2 mm., B = needle tip, C = pinch applied to receptive field with serrated forceps. (Reproduced from PERL[96] by kind permission of the author and of The Journal of Physiology)

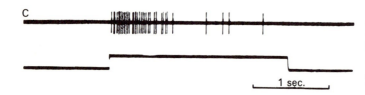
C

1 sec.

react specifically only to mechanical stimuli. When exposed to thermal stimuli – including those strong enough to destroy tissue – or to chemical stimuli, such receptors show little or no response. They are to be found in the hairless skin of man and in the hairy skin of carnivorous animals and primates[24,25,96]; they exhibit a stimulus threshold five to 1,000 times higher than that of the afore-mentioned specific mechanoreceptors having a low stimulus threshold, and they are innervated by A-delta fibres. There is another group of nociceptors which react both to mechanical and to thermal stimuli. Receptors of this kind, which are supplied with fine myelinated fibres, respond to damaging heat (i.e. heat exceeding 45°C.) as well as to harmful mechanical influences[25,55]; most of them also react to chemical stimuli. Neither of the two types of noci-ceptor to which reference has just been made displays any spontaneous activity at rest, i.e. prior to the infliction of damage to the skin.

The high-threshold nociceptors described above, which respond to strong, damaging stimuli, could quite well also be classed as pain receptors. Strictly speaking, however, this would be merely an inference and not a confirmed fact, even though the defensive reactions and other responses observed in animals subjected to stimulation of these high-threshold nociceptors are in-distinguishable from those indicative of painful sensations.

Consequently, although the experiments mentioned provide strong evidence for the existence of "pain" receptors, they afford no reliable clues to the histological characteristics of such receptors[11], which therefore still have to be inferred from older, morphologically less well-substantiated, findings implying that it is the free nerve endings which act as pain receptors[17]. The fact that pain can also be felt at sites where only free nerve endings are detectable (e.g. in the cornea) merely suggests, but does not prove, that the specific nociceptors already referred to have the same type of morphological substrate as pain receptors.

The free nerve endings in the skin usually originate from fibres of small or medium calibre, which as a rule are myelinated; very rarely, however, they also derive from thicker myelinated fibres[28]. Although, when viewed in the light microscope, they exhibit only minor differences, their ultramicroscopic structure is highly variable with respect to the axoplasmic components and cholinesterase. The submicroscopic vesicular and granular components may possibly have something to do with the production or release of transmitter substances such as acetylcholine and catecholamines[28]. The marked variability of the ultramicroscopic picture presented by these free nerve endings might also reflect differences in their mechanisms of neurochemical transmission. But no evidence has been found to indicate that any one particular ultramicroscopic or chemical configuration can be assigned to any one specific sensory function. Hence, it is not along these lines – or at least not along these lines alone – that the specificity of a given sensory modality can be accounted for[28].

Other more recent electron-microscopic studies have likewise failed to reveal with certainty any receptors which could definitely be classified as nociceptors[11], with the possible exception of nerve endings in the dental pulp, where myelinated fibres terminate in the form of free ramifications[117]. By and large, histologists still admit that it is impossible on the basis of morphological investigations to draw any conclusions about the number and distribution of nociceptors or pain receptors[37].

Precisely because of the fact that a variety of different sensations – such as awareness of movement, changes in temperature, *and* pain – can be elicited at free nerve endings of uniform structure, e.g. in the human cornea, it follows that the other ways in which WEDDELL[127] suggests that stimuli may become differentiated provide a plausible alternative, or complement, to the theory based on receptor-specific differentiation. According to this author, it is not until the distinctive spatio-temporal characteristics of the individual afferent impulses have actually been analysed in the central organ that the different and specific sensations typical of the various sensory modalities, including also that of pain, can be felt. In man, for example, WEDDELL and MILLER[128] have shown that the spatial summation of non-damaging heat stimuli is capable of producing a sensation of pain. In other words, pain may be experienced under circumstances in which a large number of impulses generated in a particular zone are transmitted to the centre from receptors that are not in fact specific for this modality[127]. WEDDELL and co-workers carried out, among other things, a meticulous histological examination of an area of skin the sensory function of which had previously been subjected to very close study; their findings not only disclosed deviations from the pattern of relationships between sensory modality and morphological substrate of the nerve endings as described above, but also revealed the presence of atypical nerve endings and showed that hairy and hairless skin, though exhibiting the same type of sensibility, nevertheless display histological differences[128].

In view of the facts presented here, it would certainly be wrong to conclude that the two interpretations outlined above are mutually exclusive. *To sum up*, the conclusion which would seem to emerge from these various observations is:
– that certain areas of skin contain receptors which, though not of uniform histological appearance, are specific for nociceptive stimuli,
– but that, under certain conditions (i.e. depending on the spatial and temporal constellations of the afferent impulses), painful sensations can also be elicited via receptors which are not (pain-)specific.

The role played by *chemical substances* in the causation of pain has recently been the subject of repeated analysis[61,130]. Histamine, 5-hydroxytryptamine (serotonin), and plasma kinins, which are involved in inflammatory processes, can also be applied in such a way as to produce pain. A similar effect has likewise been observed with acetylcholine, prostaglandins, and potassium. The production of endogenous algogenic substances of this type may be promoted as a result of the plasma coming into contact with glass or, for example, with urate crystals in patients suffering from gout. The question as to the role of chemical mediators or the formation of such chemical substances during the process by which stimuli become transformed into impulses is one that may pose itself in circumstances where prolonged changes in the sensitivity of receptors are observed or where the latter undergo very slow adaptation[25]. This is a question, however, on which no reliable information is yet available. The possibility that so-called second, "slow" pain, to which reference will be made later, might be a form of pain chemically mediated in the periphery is at present still only an hypothesis[129].

Turning now from the skin to the viscera, it should be pointed out that the stimuli giving rise to *sensations of pain in the viscera* comprise, firstly, distension of hollow organs, secondly, traction exerted on certain structures, and, thirdly, chemical irritation[36]. In the walls of hollow abdominal organs IGGO[51] succeeded in identifying tension-sensitive receptors which are coupled in series with the smooth-muscle fibres and which may be capable of mediating not only the dull sensation resulting from filling of these hollow organs, but also pain, e.g. in the presence of colic. In the gastric mucosa IGGO also found receptors sensitive to acids.

3.2. *The conduction of pain impulses to the central organ*
The impulses emanating from peripheral receptors in the skin, mucosa, deep tissue layers, and viscera are conducted by various types of fibres displaying

distinctive morphological and electrophysiological features[99]. The fibres leading from the skin (as well as from certain regions of the viscera) to the posterior spinal nerve roots comprise:

– a small group of myelinated A fibres (accounting for 20% of the total of A and C fibres), which are designated in descending order of their conduction velocity (45–15 m./sec.) and calibre (12–3 μ) as A-alpha, A-beta, A-gamma, and A-delta fibres;
– and a larger group of non-myelinated C fibres (80%) with a conduction velocity of 0.5–2 m./sec. and a calibre of less than 2 μ, whose appurtenant nerve endings respond chiefly to mechanical stimuli of low intensity.

An alternative system of classification exists in which the fibres are assigned to Groups I–IV; according to this system, the A-alpha fibres, for example, are allocated to Group I, the A-delta fibres to Group III, and the C fibres to Group IV.

Although it has not proved possible consistently to assign any one particular type of fibre to any one morphologically distinct receptor in the periphery, it has been demonstrated with regard to the conduction of pain impulses that ischaemia has the effect of interrupting conduction in the thick (A-alpha) fibres before conduction ceases in the thin (C) fibres. Hence, in animals with experimentally induced ischaemia, it can be shown that nociceptive reflexes continue to occur despite blockade of the A fibres resulting from oxygen deficiency. Similarly, under the same experimental conditions in man, pain can still be felt after sensitivity to touch and temperature has been abolished. In response to cocaine, by contrast, which acts initially by blocking the thin fibres, it is sensitivity to pain elicited by contact and deep pressure that is the first to disappear. As long ago as 1935, CLARK et al.[30] had already demonstrated in anaesthetised cats that electrical stimulation of peripheral nerve fibres provokes nociceptive autonomic reflexes only if and when the fibres in question are thin myelinated or non-myelinated ones.

In man it was found that electrical stimulation of the exposed sural nerve did not give rise to any painful sensation until the stimulus was intensified to the point where it excited not only the A-beta and A-gamma fibres but also the A-delta fibres. The pain became unbearable only when the stimulus was so strong as to excite also the C fibres. Following chordotomy, stimulation of the same intensity was well tolerated, i.e. it gave rise at the most to nothing more than an unpleasant sensation[31].

These findings all serve to indicate that the stimuli predominantly responsible for pain are those causing impulses to be transmitted to the spinal cord via thin myelinated A-delta fibres or via thin non-myelinated C fibres. This, however, by no means excludes the possibility that other types of fibre may also transmit impulses which are likewise centrally integrated and decoded in the course of the complex process of pain apperception[41]; nor, of course, does it afford any proof that – as was at one time believed – the C fibres are *exclusively* concerned with the mediation of pain. On the contrary, IGGO[49] has shown that

283

C fibres are capable of conveying impulses not only from low-threshold mechanoreceptors, but also from slowly adapting temperature-specific receptors, i.e. also from nociceptors exhibiting a high threshold for thermal and mechanical stimuli. The C fibres, which had previously been thought to mediate pain only, have thus proved to be non-specific with respect to their appreciation of stimuli[34]. In studies on isolated fibres of the cutaneous nerves of the cat, MARUHASHI et al.[75] observed that afferents from receptors responding to pressure (fibre calibre: 3–4 μ) or to cold (1.5–3 μ) may actually be of smaller calibre than afferents from nociceptors (3–11 μ).

The fact nevertheless remains that, from the purely numerical standpoint, it is the thin myelinated A-delta and the non-myelinated C fibres that primarily serve to mediate pain; also purely numerically, the C fibres account for more units belonging to nociceptive end-organs[50]. In connection with the conduction of pain impulses, differing functions have also been ascribed to these two types of fibre, and an attempt made to relate these functions to the phenomenon of so-called "double pain". It is indeed a fact that, in response to a pin-prick for instance, the sensation experienced takes the form of an immediate, sharp "first pain" followed, after a brief painless interval, by a duller, aching "second pain". It has been claimed that the first pain is mediated via the A-delta fibres, and the second pain via the C fibres. This would also appear to be borne out by the observation that, in response to ischaemia (the immediate effect of which is to block the thicker fibres), the first pain is initially abolished, whereas the second pain continues to be felt[114]. Incidentally, this observation conflicts with another hypothesis according to which the delayed onset of the second pain can be accounted for either by a time lag occurring in polysynaptic transmission within the grey matter of the spinal cord or by the release of chemical substances in the peripheral cells. Certain authors, on the other hand, have postulated that the C fibres are responsible for the dull, drawn-out second pain because of their peculiar tendency to produce protracted series of discharges which last longer than the stimulus itself[111].

In studies performed in man, TOREBJÖRK and HALLIN[120] investigated the conduction of pain impulses in afferent fibres by directly recording the flow of these impulses from a cutaneous sensory nerve. The technique they employed enabled them to register the degree of excitation provoked in the nerve in response to intradermal electrical stimulation and to correlate it with the sensations experienced by the test-subject. In this way, they furnished proof that, when C-fibre units were subjected to repetitive stimulation, increases in latency and even blockade of impulse transmission occurred, during which the test-subject reported a corresponding diminution in pain. But, when the C units were re-excited by stepping up the intensity of the stimulus, or when fresh C units were recruited, the pain increased again.

The *afferent autonomic nerves from the viscera* feature a particularly large quantity of thin fibres. Numerically predominant among the A fibres are the A-delta fibres, and the ratio of A to C fibres amounts to 1:8 or 1:9 in the visceral nerves, as compared with only 1:4 in the posterior roots[99]. In absolute terms, however, the number of visceral afferents is much smaller than that of the somatic afferents, the ratio in the cat, for example, working out at about 1:10. Despite this, the visceral fibres supply a territory which is equivalent in size to approximately one-quarter of the body surface, and from histological studies it is known that they have extensive ramifications. The sensory viscerotomes thus overlap to quite a marked degree, with the result that afferent impulses from a single region may reach the spinal cord via more than one posterior root.

From a summary review of the data currently available on pain receptors and on the transmission of afferent pain impulses from the periphery it is apparent that here the concept of fixed relationships between substrate and function is an oversimplification and, as such, no longer tenable. Findings obtained in histological studies have shown that not even with the aid of ultra-microscopy is it possible in absolute terms to establish any definite correlation between particular types of nerve endings and particular qualities of stimuli. No receptor is ever completely specific with regard to its appreciation of stimuli, and many receptors are quite non-specific in this respect. Not only is it wrong to suppose that certain afferent nerve fibres can be consistently assigned to certain end-organs, but also the notion that certain afferents are responsible for transmitting information on one particular quality of stimulus is backed only by very approximative statistical evidence. The sensation conveyed via the receptor substrate and the impulse-conducting afferent fibre is therefore a variable one. What is more, besides the fact that the sensation thus experienced depends on the nature of the substrate and is subject to variation, it is also quite conceivable that functional encoding of afferent impulses may occur within this morphological substrate. In addition, each individual element in this complex system might, as a result of exogenously or endogenously induced alterations in its ultrastructure, undergo changes in its functional properties – a possibility which it would be interesting to investigate experimentally.

We are accordingly confronted here with an extremely plastic and dynamic system, the complexity of which becomes even greater when we reach the central organ itself.

3.3. The zone of entry of pain fibres into the spinal cord and the input control system ("gate control" theory)

It is through the posterior roots that the sensory afferents reach the spinal cord. Within these posterior roots they already tend to form bundles, the thin A-delta and C fibres – which also serve to transmit pain impulses in particular – occupying the ventral part of the root. The A-alpha fibres, which are important as transmitters of epicritic impulses, are located in the dorsal portion of the posterior root. Reference to the significance of this fact from the therapeutic angle will be made later[73].

The incoming (pain) impulses, which are already highly differentiated thanks to the complex mechanisms in the periphery that have been described above, become modulated yet again in their passage through a relay system situated

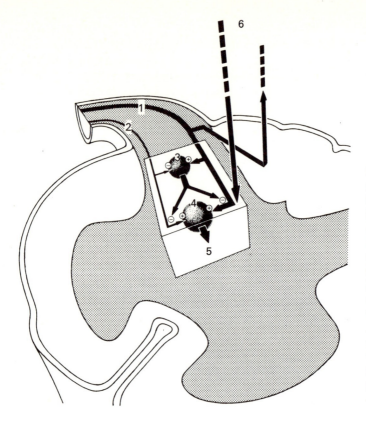

Fig. 4. Diagrammatic representation of the input control system in the posterior horn of the spinal cord. 1 = thick myelinated afferent, 2 = thin C fibre, 3 = cell in Rolando's fasciculus, 4 = original cell of the second neurone, 5 = pathway leading to higher centres, 6 = central control mechanisms (+ = activating; − = inhibiting).

in the posterior horn. In 1965 MELZACK and WALL[83] described this input control system in terms of the so-called "gate control" theory, which attempts to explain the processes occurring at this stage by reference to neurophysiological observations (Figure 4). The main features of the gate control theory are as follows:

– The cells in the posterior horn of the spinal cord are directly influenced by more than one afferent from the periphery.
– As a rule, an afferent impulse transmitted via thick myelinated fibres excites the posterior-horn cells, this excitation then being followed, however, by a protracted period of inhibition. Conversely, impulses conveyed by thin myelinated and non-myelinated afferent fibres provoke excitation followed by fairly prolonged after-discharges and facilitation. This difference is ascribed to pre-synaptic inhibition and facilitation, respectively, in which the cells of Rolando's fasciculus – i.e. of the gelatinous substance in the posterior horn of grey matter within the spinal cord – also appear to be involved. These form a dense system of interconnected cells, which are also anatomically linked together over several segments of the spinal cord by means of Lissauer's column.
– The reactivity of this whole relay system is in turn controlled by efferent central influences emanating from the spinal cord and brain.

The conclusions relevant to the pathophysiology of pain which can be drawn from this hypothesis may be *summarised* along roughly the following lines:

– The posterior-horn cells, which relay incoming impulses in a central direction, are initially activated in response to excitation of the thicker myelinated afferent fibres, but are afterwards (pre-synaptically) inhibited. On the other hand, the effect which the inflowing impulses exert on the posterior-horn cells is activated by the positive feedback mechanism of the thin fibres.

– The thinner afferent fibres, which adapt more slowly and which are chiefly responsible for providing the posterior-horn cells with a steady stream of tonic impulses at rest, serve to keep the input control system relatively open. A new stimulus or a change in the pre-existing state of stimulation in the periphery will produce excitation mainly in the thick fibres; this, in turn, will make the relay points in the input control system tend to close up. But, if the stimulus increases in intensity, the thick fibres will adapt more rapidly and the thin fibres more slowly; the relay points then open again, and the posterior-horn cells become more strongly stimulated, with the result that a sensation of pain may possibly be felt. If, however, the thick fibres are now *selectively* stimulated, this will inevitably cause the input control system to "close" once more, so that activity of the posterior-horn cells is reduced.

– Adding to the complexity of the whole picture is the fact that the membrane capacity of these same cells is also influenced by further synapses which conduct afferent impulses emanating from other segments, including segments on the contralateral side, as well as from the centre.

Pre-synaptic inhibition, for which axo-axonal synapses are responsible, is mediated by substances differing from those that are involved in post-synaptic transmission[107,109]. Consequently, although diazepam, for example, has been found to produce primary afferent depolarisation (P.A.D.), this drug exerts virtually no effect on post-synaptic inhibition. It would also appear that the convulsive activity of picrotoxin may possibly be due to the fact that it competes at the receptor sites with the substance mediating pre-synaptic inhibition.

The gate control theory of MELZACK and WALL[83] has given rise to a number of objections[107,108], which in turn have called forth further arguments in support of it[124]. One of the principal findings indicative of pre-synaptic inhibition as postulated in the gate control theory is the occurrence of negative posterior-root potentials (dorsal-root potentials = D.R.P.) in response to stimulation of thick A-alpha afferents. But other authors[39,135] were unable to confirm this finding; instead, they even observed negative dorsal-root potentials following stimulation of C fibres. Moreover, as has already been mentioned, a whole series of radically differing receptors have non-myelinated C fibres, and it therefore seems. unlikely that these fibres would behave as uniformly as suggested by the gate control theory[53].

Although, when enunciating their theory, MELZACK and WALL[83] assigned to the posterior-horn cells the role of common target cells for various afferent impulses, they nevertheless explicitly envisaged the possibility that, within the spectrum of differing responses to afferent impulses of varying quality, there might also be cells which respond solely to nociceptive impulses. Cells of this type were in fact subsequently identified by CHRISTENSEN and PERL[29] in the first lamina of the posterior horns.

Stimulation of thin afferent fibres or of nociceptors, however, does not invariably give rise to positive dorsal-root potentials[107]. It was later confirmed that in the deeper cell strata of the posterior horn, especially in the fifth lamina, the impulses from various peripheral cells converge to such an extent that these deep-lying cells respond to a very wide variety of afferent impulses. Found in this layer were cells which, for example, responded not only to impulses transmitted from the viscera by thin myelinated afferents with a high stimulus threshold but also to impulses emanating from the skin via low-threshold afferents[98]. Incidentally, one interpretation of so-called "referred pain", which will be discussed in due course, is also based on the fact that afferent impulses evoked by various qualities of visceral and cutaneous stimuli may converge in one and the same cell.

Results yielded by tests involving the stimulation of peripheral nerve stumps in patients suffering from painful conditions have been interpreted as affording confirmation that the gate control hypothesis is fundamentally correct. If it is true that a patient experiences pain because not enough afferent impulses are passing through the thicker nerve fibres, which exert an inhibitory action by causing the relay points to close, then it should in theory prove possible to relieve the pain by selectively stimulating these fibres. When such fibres, which have a low threshold for electrical stimuli, were subjected to electrical stimulation proximal to a neuroma, it was found that pain could in fact be temporarily abolished[125]. In cases of causalgia, electrical stimulation of the damaged peripheral nerves distal to the site of the damage (together with stimulation of the preponderating thin afferent fibres which were still capable of conducting) resulted in aggravation of the pain. On the other hand, when the electrical stimulus was applied proximally to the lesion, causing the patient to project mild paraesthesia into the periphery, the pain disappeared[84].

Since all those cutaneous afferents which ascend through the posterior columns of the spinal cord have collaterals running to the posterior-horn cells, studies have been undertaken in which the posterior columns were electrically stimulated so as to produce antidromic impulses causing the cells of the relay points to close up as in response to stimulation of peripheral afferents. By this means, too, it was found possible to afford effective relief from pain[85, 90, 104, 112].

Hence, though the gate control theory as originally formulated may not be acceptable in every respect, for the clinically oriented observer it does have a number of important features which still remain valid. *To sum up*, it may be assumed that an interaction between various afferents occurs within a control system operating already at the zone in which these afferents enter the posterior roots. Probably as a result of pre-synaptic inhibition mediated by interneurones in Rolando's fasciculus, excitation of thick myelinated fibres inhibits the response to afferent bursts from thin fibres which, among other things, also conduct nociceptive or pain impulses. In the spinal cord, the impulses converge on superordinate posterior-horn cells, each successive step in this process being potentially conducive to an interaction between different excitatory impulses. Intervening in this system, or in these systems, are also segmental, contralateral, or central influences which may exert either an inhibitory or a facilitatory effect. The biochemistry of the processes – including pre-synaptic ones – which occur here likewise appears to be of a non-uniform character.

3.4. The conduction of pain impulses in the spinal cord and brainstem

After having been relayed through the cells in the posterior horn of the spinal cord, the pain impulses decussate, to some extent obliquely, in the anterior grey commissure and continue in a cranial direction, entering the lateral column of the spinal cord on the opposite side at a level approximately two segments higher. In man, this is the point of origin of the lateral spinothalamic tract, which ascends directly into the ventro-posterolateral nucleus of the thalamus. Among the vertebrates, it is only in mammals that this neo-spino-thalamic tract is present. Also to be found in mammals, however, is a palaeo-spinothalamic tract, although this becomes more rudimentary the higher the type of mammal concerned[18]. The palaeo-spinothalamic tract, which is largely polysynaptic, leads from the posterior-horn cells to various structures in the brainstem, including the reticular formation in particular, and thence to the intralaminar nuclei of the thalamus[111]; here, impulses triggered off both by cutaneous and by visceral stimuli may act upon one and the same thalamic neurone. Broadly speaking, the predominantly monosynaptic or oligosynaptic neo-spinothalamic system can be equated with the lemniscal system[21]. It chiefly conducts impulses from the A-gamma and A-delta fibres, the appurtenant neurones in the ventro-posterolateral nucleus of the thalamus being arranged somatotopically. The polysynaptic palaeo-spinothalamic system, on the other hand, corresponds to the extralemniscal system[21]; it serves mainly to continue the A-delta and C fibres, and the neurones in the intralaminar nuclei of the thalamus, to which it leads, have a converging instead of a somatotopic alignment. In laboratory animals, acoustic stimuli producing an arousal reaction have been found to cause a decrease in the amplitude of evoked potentials from the extralemniscal system and – in the ventro-posterolateral nucleus of the thalamus – an increase in that of evoked potentials from the lemniscal system. The fact that pain impulses are thus conducted in the spinal cord via a dual pathway, which is only partially polysynaptic and not exclusively contralateral, may perhaps account for the observation that, in certain cases in which histologically verified bilateral chordotomy had been performed, no cutaneous sensory loss occurred[94].

In addition to these ascending tracts in the spinal cord that play such an important role in the conduction of pain impulses, descending control mechanisms of a predominantly inhibitory character[44] have also been demonstrated both in the extralemniscal system[35, 123], through which the A-delta and C fibres are continued, as well as in the lemniscal system[9]. It is reasonable to suppose that such cranio-caudal pathways might conceivably provide a means by which inflowing impulses could already be modulated at the level of the input control system, i.e. at their point of entry into the posterior roots, this modulation being effected in response to changes in alertness, emotional excitation, and other "psychic" factors. In patients undergoing stereotactic operations as treatment for Parkinson's disease, it has been reported that, following experimentally induced stimulation of the ventro-posterolateral nucleus of the thalamus, a painful cutaneous stimulus was no longer felt as strongly as before[44]. That it is indeed upon the control system in the posterior horn that this descending modulatory influence exerts its effect, has been confirmed by the results of other experiments[124]. BROWN and FRANZ[22], for example, found that individual neurones in the fourth lamina of the posterior horn normally show a differentiated response to differing stimuli. In the spinal animal, by contrast, the cells in this same zone all responded identically to these stimuli, as well as to additional stimuli which prior to spinalisation had elicited no reaction. After cold-induced blockade of the spinal cord, it has been demonstrated[124] that cells in the sixth lamina of the posterior horn become more responsive to cutaneous stimuli and also that the tributary skin zone is enlarged.

Incidentally, it should be mentioned at this point that electrical stimulation of ascending pain pathways in the spinal cord, i.e. particularly of the spino-thalamic tract, never gives rise to sensations of pain[78].

The central control mechanisms which already contribute to the influences exerted on the regulation of afferent impulses at their zone of entry into the posterior roots have also been studied from the pharmacological aspect[107, 109]. Catecholamines have been found to exercise a clear-cut influence on the presynaptic inhibition of posterior-root afferents, presumably because they act upon descending adrenergic control mechanisms in the spinal cord. LUNDBERG[71], for instance, has shown that depolarisation of the primary posterior-root afferent (primary afferent depolarisation = P.A.D.), which occurs in the ipsilateral and contralateral flexor reflex in response to discharges in other flexor-reflex afferents, was strongly diminished following intravenous administration of dopa. The posterior-root potentials in the A-alpha muscle-afferents, on the other hand, underwent no change[109].

To sum up, then, in the spinal cord the pain impulses pass through the oligo-synaptic or monosynaptic lemniscal system (A-gamma and A-delta fibres) to the ventro-posterolateral nucleus of the thalamus, and through the poly-synaptic extralemniscal system (A-delta and C fibres) to the intralaminar nuclei of the thalamus. The extralemniscal system sends out numerous collaterals, particularly to the reticular formation of the brainstem. In addition, the spinal cord has been found to conduct descending impulses which impinge on the posterior-horn cells. These impulses are a feature of supraspinal modulatory control mechanisms which also assume special significance from the pharmacological standpoint.

3.5. The thalamus as a receiving station for pain impulses

As has already been mentioned above, the pathway for the conduction of pain impulses consists both of the somatotopically organised lemniscal system ending in the ventro-posterolateral nucleus of the thalamus as well as of the extralemniscal system terminating in the intralaminar nuclei of the thalamus. With the aid of implanted electrodes it can be demonstrated that in the cells of the intralaminar nuclei the response to extralemniscal impulses can be inhibited by arousal stimuli. In the somatotopic cells of the ventro-posterolateral nucleus of the thalamus, by contrast, such arousal stimuli either produce no change or may actually reinforce the specific somataesthetic reactions[99]. Here, on the other hand, cellular activities evoked by stimulation of certain cutaneous regions can be inhibited by simultaneously stimulating another zone. The individual sensory modalities, which remain so clearly separated in the spinal cord, appear to converge and overlap again in the thalamus, with the result that lesions of the thalamus – unlike certain spinal-cord lesions – never give rise to a sharply dissociated sensory disturbance[36].

It is a widely accepted view that the thalamus constitutes the integrating terminal station of the pain pathways. Although at one time nobody disputed the notion that the thalamus is the last site at which, for example, pain can be provoked by electrical stimulation, recent findings have cast doubt on the correctness of this assumption. It now seems that whether or not pain can be elicited from the thalamus depends on the precise point at which the stimulus is applied[7]: whereas stimulation of the ventro-posterolateral nucleus itself (in the course of stereotactic operations) was not found to cause pain[6], stimuli applied immediately ventral to this nucleus[46] and stimulation of the cortico-dependent nucleus limitans[45] did give rise to pain; complete destruction of the nucleus limitans, however, resulted in freedom from pain[45].

It is upon neurophysiological findings of this kind that stereotactic operations on the thalamus for the relief of pain are based[110]. Effective relief from pain can in fact be afforded by inflicting relatively circumscribed damage on the centromedian nucleus of the thalamus, the nucleus limitans, the nucleus parafascicularis, or the medial portion of the nucleus dorsomedialis[74]. Pain can also be successfully relieved by administering stimuli via electrodes implanted in the ventro-posterolateral nucleus[78].

When considering the role played by the thalamus in the sensation of pain, it should of course be borne in mind that a further contribution towards discrimination of the intensity of pain, and especially of its localisation, is made at a cortical level by thalamoparietal projections[67].

3.6. The cortical elements of pain

From the thalamus the last – usually the third – neurone leads to the sensory cortex. The ventro-posterolateral nucleus of the thalamus projects somatotopically to the primary sensory zone (S I), i.e. to the post-central gyrus of the parietal lobe, where 40–50% of the cells respond both to lemniscal and to extralemniscal impulses[99]. Emanating from the centromedian nucleus of the thalamus are diffuse projections into widespread regions of the cortex; these projections are to some extent polysynaptic – a fact which accounts for the relatively prolonged latency of the responses to stimulation of the centromedian nucleus. Projection into the superior frontal gyrus, on the other hand, appears to be monosynaptic[20]. In severely painful conditions, the effect produced by ablation of this gyrus is that the patient, although still aware of the pain, no longer finds it tormenting. Into the secondary sensory zone (S II), as first identified by ADRIAN[2] in the cat, both lemniscal and extralemniscal impulses are projected[10], their topographical pathways being only partially superposable.

Two electrophysiologically different types of neurone can be distinguished in the sensory zone of the cortex[33]. One type responds only to stimulation of small, well-circumscribed areas in the periphery, particularly in the extremities. These neurones are located chiefly in the primary sensory zone within the post-central gyrus of the parietal lobe. Neurones of the second type respond to stimulation of more extensive peripheral areas and are predominantly to be found in the secondary sensory cortex[87]. It is mainly via the lateral columns of the spinal cord that the impulses reach these neurones, and via the posterior columns that they reach neurones of the first type[10]. With regard to the sensation of pain in particular, MELZACK and HAUGEN[80] found that in the cat painful stimuli produced by micro-electrodes applied to the teeth evoked potentials in both the primary (S I) and the secondary (S II) sensory zones of the cortex[99]. The cortical sensory neurones perform highly complex interpretative and analytical functions. Certain neurones in S I, for example, not only respond to a punctiform cutaneous stimulus but can also be induced to emit high-frequency discharges by stroking the same area of skin with a hair or a fine brush. These discharges, however, occur only when the skin is stroked in one particular direction; stroking in a different direction results in a decrease in the frequency of the discharges. There are other cortical neurones that are also sensitive to the speed at which the skin is stroked[131]. In the sensory cells of the cortex the characteristics of a given peripheral stimulus are individually analysed, i.e. broken down into their separate components; after the various single cortical neurones have each reacted to whichever component they are competent to analyse, the individual reactions are integrated, and it is the sum of them which then gives rise to the appropriate sensation, including presumably the sensation of pain as well.

With the aid of suitable apparatus – including especially equipment capable of summating individual discharges – it is also possible for evoked potentials occurring in response to painful stimuli to be recorded extracranially[115]. The cortical response to painful stimuli takes the form of a positive fluctuation in potential, the duration of which ranges from 50 to 200 msec., depending on the intensity of the stimulus; the primary component of these evoked potentials has a latency of 75–120 msec. But, when the electrodes are left in the same position, even a stimulus not strong enough to cause pain still gives rise to fluctuations lasting 60 msec., the primary component showing a latency of only 50 msec. In the laboratory of our own clinic FIERZ and LUDIN (personal communication, 1974) have likewise succeeded in recording clearly measurable and reproducible cortical responses to painful stimuli. This method might well prove useful when studying the phenomenon of pain and its psychophysical correlations, as well as when testing forms of analgesic treatment.

It was already reported by FOERSTER[38] in 1936, and later confirmed by PENFIELD and RASMUSSEN[95] and other authors, that stimulation of the cortex in the region of the post-central gyrus may elicit paraesthesia, feelings of "electrification", or other more specific sensations in the periphery, but that it never produces pain[68]. Conflicting to some extent with this claim that painful sensations cannot be provoked by cortical stimulation are the results of investigations undertaken by WHITE and SWEET[132] in which patients did experience pain in response to stimulation of the post-central gyrus; it should be added, however, that the patients in question were already suffering from spontaneously painful conditions. By way of contrast, it was found that phantom-limb pain could be eliminated by injecting procaine subcortically into the zone in which this somatosensory quality was represented.

3.7. Pain and the reticular formation
Although the reticular formation is located in the brainstem and is thus, topographically speaking, one of the "lower" stations through which pain impulses pass, discussion of its role in connection with pain has been postponed to this point because of the bearing that the reticular formation also has on the important problem of the subjective experience of pain, the part played by analgesia, and the relationships between "psyche" and pain, which have yet to be dealt with. It has already been mentioned that the reticular formation receives collaterals from the ascending extralemniscal system, which is polysynaptic and serves chiefly to continue the A-delta and C fibres. This complex network of neurones sends out centripetal ascending and centrifugal descending efferents, which enable inhibitory influences in particular to be exerted on those structures that conduct pain impulses, irrespective of the level at which they are located. It has been demonstrated that analgesia can be induced in the rat[77,103], as well as in the cat[70], by subjecting the central grey matter to electrical stimulation. This stimulation was observed to exert an inhibitory effect on the interneurones of the spinal cord. Damage to the central grey matter may, incidentally, result in hyperalgesia[82]. The analgesia occurring in response to electrical stimulation of the central grey matter sets in only gradually over a period of about five minutes (Figure 5)[81] and outlasts the stimulus by approximately five minutes[79]. The fact that this analgesic response is of delayed onset and lasts longer than the stimulus itself may, of course, be attributable purely and simply to electrophysiological factors (i.e. to recruitments and to the presence of self-sustaining circuits of circulating impulses); but it might also be interpreted as evidence suggesting the release of a transmitter substance. The areas which were stimulated as described above are particularly sensitive to locally applied morphine[56], and their response to electrical stimuli can, moreover, be modified as a result of changes in the serotonin level in the blood[5].

3.8. Pain and the "psyche"
In certain respects a study of the phenomenon of pain inevitably necessitates consideration of the psyche as well[13,23,26,36,57,65,66,126]. Quite apart from its

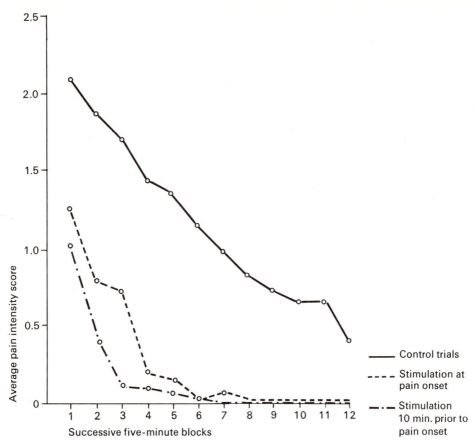

Fig. 5. Effect of electrical stimulation of the reticular formation (central grey matter and central tegmental tract) on pain produced in the rat by injection of formal saline under the skin of the paw. In the control trials no stimulation was applied to the brain. The pain intensity score was based on the following criteria: 3 points – paw held near the mouth and bitten or licked; 2 points – paw held in the air; 1 point – paw alternately lifted and set down on the floor; 0 points – paw kept on the floor. Average scores are shown for successive five-minute blocks. (Reproduced from MELZACK and MELINKOFF[81] by kind permission of the authors and of Academic Press, Inc.)

physical aspects, pain is something even the mention of which may give rise to feelings of unease (Figure 6). The intensity with which physical pain is experienced varies greatly from person to person, depending on the individual's state of mind. This well-known fact has also been conclusively confirmed by scientific analysis. During the Second World War, for example, BEECHER[15] found that, in soldiers who had been severely wounded at the Anzio bridge-head and had been exposed to enemy fire day and night, the feeling of safety and security they experienced upon finally reaching the army hospital was such that, out of a total of 215, only 25% accepted the offer of a pain-relieving injection; in contrast with this, he subsequently observed in the case of civilians with only moderately large wounds that 80% of them actually asked to be

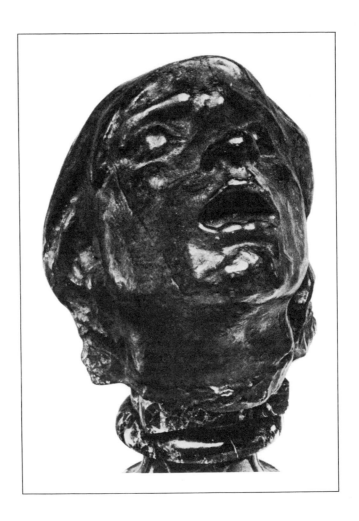

Fig.6. *"La douleur"*
by Auguste Rodin.

given an analgesic. Chronic pain is also liable to cause marked changes in behaviour, including not only severe behavioural disturbances as such, but even frank depression. On the other hand, it has been reported that, among prisoners of war who had been subjected to torture over a three-year period, there were some in whom a genuine state of anaesthesia had developed[36].

Ethnic differences, which are known to exist with respect to pain tolerance, have been quantified by STERNBACH and TURSKY[116] in experiments performed on housewives; these women showed a progressive increase in sensitivity to pain, depending – in the following order – on whether they were "Yankees", Jewish, Irish, or Italian (Figure 7). The fact that men differ from women in their sensitivity to pain (women being more sensitive than men in this regard) has also been demonstrated experimentally, both in normal subjects as well as in persons with mental disorders[93]. Incidentally, it is also possible to detect individual differences in pain tolerance by means of the LIBMAN test[69], for example, and in this way to make a more accurate assessment of the pain of which a patient complains[1].

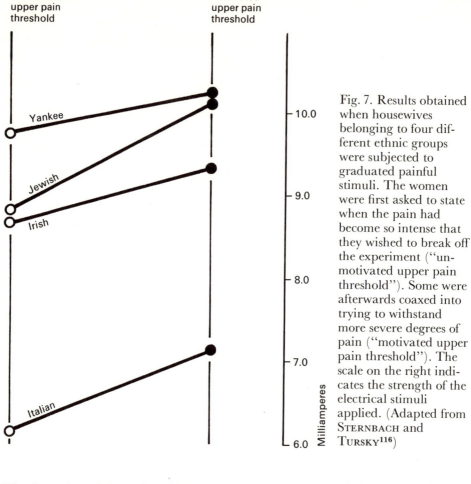

Fig. 7. Results obtained when housewives belonging to four different ethnic groups were subjected to graduated painful stimuli. The women were first asked to state when the pain had become so intense that they wished to break off the experiment ("unmotivated upper pain threshold"). Some were afterwards coaxed into trying to withstand more severe degrees of pain ("motivated upper pain threshold"). The scale on the right indicates the strength of the electrical stimuli applied. (Adapted from STERNBACH and TURSKY[116])

The intensity of the pain which a person experiences, and hence the significance he ascribes to it, thus depend not simply on the nature of the painful stimulus as such, but on the global constellation of all the stimuli to which he is exposed, on his constitution, and on his individual "attunement". Of particular interest in this connection is the neurophysiological basis responsible for determining how the painful stimulus is individually modulated and the pain subjectively apperceived. One basic factor which springs to mind at this point, and to which reference has already been made earlier, is the emission of inhibitory influences from the reticular formation of the brainstem to the interneurones in the posterior horn of the spinal cord. In addition, however, the reticular formation is also the almost exclusive source of afferent signals for the limbic system[3,4,66]. The limbic system, comprising the hippocampus, the gyrus cinguli, the amygdaloid nucleus, and a few secondary structures, has fibres which maintain important links with the hypothalamus and thus with the endocrine and autonomic nervous control systems as well (Figure 8). From the thalamic nuclei, in turn, efferents also travel to the limbic system. Bearing in mind the role played by the limbic system and especially by the hippocampus

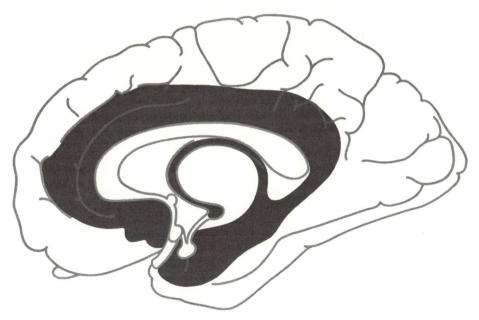

Fig. 8. Diagrammatic representation of the limbic system. (Reproduced from Akert[3] by kind permission of the publishers, S. Karger AG, Basle)

in connection with the function of memory, it seems reasonable to suppose that here, too, must also be located the relaying and mediating centre which accounts both for the influence exerted by pain on the psyche and for the repercussions that psychic factors, previous experiences, etc. have on the apperception of pain.

In summary, it may be concluded that pain is an experience whose intensity and significance for the individual display certain ethnic variations, as well as very pronounced differences from person to person and from situation to situation. The anatomical relationships existing between the ascending polysynaptic extralemniscal system and the reticular formation enable the latter to integrate various sensory afferents. As a result of this process of integration, descending inhibitory impulses may be emitted, which affect the system controlling the entry of afferents into the posterior roots. Finally, thanks to the presence of links between the reticular formation and the limbic system, it is possible for the psyche to influence the apperception of pain and, conversely, for pain afferents to exert repercussions on the psyche.

4. The pathology of pain and the pathophysiological rationale of various forms of analgesic treatment

4.1. General considerations

The very existence of specific nociceptors indicates that pain is not a primarily pathological phenomenon; on the contrary, it fulfils an important protective function. A sensation of pain – even though it may not be felt until the noxious stimulus provoking it has already resulted in damage to the tissues – serves to prevent the person concerned from sustaining a more severe lesion which might have serious or even life-threatening consequences.

This can be most impressively demonstrated by reference to pathological conditions associated with loss of pain. One case in point is that of syringomyelia, in which the conduction of pain impulses is interrupted in the spinothalamic pathways of the spinal cord, i.e. as a result of damage to the axons which decussate in the anterior grey commissure. Further examples of pathological states in which the sensation of pain is absent include hereditary sensory radicular neuropathy[32], familial dysautonomia[105], congenital sensory neuropathy with anhidrosis[97,118,122], and congenital indifference to pain[12,72]. The pathologico-anatomical substrate implicated in congenital indifference to pain has not yet been established with certainty and is probably not a uniform one; although, in one case of this kind, a decrease was noted in the number of myelinated fibres in the fasciculus subcallosus, the precise significance of this finding is unclear[72]. In two sisters suffering from confirmed congenital indifference to pain, APPENZELLER and KORNFELD[12] found signs indicative of a chronic peripheral neuropathy. But polyneuropathies of early onset, which are understandably difficult to distinguish from a congenital neuropathy, can also give rise to similar clinical pictures in children[59]. All these conditions have more or less serious indirect consequences, among which are frequent injuries, burns, mutilations, infections, and other secondary complications.

Besides serving a warning and protective function, however, *pain may* under certain circumstances also *become a disease in itself*. This is the case, for example, in instances where – as in patients suffering from cancer – the cause of the pain is such that it can be neither avoided nor eliminated. In addition, there are also certain types of injury or disease which, though not necessarily painful in themselves, have particularly adverse repercussions on peripheral or central nervous structures, thereby giving rise secondarily to distinctive clinical pictures in which the pain is often so refractory that they could quite justifiably be termed "pain syndromes".

Treatment for chronic pain attributable to a demonstrably serious cause, such as a malignant tumour for instance, may take the form either of drug therapy or of surgery. Surgical treatment consists in principle in the temporary or permanent interruption of peripheral or central pathways conducting pain impulses[19,36,43,65,110,132] or in the ablation of thalamic nuclei or cortical structures.

A more recent surgical approach to the treatment of chronically painful conditions, particularly in cases of cancer, is that known as radiculotomy[73], which is likewise based on anatomical and physiological considerations as already outlined earlier in the present paper. Here, it was explained that the thin A-delta and C fibres, which conduct pain impulses and which activate the input control system in the posterior horn, enter the spinal cord in the ventrolateral part of the posterior root. The thicker, myelinated fibres run through the dorsomedial portion of the root. Selective transection of the ventrolateral part of the posterior root, performed using microsurgical techniques, is indeed capable of eliminating pain. In contrast to radicotomy, however, this operation does not abolish epicritic sensibility, and it may also serve to relieve muscle spasm[73].

Now for a brief discussion of those painful conditions which are of such a distinctive type that they can be regarded as genuine "pain syndromes".

4.2. "Neuralgias" and tic douloureux

The term "neuralgia" tends to be very loosely employed[57, 58, 101]. Though invariably indicating that the pain is of a localised nature, it by no means always implies that this pain is of uniform character or pathogenesis – as exemplified, for instance, by the difference in the quality of the pain occurring during the sudden, brief, but excruciating attacks of trigeminal "neuralgia" and the dull, burning, and boring sensations experienced in the "neuralgia" associated with herpes zoster. That the expression "neuralgia" also embraces conditions lacking a common pathogenetic denominator is apparent, for example, from the fact that so-called intercostal neuralgia is usually due to mechanical causes, that Horton's "neuralgia" is of vasomotor origin, and that even rheumatic affections are often labelled right from the start as "neuralgias".

If the term "neuralgia" is to be retained at all, it is essential that it be employed in a more restrictive sense. As suggested by REISNER[101], for instance, it could be reserved for those painful conditions in which a consistently localised pain is attributable to disease of a peripheral sensory nerve, e.g. of the spinal root, of the plexus, or of the peripheral nerve trunk. In such conditions the pain is either paroxysmal – and is then generally of brief duration, sharp, and very severe – or, alternatively, persistent – in which case it usually has a dull, boring, and deep-seated quality. If this were to be accepted as the definition of "neuralgia", other painful conditions of a distinctive character (referred to below) would have to be differentiated from it. With regard to the pathogenesis of "neuralgia" as defined in this manner, one possibility is that the process might be of mechanical origin, i.e. due in most cases to a chronic mechanical lesion of the nerve or of the root. Examples include chronic compression syndromes involving peripheral nerves (e.g. ilio-inguinal syndrome, tarsal-tunnel syndrome, Morton's metatarsalgia, etc.) in which demyelination of peripheral axons occurs. The thicker myelinated axons are more sensitive to mechanical pressure than the thin axons which chiefly serve to conduct pain impulses. Consequently, the input control stations in the posterior horn of the spinal cord fail to receive inhibitory impulses from the thicker fibres, with the result that pain afferents from the A-delta and C fibres may preponderate. Often, on the other hand, the cause of the neuralgia is not mechanical, but has to be sought in the fine structure – usually in the ganglion. An example in point is trigeminal neuralgia, in which the myelin sheaths show microscopic evidence of damage[64]; since the patients concerned are as a rule elderly people, these microscopic lesions may perhaps be caused by the pulsations of a sclerosed carotid artery[63].

The afferents in the root of the trigeminal nerve terminate in two nuclear zones: firstly, the descending root, which plays a role similar to that of Rolando's fasciculus in the posterior horn of the spinal cord, and, secondly, the main sensory nucleus, which fulfils the same epicritic functions as the posterior-root nuclei in the spinal cord[27]. Inhibitory impulses are conveyed to the neurones of the descending root via collaterals. The presence of lesions in the thick myelinated fibres – lesions which may, for example, also arise from external pressure – leads to a preponderance of impulses from the thin fibres. The resultant excitation of a large number of neurones in the descending root is further aggravated by the fact that the inhibitory impulses mentioned above are no longer being received. Another possibility currently under discussion is that, at sites where a pathological loss of myelin has occurred, tactile impulses may jump over to the thin fibres, with the result that the preponderance of impulses from these thin fibres becomes even greater. A pool of activated neurones would thus eventually build up, in which some additional, e.g. tactile, stimulus may then trigger off an "epileptiform" discharge experienced in the form of an acute attack of pain. It is here that a membrane-stabilising drug could be expected to have its site of attack.

4.3. Neuroma pain and "algie diffusante"
In a cicatricial neuroma, the confused network of overgrown and matted axons is shot through with proliferating Schwann cells and fibroblasts, as well as capillaries. This structure is such that mechanical stimulation of the axons may occur even in response to external influences of a minor character. Acute pain, setting in synchronously with the mechanical stimulus and as a rule of the same duration as the latter, is then experienced, this pain being projected into the region that had originally been innervated by the severed nerve. Since all the axons in the segment of nerve concerned have been interrupted, the tactile impulses which under normal circumstances would have been steadily flowing in from the peripheral zone supplied by it are no longer transmitted. This, however, means that in addition the inhibitory effect on the input control system in the posterior root is abolished. The numerous afferents excited by the mechanical stimulus to which the neuroma has been subjected find this control system wide open – also to pain impulses from the thin fibres. Excision of the neuroma does, it is true, afford temporary freedom from pain, because the site of the stimulus causing the pain, i.e. the matted network of overgrown axons, is thus eliminated. But, since the steady stream of inhibitory impulses which should be entering the input control system through the thick fibres is still interrupted, this system continues to remain open. In most cases a fresh neuroma soon develops, and, because the pathophysiological conditions are essentially the same as before, it proves just as painful as the previous one. It is this which explains why repeated neuroma excisions following injuries to the peripheral nerves tend to yield disappointing results[119].
The sequelae resulting from peripheral nerve damage include not only neuroma pain as such, but quite often also a form of hyperpathia referred to as *post-traumatic neuralgia*[33]. The latter, which is exclusively confined to the distal

ends of the extremities, differs from causalgia in that it occurs only where the nerves have been completely transected. Post-traumatic neuralgia is liable to set in at a very early stage, i.e. it may develop in the marginal zone of the insensitive area before any regeneration in the form of budding of the severed nerves has taken place; alternatively, it may manifest itself in the previously anaesthetic area at a later stage when regeneration is already in progress. Here, again, it must be assumed that the denervated zone no longer emits the normal steady stream of epicritic impulses. In the posterior-root cells upon which the fibres converged prior to transection, this absence of epicritic impulses leads to a deficiency of inhibitory afferents and a corresponding increase in the excitatory impulses reaching these cells via other (neighbouring) nerve branches. It is conceivable that the structural peculiarities of the regenerating axons may perhaps also play a role in this connection by resulting in a change in the nociceptive code. How far the hyperaesthesia extends beyond the autonomous innervation zone of the damaged nerve will depend on the degree to which the adjacent cutaneous innervation zones overlap. It might possibly depend, too, on the extent to which those cells in the posterior horn of the spinal cord appertaining to the injured nerve are also reached by short collaterals from the innervation zones of other nerves. In extreme cases, spreading of the hyperpathia over an extensive area would result in what the French refer to as "*algie diffusante*".

In patients suffering from neuroma pain – as well as in cases of phantom-limb pain (see below) – the successful responses which have been obtained by electrically stimulating the thick fibres responsible for epicritic sensibility suggest that the pathogenesis of such pain can also be accounted for in terms of the gate control theory [84, 125].

4.4. Causalgia

As already observed by MITCHELL[86] in 1872, causalgia is encountered chiefly as a sequel to war wounds. Its onset often occurs within only hours of the injury, the lesion in question being invariably an incomplete one which almost always involves either the median nerve or the medial popliteal nerve. Typical of causalgia is an intense and continuous burning pain; this pain, which is greatly aggravated by touch and which can be relieved by the application of wet dressings, causes the patient to resort to protective immobilisation of the extremity and finally induces in him a peculiarly anxious, psychopathologically distinctive mode of behaviour [33, 121, 124]. Marked dystrophic changes of the skin and soft tissues in the affected area, even culminating sometimes in Sudeck's atrophy, are an invariable accompaniment.

The explanation for the pathophysiology of causalgia [121] suggested by GRANIT et al. [42] is that, after a mixed nerve has sustained injury, efferent sympathetic impulses which normally switch over to afferent sensory fibres ("cross-stimulation") do so even more readily. JUNG [60], on the other hand, postulates that the presence of pathological ephapses at the site of the lesion causes excitatory impulses to jump from one afferent to another; this, it is claimed, also applies to excitatory impulses from sympathetic efferents, which switch over most easily of all to C fibres. While this would account for the fact that the nerves predominantly involved in cases of causalgia are the median nerve and the medial popliteal nerve, which are particularly rich in sympathetic fibres, it does not explain why the causalgia itself cannot be eliminated by completely severing the damaged peripheral nerve or by amputating the limb. Presumably, the pathological process occurring in the periphery must have the effect of activating in the central nervous system an excitatory circuit which then becomes self-perpetuating. That sympathetic efferents do play a role in this connection would seem to be borne out by the fact that sympathetic blockade is the only effective form of treatment for causalgia.

4.5. Deep visceral pain and referred pain (Head's zones)
Deep visceral pain is a dull, boring, and tormenting pain which it is difficult to locate exactly[99]. It arises in response to distension of hollow organs, to traction exerted on their ligaments and attachments, to inflammation, and to the endogenous production of chemical substances. Sensitivity to pain is greatest in the parietal serous membranes. Patients suffering from painful diseases of the internal organs experience additional pain – usually of a dull quality – in certain specific regions of the body surface, the areas of skin concerned being also hypersensitive to touch. These areas, named Head's zones after the British neurologist Sir HENRY HEAD, are of major importance in clinical diagnosis. This phenomenon of so-called "referred pain"[129] can be accounted for in the light of facts already dealt with in the present paper (cf. Chapter 3 in particular): the visceral afferents converge on the same cells in the posterior horns of the spinal cord as the segmentally corresponding cutaneous afferents. In response to the arrival in the posterior horns of impulses triggered off by painful stimuli in the viscera, the pain is projected in the patient's consciousness to the area from which sensory impulses most frequently flow, i.e. to the segmentally appurtenant skin zones. Furthermore, the steady stream of impulses passing through the predominantly thin, visceral afferents[99] exerts a facilitatory influence on the input control system of the posterior horns; consequently, impulses converging on the same system in response to stimuli applied to the skin give rise to exaggeratedly unpleasant, dysaesthetic sensations. Evidence in support of this interpretation of the pathophysiology of referred pain is provided by the finding that anaesthetisation of the painful skin zones serves to relieve or even to eliminate the corresponding visceral pain[124]. Since the local anaesthetic employed for this purpose takes effect mainly by putting the thin fibres out of action, it diminishes the inflow of facilitatory afferent impulses converging from the skin zone on the same posterior-horn cells as the visceral impulses. The inhibitory impulses from this skin zone which are still arriving via the thick myelinated fibres of the cutaneous nerves (because these thick fibres are less sensitive to anaesthetics than the thin ones) now become sufficient to offset the afferent impulses emanating from the viscera. In this connection, it is interesting to speculate to what extent the successful results obtained with *acupuncture* in chronically painful conditions involving the internal organs may be at least partially accountable for in terms of this inter-

pretation of the pathophysiology of referred pain; it is possible that the stimulus produced by inserting a metal needle at the appropriate skin site and then gently moving it might send a series of impulses through the myelinated epicritic fibres to the posterior horn, and that these additional inhibitory impulses might suffice to counter the relative preponderance of excitatory impulses from the thin visceral afferents.

Besides these interpretations based on mechanisms of a largely peripheral or spinal character, it may be that central phenomena also play a role: convergence of cutaneous and visceral neurones has, for example, been demonstrated in the cells of the sensory cortex[8, 91, 131]; and it has also been found that, following mechanical stimulation of the skin, the response with which a cortical cell reacts to electrical stimulation of the splanchnic nerve is appreciably diminished.

4.6. Pain associated with herpes zoster
After the virus responsible for herpes zoster has invaded the sensory spinal ganglia or the gasserian ganglion, the patient – particularly if he happens to be an elderly person – may often find himself left with an extremely intractable pain of the burning, boring type. Sometimes, lightning paroxysms of pain occur later. In the affected zone, which is hypersensitive to touch, the patient has a feeling of severe soreness. Insofar as there is evidence that it is thick myelinated fibres which are preferentially involved, the pathophysiology of the pain associated with herpes zoster is comparable with that of trigeminal neuralgia.

In biopsy studies on intercostal nerves from segments affected by herpes zoster, NOORDENBOS[92] did in fact observe quite a marked decrease in the thick myelinated fibres, coupled with a significant relative increase in both the myelinated and non-myelinated thin fibres[99]. Under these circumstances, the assumption that a lack of inhibitory impulses from the A-alpha fibres leads to a relative increase in pain impulses from the thin fibres appears very plausible. In a few cases of post-herpetic pain, MAZARS et al.[78] succeeded in eliminating the pain by stimulating Reil's ribbon; though this suggests that in pain attributable to herpes zoster a central plane may also be involved, it fails to shed any light on the latter's specific role.

4.7. Pain due to deafferentation
Following transection of a posterior spinal nerve root, as performed during radicotomy, stimulation of neighbouring dermatomes may cause a sudden onset of lightning pain. Radicotomy has the effect of depriving the segmental posterior-horn cells of their epicritic afferents, which exert an inhibitory influence on the input control system. Through ascending and descending collaterals, however, these same cells continue to receive impulses from the less segmentally arranged, thin protopathic afferents of adjacent nerve roots, to which they respond uninhibitedly[27]. This has been confirmed by WALL and SWEET[125], who found that the lightning pain mentioned above could be abolished by applying a mild electrical stimulus to the proximal stump of the

severed posterior root – a stimulus to which the thick, myelinated, inhibitory root fibres are the first to respond.

4.8. Phantom-limb pain

Some 10% of all patients who have had a limb amputated suffer from pain syndromes[43] consisting chiefly of neuroma pain or of phantom-limb pain. The latter usually sets in either spontaneously or merely in response to active movement of the stump of the limb. It is of a burning type and may take the form of continuous pain, acute attacks of pain, or a combination of both. A peculiar feature of this condition is the impression the patient has that the pain originates from the missing portion of the limb. This curious phenomenon may be attributable to the fact that those cells – located in the spinal cord and further towards the centre – which receive excitatory impulses still "impute" them topographically to the regions of the body whence they were accustomed to receiving their main inflow of excitatory impulses in the past. As a result of the amputation, however, these cells have been deprived of their epicritic afferents, with the result that no inhibitory influence is now exerted on the input control system. Consequently, even relatively minor stimuli emanating from the region of the stump itself or from other areas within the remaining portion of the limb are sufficient to excite the pool of cells, which in turn may possibly cause them to produce hypersynchronous mass-discharges.

Evidence in favour of this interpretation is afforded by the observation that phantom-limb pain disappears following electrical stimulation of the nerve trunks – and thus of the thick, myelinated, inhibitory afferent fibres – in the stump of the limb[84, 125]. But the fact that here, too, some abnormal mechanism or mechanisms must also be operative on a central plane, is suggested in particular by those cases in which stimulation of the posterior columns of the spinal cord has been found to elicit a good therapeutic response[85].

4.9. Pain believed to originate in the reticular formation

As has already been explained earlier (cf. Section 3.7.), the reticular formation of the brainstem exerts chiefly a depressant influence on the conduction of pain impulses[70, 77, 79, 103]. Moreover, damage to the reticular formation results in hyperalgesia[82]. It therefore seems by no means unlikely that certain types of painful attack occurring spontaneously and confined to one half of the body may be attributable to a lesion in the reticular formation. The connection existing between unilateral tonic (motor) seizures and lesions of the reticular formation has been well established[89]; the cases in question included very many in which these tonic seizures were accompanied by pain, whereas cases featuring attacks of pain only, with no motor involvement, were rarely encountered. Other types of paroxysmal motor seizure, taking the form of paroxysmal dysarthria and ataxia, have also been observed in multiple sclerosis patients with foci in the region of the brainstem[134]. The fact that carbamazepine (®Tegretol) and other anti-epileptic agents have been found to yield good results in such cases suggests that local hypersynchronous discharges probably play a role here; since in all these cases, however, the electro-encephalographic findings remain normal, no cortical projection of these discharges evidently occurs.

4.10. Thalamic pain

It has already been mentioned earlier in the present paper (cf. Section 3.5.) that stimulation of the thalamus may elicit or abolish pain, depending on the site in the thalamus at which the stimulus is applied. In view of this, it is not surprising that, particularly after a cerebrovascular accident, a painful thalamic syndrome may set in, even where no attempts at treatment have been made[43]. On the side of the body opposite the lesion, the patient suffers from intractable, burning pains whose topographical distribution is difficult to pinpoint. Touch acts as a stimulus eliciting an unpleasant sensation which is of delayed onset and which outlasts the stimulus itself. Though sensibility is also disturbed in other respects, and is to some extent dissociated, it is never so clearly dissociated as in patients with spinal-cord lesions. In these cases of thalamic syndrome, sensory stimuli and emotional reactions are likewise liable to trigger off attacks of pain. A syndrome of this kind may, incidentally, also develop following stereotactic operations on the thalamus[99], but never after stereotactic surgery involving only the centromedian nucleus[76].

4.11. Cortical pain?

Reference has been made earlier on (cf. Section 3.6.) to the fact that stimulation of the cerebral cortex may produce painful sensations, but only in patients already suffering from spontaneous pain[132]. That pain of cortical origin may also occur spontaneously is therefore conceivable, although such cases appear to be extremely rare. WILKINSON[133] has reported on a patient in whom "epileptic pain" was successfully eliminated by extirpating a metastatic tumour located deep in the contralateral parietal sulcus.

5. Concluding remarks

The substrate involved in the perception, sensation, and interpretation of pain is a system organised in an extremely complex manner, operating on various functional planes and featuring numerous control and feedback mechanisms. Such, indeed, is the complexity of this system, and of all the interrelationships on which its functioning depends, that, despite the wealth of material already published on the subject, only certain aspects of the neurophysiology of pain have yet been elucidated. A well-documented general picture is nevertheless now beginning to emerge, on the basis of which it is possible to gain a better understanding of certain clinical phenomena. What is more, the results of recent neurological research have also opened up new approaches to treatment. The review which has been presented here will, it is hoped, have served to shed light on some of these fundamental aspects that are of both clinical and therapeutic importance.

6. Summary

An outline, based on data contained in the relevant literature, is first of all given of the functional organisation of pain at the various levels. Located in the periphery are certain cutaneous zones containing receptors which, though specific for nociceptive stimuli, do not constitute a uniform histological substrate. Depending on the temporal and spatial constellation of the afferent impulses, however, painful sensations can also be elicited via receptors which are not (pain-)specific. It is chiefly through thin myelinated A-delta fibres and non-myelinated C fibres that pain impulses are transmitted to the central organ. But it is impossible to establish any absolute correlation between certain specific end-organs and certain specific fibres, especially since it is also conceivable that functional encoding of afferent impulses may occur within a particular morphological substrate. Neurophysiological findings suggest that there is a first input control system in the zone at which pain fibres enter the posterior roots in the spinal cord. Although not all the implications of the "gate control" hypothesis of MELZACK and WALL[83] are acceptable from the neurophysiological standpoint, it is a useful theory and not incompatible with clinical and therapeutic observations. Probably as a result of pre-synaptic inhibition mediated by interneurones in Rolando's fasciculus, excitation of thick myelinated fibres inhibits the response to afferent bursts from thin fibres which, among other things, also conduct nociceptive or pain impulses. In the spinal cord, the impulses converge upon superordinate posterior-horn cells, each successive step in this process being potentially conducive to an interaction between different excitatory impulses. Intervening in this first input control system are also segmental as well as contralateral and central impulses which may exert either an inhibitory or a facilitatory effect.

In the spinal cord, most of the pain impulses pass through the monosynaptic neo-spinothalamic tract into the ventro-posterolateral nucleus of the thalamus, whereas some enter the intralaminar nuclei of the thalamus via the polysynaptic palaeo-spinothalamic tract. The latter sends out collaterals to the reticular formation of the brainstem. In view not only of the connections linking the reticular formation with the thalamus and cerebrum, but also of the feedback mechanisms operating between the reticular formation and the spinal cord, it must be assumed that the reticular formation is the site of a relay centre through which pain may have repercussions on psyche and behaviour and through which, on the other hand, external influences and psychic factors can affect the apperception of pain. The role played by the thalamus and by cortical (parietal) neurones in the interpretation of pain is also outlined.

On the basis of this analysis of the functional organisation of pain, the pathophysiology of painful diseases is examined and an attempt made to explain the rationale of various forms of treatment for such diseases. Discussed in this connection are the "neuralgias", tic douloureux, neuroma pain, "algie diffusante", causalgia, deep visceral pain, Head's zones, herpetic pain, pain due to deafferentation, phantom-limb pain, pain believed to originate in the reticular formation, thalamic pain, and the possibility of cortical pain.

1 ADLER, R., LOMAZZI, F.: Die Bedeutung der individuellen Schmerzempfindlichkeit für die Beurteilung von Schmerzzuständen. Der Libman-Test als klinisches Hilfsmittel. Schweiz. med. Wschr. *104*, 1192–1195 (1974)

2 ADRIAN, E. D.: Afferent discharges to the cerebral cortex from peripheral sense organs. J. Physiol. (Lond.) *100*, 159–191 (1941)

3 AKERT, K.: Das limbische System und seine funktionelle Bedeutung. Relaxation und Sedation des menschlichen Uterus, IInd Symp., Berne 1963. Fortschr. Geburtsh. Gynäk., Vol. XIX, pp. 4–17 (Karger, Basle 1964)

4 AKERT, K., HUMMEL, P.: Anatomie und Physiologie des limbischen Systems, 2nd Ed. (Hoffmann-La Roche, Basle 1968)

5 AKIL, H., MAYER, D.J.: Antagonism of stimulation-produced analgesia by p-CPA, a serotonin synthesis inhibitor. Brain Res. *44*, 692–697 (1972)

6 ALBE-FESSARD, D., ARFEL, G., DEROME, P., DONDEY, M.: Electrophysiology of the human thalamus with special reference to trigeminal pain. In Hassler, R., Walker, A. E. (Editors): Trigeminal neuralgia. Pathogenesis and pathophysiology, pp. 139–148 (Thieme, Stuttgart 1970)

7 ALBE-FESSARD, D., BESSON, J.-M.: Convergent thalamic and cortical projections – the non-specific system, loc. cit. [54], pp. 489–560

8 AMASSIAN, V. E.: Interaction in the somatovisceral projection system. Res. Publ. Ass. nerv. ment. Dis. *30*, 371–402 (1952)

9 ANDERSEN, P., ECCLES, J. C., SEARS, T. A.: Cortically evoked depolarization of primary afferent fibers in the spinal cord. J. Neurophysiol. *27*, 63–77 (1964)

10 ANDERSSON, S.A.: Projection of different spinal pathways to the second somatic sensory area in cat. Acta physiol. scand. *56*, Suppl. 194 (1962)

11 ANDRES, K. H., DÜRING, M. VON: Morphology of cutaneous receptors, loc. cit. [54], pp. 3–28

12 APPENZELLER, O., KORNFELD, M.: Indifference to pain. Arch. Neurol. (Chic.) *27*, 322–339 (1972)

13 AUERSPERG, A.: Schmerz und Schmerzhaftigkeit (Springer, Berlin/Göttingen/Heidelberg 1963)

14 BARRAQUER-BORDAS, L., JANÉ-CARRENCÁ, F.: El dolor. Anatomofisiología clínica y terapéutica farmacológica (Paz Montalvo, Madrid 1968)

15 BEECHER, H. K.: Anästhesiologie. Med. Prisma No. 14 (1963)

16 BESSOU, P., BURGESS, P. R., PERL, E. R., TAYLOR, C. B.: Dynamic properties of mechanoreceptors with unmyelinated (C) fibers. J. Neurophysiol. *34*, 116–131 (1971)

17 BISHOP, G. H.: Responses to electrical stimulation of single sensory units of skin. J. Neurophysiol. *6*, 361–382 (1943)

18 BISHOP, G. H.: The relation between nerve fiber size and sensory modality: phylogenetic implications of the afferent innervation of cortex. J. nerv. ment. Dis. *128*, 89–114 (1959)

19 BONICA, J.J.: The management of pain. With special emphasis on the use of analgesic block in diagnosis, prognosis and therapy (Lea & Febiger, Philadelphia 1953)

20 BOWSHER, D.: Les relais des sensibilités somesthésique et douloureuse au niveau du tronc cérébral et du thalamus. Toulouse méd. *64*, 965–983 (1963)

21 BOWSHER, D., ALBE-FESSARD, D.: Patterns of somatosensory organization within the central nervous system, loc. cit. [62], pp. 107–122

22 BROWN, A. G., FRANZ, D. N.: Responses of spinocervical tract neurones to natural stimulation of identified cutaneous receptors. Exp. Brain Res. *7*, 231–249 (1969)

23 BÜRGER-PRINZ, H.: Zur Psychologie des Schmerzes. Nervenarzt *22*, 376–380 (1951)

24 BURGESS, P. R., PERL, E. R.: Myelinated afferent fibres responding specifically to noxious stimulation of the skin. J. Physiol. (Lond.) *190*, 541–562 (1967)

25 Burgess, P.R., Perl, E.R.: Cutaneous mechanoreceptors and nociceptors, loc. cit. [54], pp. 29–78

26 Buytendijk, F.J.J.: Über den Schmerz (Huber, Berne 1948)

27 Cambier, J., Dehen, H.: Les douleurs fulgurantes. Etiologie et physiopathologie. Presse méd. *79*, 1419–1422 (1971)

28 Cauna, N.: Fine structure of the receptor organs and its probable functional significance, loc. cit. [102], pp. 117–127

29 Christensen, B.N., Perl, E.R.: Spinal neurons specifically excited by noxious or thermal stimuli: marginal zone of the dorsal horn. J. Neurophysiol. *33*, 293–307 (1970)

30 Clark, D., Hughes, J., Gasser, H.S.: Afferent function in the group of nerve fibers of slowest conduction velocity. Amer. J. Physiol. *114*, 69–76 (1935)

31 Collins, W.F., Jr., Nulsen, F.E., Randt, C.T.: Relation of peripheral nerve fiber size and sensation in man. Arch. Neurol. (Chic.) *3*, 381–385 (1960)

32 Denny-Brown, D.: Hereditary sensory radicular neuropathy. J. Neurol. Neurosurg. Psychiat. *14*, 237–252 (1951)

33 Denny-Brown, D.: The release of deep pain by nerve injury. Brain *88*, 725–738 (1965)

34 Douglas, W.W., Ritchie, J.M.: Mammalian nonmyelinated nerve fibers. Physiol. Rev. (Lond.) *42*, 297–334 (1962)

35 Feltz, P., Krauthamer, G., Albe-Fessard, D.: Neurons of the medial diencephalon. I. Somatosensory responses and caudate inhibition. J. Neurophysiol. *30*, 55–80 (1967)

36 Finneson, B.E.: Diagnosis and management of pain syndromes, 2nd Ed. (Saunders, Philadelphia/London/Toronto 1969)

37 Fleischhauer, K.: Zur Morphologie der Schmerzrezeptoren, loc. cit. [57], pp. 8–11

38 Foerster, O.: Sensible corticale Felder. In Bumke, O., Foerster, O. (Editors): Handbuch der Neurologie, Vol. VI, pp. 358–448 (Springer, Berlin 1936)

39 Franz, D.N., Iggo, A.: Dorsal root potentials and ventral root reflexes evoked by nonmyelinated fibres. Science *162*, 1140–1142 (1968)

40 Frey, M. von: Beiträge zur Sinnesphysiologie der Haut. Dritte Mitteilung. Ber. Verh. sächs. Ges. Wiss. Leipzig, mathem.-phys. Kl. *47*, 166–184 (1895)

41 Gooddy, W.: On the nature of pain. Brain *80*, 118–131 (1957)

42 Granit, R., Leksell, L., Skoglund, C.R.: Fibre interaction in injured or compressed region of nerve. Brain *67*, 125–140 (1944)

43 Guillaume, J., Sèze, S. de, Mazars, G.: Chirurgie cérébro-spinale de la douleur (Presses Universitaires de France, Paris 1949)

44 Gybels, J., Carton, H., Cosyns, P., Peluso, F.: Die supraspinale Kontrolle experimentell erzeugter Schmerzempfindung beim Menschen, loc. cit. [58], pp. 137–140

45 Hassler, R.: Die zentralen Systeme des Schmerzes. Acta neurochir. (Vienna) *8*, 353–423 (1960)

46 Hassler, R.: Interrelationship of cortical and subcortical pain systems. In Lim, R.K.S., et al. (Editors): Pharmacology of pain, pp. 219–229 (Pergamon Press, Oxford etc. 1968)

47 Hensel, H.: Cutaneous thermoreceptors, loc. cit. [54], pp. 79–110

48 Hensel, H., Huopaniemi, R.: Static and dynamic properties of warm fibres in the infraorbital nerve. Europ. J. Physiol. *309*, 1–10 (1969)

49 Iggo, A.: Cutaneous mechanoreceptors with afferent C fibres. J. Physiol. (Lond.) *152*, 337–353 (1960)

50 Iggo, A.: Pain and pain receptors (concluding discussion), loc. cit. [102], pp. 360–366

51 Iggo, A.: Physiology of visceral afferent systems. Acta neuroveg. (Vienna) *28*, 121–134 (1966)

52 Iggo, A.: Beweise für die Existenz von «Schmerz»-Rezeptoren, loc. cit. [58], pp. 64–71

53 Iggo, A.: Kritische Bemerkungen zur Gate-Control-Theorie, loc. cit. [58], p. 136

54 IGGO, A. (Editor): Somatosensory system. Handbook of sensory physiology, Vol. II (Springer, Berlin/Heidelberg/New York 1973)

55 IGGO, A., OGAWA, H.: Primate cutaneous thermal nociceptors. J. Physiol. (Lond.) *216*, 77P–78P (1971); abstract of paper

56 JACQUET, Y. F., LAJTHA, A.: Morphine action at central nervous system sites in rat: analgesia or hyperalgesia depending on site and dose. Science *182*, 490–492 (1973)

57 JANZEN, R. (Editor): Schmerzanalyse als Wegweiser zur Diagnose (Thieme, Stuttgart 1966)

58 JANZEN, R., KEIDEL, W. D., HERZ, A., STEICHELE, C. (Editors): Schmerz. Grundlagen – Pharmakologie – Therapie (Thieme, Stuttgart 1972)

59 JOHNSON, R. H., SPALDING, J. M. K.: Progressive sensory neuropathy in children. J. Neurol. Neurosurg. Psychiat. *27*, 125–130 (1964)

60 JUNG, R.: Allgemeine Neurophysiologie. In Bergmann, G. von, et al. (Editors): Handbuch der inneren Medizin, 4th Ed., Vol. V/1: Neurologie, pp. 1–181; pp. 68–69: Pathologische und künstliche Synapsen (Springer, Berlin/Göttingen/Heidelberg 1953)

61 KEELE, C. A.: Measurement of responses to chemically induced pain, loc. cit. [102], pp. 57–72

62 KEELE, C. A., SMITH, R. (Editors): The assessment of pain in man and animals, Proc. int. Symp., London 1961 (Livingstone, Edinburgh/London 1962)

63 KERR, F. W. L.: The etiology of trigeminal neuralgia. Arch. Neurol. (Chic.) *8*, 15–25 (1963)

64 KERR, F. W. L., MILLER, R. H.: The pathology of trigeminal neuralgia. Electron microscopic studies. Arch. Neurol. (Chic.) *15*, 308–319 (1966)

65 KRAYENBÜHL, H., STOLL, W. A.: Psychochirurgie bei unerträglichen Schmerzen. Acta neurochir. (Vienna) *1*, 1–41 (1950)

66 LECHNER, H.: Der Lobus limbicus und seine funktionellen Beziehungen zur Affektivität. Wien. Z. Nervenheilk. *16*, 281–320 (1959)

67 LECHNER, H., KUGLER, J., FONTANARI, D. (Editors): Die kranialen und zervikobrachialen Neuralgien (Huber, Berne/Stuttgart/Vienna 1973)

68 LIBET, B.: Electrical stimulation of cortex in human subjects, and conscious sensory aspects, loc. cit. [54], pp. 743–790

69 LIBMAN, E.: Observations on individual sensitiveness to pain. J. Amer. med. Ass. *102*, 335–341 (1934)

70 LIEBESKIND, J. C., GUILBAUD, G., BESSON, J.-M., OLIVERAS, J.-L.: Analgesia from electrical stimulation of the periaqueductal gray matter in the cat: behavioral observations and inhibitory effects on spinal cord interneurons. Brain Res. *50*, 441–446 (1973)

71 LUNDBERG, A.: The supraspinal control of transmission in spinal reflex pathways. Electroenceph. clin. Neurophysiol. Suppl. 25: 35–46 (1967)

72 MAGEE, K. R.: Congenital indifference of pain. An anatomicopathologic study. Arch. Neurol. (Chic.) *9*, 635–640 (1963)

73 MANSUY, L., SINDOU, M., FISCHER, G., GERIN, P.: Etat actuel de la physiologie de la douleur au niveau médullaire. Applications neurochirurgicales. Nouv. Presse méd. *3*, 313–317 (1974)

74 MARTINS, L. F., UMBACH, W.: Klinisch-anatomischer Vergleich zwischen Läsionstopik und Schmerzverbesserung bei stereotaktischer Ausschaltung. Neurochirurgia (Stuttg.) *17*, 77–83 (1974)

75 MARUHASHI, J., MIZUGUCHI, K., TASAKI, I.: Action currents in single afferent nerve fibres elicited by stimulation of the skin of the toad and the cat. J. Physiol. (Lond.) *117*, 129–151 (1952)

76 MASPES, P. E., PAGNI, C. A.: Studio critico degli interventi stereotassici eseguiti a livello talamico per il trattamento dei dolori incoercibili. Atti XV Congr. naz. Soc. ital. Neurol.; Riv. Pat. nerv. ment. (1965); quoted in [99]

77 Mayer, D.J., Wolfle, T.L., Akil, H., Carder, B., Liebeskind, J.C.: Analgesia from electrical stimulation in the brainstem of the rat. Science *174*, 1351–1354 (1971)

78 Mazars, G., Merienne, L., Cioloca, C.: Traitement de certains types de douleurs par des stimulateurs thalamiques implantables. Neuro-Chirurgie *20*, 117–124 (1974)

79 Melzack, R.: The puzzle of the brain (Basic Books, New York 1973)

80 Melzack, R., Haugen, F.P.: Responses evoked at the cortex by tooth stimulation. Amer. J. Physiol. *190*, 570–574 (1957)

81 Melzack, R., Melinkoff, D.F.: Analgesia produced by brain stimulation: evidence of a prolonged onset period. Exp. Neurol. *43*, 369–374 (1974)

82 Melzack, R., Stotler, W.A., Livingston, W.K.: Effects of discrete brainstem lesions in cats on perception of noxious stimulation. J. Neurophysiol. *21*, 353–367 (1958)

83 Melzack, R., Wall, P.D.: Pain mechanisms: a new theory. Science *150*, 971–979 (1965)

84 Meyer, G.A., Fields, H.L.: Causalgia treated by selective large fibre stimulation of peripheral nerve. Brain *95*, 163–168 (1972)

85 Miles, J., Liptons, S., Hayward, M., Bowsher, D., Mumford, J., Molony, V.: Pain relief by implanted electrical stimulators. Lancet *1974/I*, 777–779

86 Mitchell, S.W.: Injuries of nerves and their consequences (Smith, Elder, London/Lippincott, Philadelphia 1872)

87 Mountcastle, V.B., Powell, T.P.S.: Neural mechanisms subserving cutaneous sensibility, with special reference to the role of afferent inhibition in sensory perception and discrimination. Bull. Johns Hopk. Hosp. *105*, 201–232 (1959)

88 Müller, J.: Handbuch der Physiologie des Menschen für Vorlesungen (Hölscher, Koblenz 1840); quoted in [99], p. 115

89 Mumenthaler, M., Hecker, A.: Klinik und Zuordnung tonischer Hirnstammanfälle anhand von 27 eigenen Beobachtungen. Fortschr. Neurol. Psychiat. *41*, 623–639 (1973)

90 Nashold, B.S., Jr., Friedman, H.: Dorsal column stimulation for control of pain. Preliminary report on 30 patients. J. Neurosurg. *36*, 590–597 (1972)

91 Newman, P.P.: Single unit activity in the viscero-sensory areas of the cerebral cortex. J. Physiol. (Lond.) *160*, 284–297 (1962)

92 Noordenbos, W.: Pain (Elsevier, Amsterdam etc. 1959)

93 Notermans, S.L.H., Tophoff, M.M.W.A.: Sex difference in pain tolerance and pain apperception. Psychiat. Neurol. Neurochir. (Amst.) *70*, 23–29 (1967)

94 Osácar, E.M., Meyer, A.E., Jakab, I.: A histologically verified bilateral anterolateral chordotomy without cutaneous sensory loss. A case report. Acta neurochir. (Vienna) *9*, 525–537 (1961)

95 Penfield, W., Rasmussen, T.: The cerebral cortex of man (Macmillan, New York 1950)

96 Perl, E.R.: Myelinated afferent fibres innervating the primate skin and their response to noxious stimuli. J. Physiol. (Lond.) *197*, 593–615 (1968)

97 Pinsky, L., DiGeorge, A.M.: Congenital familial sensory neuropathy with anhidrosis. J. Pediat. *68*, 1–13 (1966)

98 Pomeranz, B., Wall, P.D., Weber, W.V.: Cord cells responding to fine myelinated afferents from viscera, muscle and skin. J. Physiol. (Lond.) *199*, 511–532 (1968)

99 Procacci, P.: A survey of modern concepts of pain. In Finken, P.J., Bruyn, G.W. (Editors): Handbook of clinical neurology, Vol. I, pp. 114–146 (North Holland, Amsterdam 1969)

100 Quilliam, T.A.: Structure of receptor organs. Unit design and array patterns in receptor organs, loc. cit. [102], pp. 86–112

101 Reisner, H.: Zum Begriff der Neuralgie, loc. cit. [67], pp. 7–12

102 Reuck, A.V.S. de, Knight, J.: (Editors): Touch, heat and pain, Ciba Found. Symp. (Churchill, London 1966)

103 Reynolds, D.V.: Surgery in the rat during electrical analgesia induced by focal brain stimulation. Science *164*, 444–445 (1969)

104 Riechert, T., Kapp, H., Krainick, J.-U., Schmidt, C.L., Thoden, U.: Die operative Behandlung chronischer Schmerzzustände durch elektrische Hinterstrangreizung. Dtsch. med. Wschr. *98*, 1130–1131 (1973)

105 Riley, C.M.: Familial dysautonomia. Advanc. Pediat. *9*, 157–190 (1957)

106 Sato, M., Ozeki, M.: Initiation of impulses by mechanosensory nerve terminals, loc. cit. [102], pp. 203–226

107 Schmidt, R.F.: Presynaptic inhibition in the vertebrate central nervous system. Ergebn. Physiol. *63*, 19–101 (1971)

108 Schmidt, R.F.: Die Gate-Control-Theorie des Schmerzes: eine unwahrscheinliche Hypothese, loc. cit. [58], pp. 133–135

109 Schmidt, R.F.: Control of the access of afferent activity to somatosensory pathways, loc. cit. [54], pp. 151–206

110 Schürmann, K.: Grundlagen der operativen Schmerzbehandlung, loc. cit. [58], pp. 194–206

111 Shealy, C.N.: Implications of central projection of C fibers in sensory perception. In Curtis, D.R., McIntyre, A.K. (Editors): Studies in physiology, pp. 253–258 (Springer, Berlin/Heidelberg/New York 1965)

112 Shealy, C.N., Mortimer, J.T., Hagfors, N.R.: Dorsal column electroanalgesia. J. Neurosurg. *32*, 560–564 (1970)

113 Sherrington, C.S.: The integrative action of the nervous system (Scribner's Sons, New York 1906)

114 Sinclair, D.C., Stokes, B.A.R.: The production and characteristics of "second pain". Brain *87*, 609–618 (1964)

115 Spreng, M., Ichioka, M.: Langsame Rindenpotentiale bei Schmerzreizung am Menschen. Europ. J. Physiol. *279*, 121–132 (1964)

116 Sternbach, R.A., Tursky, B.: Ethnic differences among housewives in psychophysical and skin potential responses to electric shock. Psychophysiology *1*, 241–246 (1965)

117 Stockinger, L., Pritz, W.: Morphologische Aspekte der Schmerzempfindung im Zahn. Dtsch. zahnärztl. Z. *25*, 557–565 (1970)

118 Swanson, A.G.: Congenital insensitivity to pain with anhidrosis. Arch. Neurol. (Chic.) *8*, 299–306 (1963)

119 Teuscher, J.: Schmerzsyndrome nach Verletzung peripherer Nervenäste an den oberen Extremitäten. Klinisch-therapeutische Aspekte. Z. Unfallmed. Berufskr. *66*, 206–227 (1973)

120 Torebjörk, H.E., Hallin, R.G.: Responses in human A and C fibres to repeated electrical intradermal stimulation. J. Neurol. Neurosurg. Psychiat. *37*, 653–664 (1974)

121 Trostdorf, E.: Die Kausalgie (Thieme, Stuttgart 1956)

122 Vassella, F., Emrich, H.M., Kraus-Ruppert, R., Aufdermaur, F., Tönz, O.: Congenital sensory neuropathy with anhidrosis. Arch. Dis. Childh. *43*, 124–130 (1968)

123 Wall, P.D.: The laminar organization of dorsal horn and effects of descending impulses. J. Physiol. (Lond.) *188*, 403–423 (1967)

124 Wall, P.D.: Dorsal horn electrophysiology, loc. cit. [54], pp. 253–270

125 Wall, P.D., Sweet, W.H.: Temporary abolition of pain in man. Science *155*, 108–109 (1967)

126 Weber, A.: Zur Physiologie und Psychologie des Schmerzes. Schweiz. med. Wschr. *98*, 342–344 (1968)

127 Weddell, A.G.M.: Observations on the anatomy of pain sensibility, loc. cit. [62], pp. 47–59

128 WEDDELL, A.G.M., MILLER, S.: Cutaneous sensibility. Ann. Rev. Physiol. *24*, 199–222 (1962)

129 WEISS, C.: Oberflächen- und Tiefenschmerz. Auslösung und Leitung der Erregung, loc. cit. [57], pp. 12–19

130 WERLE, E.: Über körpereigene schmerzerzeugende Substanzen unter besonderer Berücksichtigung der Plasmakinine, loc. cit. [58], pp. 92–99

131 WERNER, G., WHITSEL, B.L.: Functional organization of the somatosensory cortex, loc. cit. [54], pp. 621–700

132 WHITE, J.C., SWEET, W.H.: Pain. Its mechanisms and neurosurgical control (Thomas, Springfield, Ill. 1955)

133 WILKINSON, H.A.: Epileptic pain. An uncommon manifestation with localizing value. Neurology (Minneap.) *23*, 518–520 (1973)

134 WOLF, P., ASSMUS, H.: Paroxysmale Dysarthrie und Ataxie. Ein pathognomonisches Anfallssyndrom bei multipler Sklerose. J. Neurol. (Berl.) *208*, 27–38 (1974)

135 ZIMMERMANN, M.: Dorsal root potentials after C-fiber stimulation. Science *160*, 896–898 (1968)

Discussion

W. BIRKMAYER: I think that for the clinician the paper Dr. MUMENTHALER has presented, covering the entire range from the purely theoretical aspects to their practical clinical implications, provides an excellent digest of the whole topic. The way in which he built up his review, taking us step by step through the various synaptic segments, struck me as particularly useful from the standpoint of the clinician.

H. PETSCHE: As a neurophysiologist I feel that it only remains for me to congratulate Dr. MUMENTHALER. Seldom have I met a clinician who evinced such an understanding of the neurophysiological and morphological problems with which this whole field bristles or who displayed such skill in explaining their nature. The selection he presented from his voluminous manuscript was also extraordinarily well chosen.
I should merely like here to add a few words on the gate control theory, of which most clinicians will already have heard. I thought, Dr. MUMENTHALER, that you explained the gate control theory with admirable clarity while at the same time subjecting it to critical analysis. The reproach is often levelled against the neurophysiologist – and perhaps not without some justification – that his work tends to be regarded as *l'art pour l'art* by those concerned with the more practical aspects of medicine. It is true that, once a neurophysiologist has discovered an interesting phenomenon, he is apt to concentrate on it so intensively and to wax so enthusiastic about it that he becomes blind to everything else and completely forgets the problems of clinical reality. But in the case of the gate control theory it is already apparent today that, though certain features of the theory may still be contestable, it opens up a remarkably promising approach to the treatment of causalgia and other refractory types of peripheral pain. You also referred to this point in your paper, Dr. MUMENTHALER. During the past few years, notable successes have been achieved by implanting electrodes in Rolando's substance. The patients were able to control the pain themselves by means of radio signals causing weak electrical stimuli to be emitted from the electrodes, which remained permanently *in situ*. These experiments may sound rather heroic to some, but perhaps they are not really so heroic as was at one time chordotomy, which is now generally accepted.
But how frightfully complicated the morphology of Rolando's substance is, and how little we yet know about the processes occurring within it, is impressively demonstrated by the findings RÉTHELYI and SZENTÁGOTHAI* obtained in a series of investigations on Golgi preparations. The pictures they have published reveal such a complexity of morphological links and interconnections that any attempt at unravelling them would at first sight appear doomed to failure. It is nevertheless certainly worth our while to try and tackle these problems, because occasionally, as experience has shown, studies of this kind lead to the elaboration of theories that are also of great clinical importance.

W. BIRKMAYER: I should also like to add a personal vote of congratulation and thanks to Dr. MUMENTHALER for having promoted the reticular formation to an object worthy of clinical attention. We have been studying the reticular formation for some 20 years now, chiefly in connection with the arousal reaction, but also because it is known to have a very high concentration of biogenic amines, including serotonin in particular. If I remember rightly, Dr. REISNER recently pointed out, at a small morning refresher course held in Vienna, that states characterised by pain alone can be very effectively controlled by major tranquillisers. This pain-sedating effect is undoubtedly attributable to the action such drugs exert on the reticular formation, an action which, as it were, serves to mitigate the emotional element involved in the experience of pain.

---

* RÉTHELYI, M., SZENTÁGOTHAI, J.: Distribution and connections of afferent fibres in the spinal cord. In Iggo, A. (Editor): Handbook of sensory physiology, Vol. II: Somatosensory system, p. 207 (Springer, Berlin/Heidelberg/New York 1973)

H. J. BEIN: You have just mentioned, Mr. Chairman, that major tranquillisers can produce an analgesic effect, and you have related this effect to the reticular formation. In the case of psycho-active drugs and other centrally acting preparations, including also anti-epileptic agents for example, there is a strong temptation to assume that the site of attack responsible for the drug's analgesic component is located – like the sites of attack for other cerebral effects – in the central nervous system. But this is by no means so certain; on the contrary, we must proceed on the assumption that not only central but also peripheral sites of attack are involved in the production of an analgesic effect. This even applies to morphine, the classic centrally acting analgesic. Dr. MU-MENTHALER mentioned various afferent pathways. I have undertaken detailed studies on the influence which drugs exert upon such afferent pathways. Here, I have found, for instance, that the potentials registered in the corresponding afferent nerves in response to stimulation of an intestinal loop disappear following small doses of intravenously injected morphine. This, moreover, is not the only evidence to suggest that morphine also has a direct peripheral site of attack. The clinically observable analgesic effects of major tranquillisers and antidepressants, too, are not necessarily attributable solely to a site of attack located in the brain. Antidepressants, for instance, influence catecholamine metabolism in the periphery, not only in animals but also in man. It is therefore quite conceivable that such biochemical changes occurring in the periphery and/or in the spinal cord may induce in the complicated system described by Dr. MUMENTHALER certain modifications which ultimately affect the sensation of pain. Finally, just another word or two about the reticular formation: it provides an excellent object for neurophysiological demonstration purposes; one snag, however, is the fact that there are various effects – such as inhibition of interspinal neurones – which can be demonstrated only in the anaesthetised animal.

W. BIRKMAYER: May I just add that the antidepressants do, of course, have the effect of normalising – or at least favourably influencing – not only the peripheral catecholaminergic neurones but also the indolaminergic, i.e. serotoninergic, neuronal chains.

W. P. KOELLA: I, too, wish to congratulate Dr. MUMENTHALER on his excellent paper dealing with a topic that is of great interest to us neurophysiologists. I should also like to add a few words on just one aspect of the reticular formation, an aspect which once again illustrates the complexity of the repercussions which this important system has on the functioning of the brain. We know that, when a lightly anaesthetised or a non-anaesthetised animal is subjected to individual painful stimuli, a marked arousal reaction occurs. Painful stimuli are in fact probably the best arousal-inducers. That the whole process involved is an extremely complex one, however, is revealed by the following experiment: not only in the animal, as we ourselves have demonstrated, but also in man, repeated painful stimuli administered with monotonous regularity may actually produce the opposite of arousal, namely, a damping effect or even a typical state of somnolence – as reported by OSWALD*, for example. It would thus appear that stimuli of this kind not only generate impulses reaching the reticular formation but also activate other control circuits, and that these circuits in turn emit inhibitory impulses which, provided they are encoded in the correct temporal sequence, can induce the opposite of arousal, i.e. sedation and sleep.

W. BIRKMAYER: I think the point you've just made, Dr. KOELLA, is also an important one, because it is believed, for example, that hypnosis – and possibly acupuncture too – exert an influence on inhibitory neuronal units in the reticular formation.

H. REISNER: It must have been a very intriguing, but at the same time very difficult challenge, Dr. MUMENTHALER, to cover such a vast topic as succinctly as you have succeeded in doing. I should like to revert to one question you raised, namely, that of

* OSWALD, I.: Sleeping and waking. Physiology and psychology, p. 149 (Elsevier, Amsterdam/New York 1962)

phantom-limb pain, because I have already been studying this problem for decades. It would interest me very much to hear more about your views on phantom-limb pain. We all know that, when a patient suffering from this type of pain is referred to a neurosurgeon, he is liable to return to us afterwards bearing surgical scars at a wide variety of different sites. There is indeed hardly any structure in the peripheral autonomic nervous and central nervous systems from which it is not possible to influence phantom-limb pain. Consider, for example, the possibilities of psychosurgery, or the fact that one can also relieve phantom-limb pain by operating on the autonomic nervous system. We have had cases, for instance, in which stellectomy or sympathectomy afforded temporary relief from such pain. Incidentally, among all the patients I have seen during the past 15 years with phantom-limb pain originating from the Second World War, I have not encountered a single one who was not also suffering from some form of addiction, and I therefore do not consider it advisable to refer such cases to a neurosurgeon. But now I come to my first question, Dr. MUMENTHALER. Do you believe that it is indeed possible to relieve phantom-limb pain by exerting an influence on the autonomic nervous system in the periphery? Secondly, we know that pain entails a complex interplay of factors operating at all levels from the periphery to the centre, and that – as you yourself have emphasised – a very important role is also played by the interaction between pain and psyche. We can certainly determine the point from which pain originates, as illustrated by the example of toothache. But do you really think that, bearing in mind the vast area involved, it is possible to localise pain at a particular level, e.g. in the reticular formation or in the posterior root? I rather doubt whether this is feasible.

M. MUMENTHALER: I'd like to begin by answering the questions that Dr. REISNER has asked. In the case of phantom-limb pain, it must be assumed that, following amputation of a limb, the pool of posterior-horn cells which would normally be receiving a steady stream of impulses from the periphery is simply deprived of this continuous afferent flow. When impulses are then emitted from the small portion of the limb that still remains, i.e. from the stump, they probably consist mainly of epicritic impulses which have the effect of opening the gate control system. These afferent impulses are registered as painful and are projected into that region of the periphery from which the brain had previously been accustomed to receiving them, i.e. into the phantom limb. If this hypothesis is correct, one should be able to relieve phantom-limb pain by stimulating those fibres of which there are not enough in the region concerned, namely, the thick myelinated A-alpha and A-beta fibres; and this is indeed possible. If the stump is of sufficient size for an electrode to be applied to a large nerve trunk, and if this peripheral nerve trunk is now subjected to electrical stimulation that is just strong enough to activate only the thick myelinated fibres, then the pain does in fact disappear*. This affords proof that, at least at a certain stage, phantom-limb pain is attributable to a disequilibrium between impulses flowing in through the thick and thin fibres.

Regarding the question of the role played by autonomic nervous afferents, I'm afraid I cannot supply any cut-and-dried answer. As in the case of neuroma pain, it has repeatedly been suggested that the existence of pathological ephapses may cause efferent sympathetic impulses to jump across to afferent pathways which lead back to the centre, and that such short-circuiting may partly account for the fact that autonomic nervous excitation can exert an influence on phantom-limb pain.

Turning to the other contributions that have been made to this discussion, I should like to thank Dr. PETSCHE for his interesting comments. I believe that, regardless of whether or not the gate control theory is contestable on neurophysiological grounds,

* WALL, P. D., SWEET, W. H.: Temporary abolition of pain in man. Science *155*, 108 (1967)

MEYER, G. A., FIELDS, H. L.: Causalgia treated by selective large fibre stimulation of peripheral nerve. Brain *95*, 163 (1972)

it certainly has important practical implications in the realm of treatment. I have already mentioned one therapeutic possibility in my answer to Dr. REISNER. Another consists in stimulating the dorsal columns, a procedure referred to as D.C.S. (dorsal column stimulation). Here, electrical stimuli of appropriate intensity are applied to the patient's spinal cord at a site cranial to a painful lesion. This evokes an emission of efferent impulses which travel via the descending control system to corresponding segments of the spinal cord and which relieve pain at least as effectively as chordotomy does. What is more, dorsal column stimulation is not such a radical measure as chordotomy. Further confirmation of the clinical value of the gate control theory is provided by the good responses elicited by radiculotomy, in which, as already mentioned in my paper, relief from pain is produced by selectively transecting, in the ventrolateral part of the posterior root, the thin afferents conveying impulses which open the gate control system. The latest development, about which I recently learned from a colleague of mine who is a neurosurgeon, is based on a technique designed to produce local cooling: for this purpose, a special probe is employed which freezes and coagulates the thin afferents, leaving the thicker and more resistant myelinated fibres unimpaired. This, too, is a method for the segmental relief of pain that inflicts very little harm on the patient. I therefore believe that the gate control theory, from which so many useful clinical inferences have already been drawn, deserves our continued attention, even though it may not be quite perfect from the neurophysiological angle.

What Dr. BEIN said was to some extent new to me. Listening to him, I was reminded of certain findings obtained with diazepam, which is known to have not only central but also peripheral sites of attack, e.g. on the muscle fibres. As LUDIN and co-workers*, among others, have pointed out, investigators tend to be so concerned with central drug effects that they are apt to neglect findings of the type to which Dr. BEIN has referred; and I am therefore grateful to him for having raised the points he did. His objection that results obtained when the reticular formation is stimulated in anaesthetised animals are not applicable to the non-anaesthetised animal is undoubtedly a valid one so far as experimental research is concerned. On the other hand, however, I would like to recall in this connection that, for example, in non-anaesthetised patients undergoing stereotactic operations it has been found possible to reduce the sensation of pain by stimulating certain centres in the thalamus**; consequently, by analogy with this, it seems safe to conclude that pain can also be influenced in the non-anaesthetised organism by stimulating central structures.

Dr. KOELLA's reference to the fact that painful stimuli initially produce arousal, but, if regularly repeated, tend if anything to have a somnifacient effect, only serves to emphasise once again how complex the whole phenomenon of pain is.

Finally, a brief word or two about acupuncture, to which our Chairman made a passing reference. The gate control theory offers at least a partial scientific explanation for acupuncture too. The insertion of a needle, which is then made to rotate gently, presumably acts as a painless, i.e. non-nociceptive, stimulus which sets up impulses passing through thick myelinated afferents to the spinal cord. These impulses would have the effect of blocking the input of painful afferences into the gate control system. Under these circumstances it seems quite understandable that certain painful stimuli produced segmentally or parasegmentally in the appurtenant viscerotome – in the course of an abdominal operation, for example – would prove less painful for the patient.

---

* LUDIN, H. P., DUBACH, K.: Action of diazepam on muscular contraction in man. J. Neurol. (Berl.) *199*, 30 (1971)

LUDIN, H. P., ROBERT, F.: The action of diazepam on human skeletal muscle. Europ. Neurol. (Basle) *11*, 345 (1974)

** GYBELS, J., CARTON, H., COSYNS, P., PELUSO, F.: Die supraspinale Kontrolle experimentell erzeugter Schmerzempfindung beim Menschen. In Janzen, R., Keidel, W. D., Herz, A., Steichele, C. (Editors): Schmerz. Grundlagen – Pharmakologie – Therapie, p. 137 (Thieme, Stuttgart 1972)

Trigeminal neuralgia in comparison with other forms of lightning pain

by J. Cambier and H. Dehen*

Among the various types of pain met with in neurological diseases, lightning pain is characterised by an extremely precise symptomatology: it is a sensation of sudden onset and brief duration, which occurs, as the name suggests, like a flash of lightning, or in short, sharp bursts. The site of the pain can be accurately pinpointed by the patient, who is able not only to indicate its site but also to trace its exact course. It may develop spontaneously, or else it may be induced by stimulation of a limited area of skin ("trigger zone"). The tactile stimulus required to produce it is not nociceptive; on the contrary, it consists simply of stroking the skin. The pain can be terminated by suppressing the relevant afferent impulses. Finally, all forms of lightning pain are followed by a refractory period during which stimulation of the trigger zone fails to elicit the pain. This refractory period therefore modulates the rhythm of lightning pain.

So much for the features consistently encountered in this type of pain, which may also be associated with brief motor activity (facial tic, limb withdrawal) or vasomotor activity localised in the same area as the pain and displaying the same segmental distribution as the neuronal discharge.

This description fits in perfectly with the symptomatological analysis of tabetic lightning pain which Alajouanine et al.[1] published in 1936, but it also applies equally well to essential trigeminal neuralgia. The same type of pain may also be caused by other pathological conditions; we, for example, have observed lightning pain in the course of certain cases of diabetic neuropathy, in neuropathies associated with neoplasms, and in some degenerative neuropathies[3]. Furthermore, a "lightning" component is often found in post-herpetic pain syndromes and in pain syndromes subsequent to amputation or to traumatic rupture of nerve plexuses. We ourselves have made a particular study of lightning pains developing after radicotomy.

The fact that the basic features of lightning pain remain identical in such diverse aetiological circumstances shows that this type of pain is not due to one specific cause or even to one specific anatomical lesion, but that it is an indicator of a pathophysiological mechanism common to various causes. This existence of a common pathophysiological background has been confirmed by studies on the treatment of lightning pain[4,7]; and we, too, have demonstrated, for example, that hydantoins and carbamazepine (®Tegretol) prove completely or partially effective in lightning pain irrespective of its aetiology.

Lightning pain as a sequel to radicotomy[3] represents a simplified and almost experimental model which makes it easier to understand this pathophysio-

---

* Clinique neurologique de la Faculté Xavier Bichat, Hôpital Beaujon, Clichy, France.   317

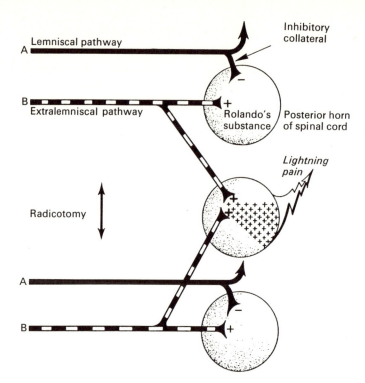

Fig. 1. Schematic representation of lightning pain following radicotomy. The region of the deafferented posterior horn remains subject to excitatory afferent impulses conducted along the extralemniscal pathway and reaching the spinal cord via the nerve roots just above and just below the transected root.

logical mechanism (Figure 1). In this model the pain occurs irregularly following surgical section or following destruction of one or two neighbouring roots by a pathological process. The lightning pain develops a few weeks or months afterwards. It is confined to a very limited region, in which a sensory deficit can be observed. It can consistently be induced by stroking the skin in the dermatomes abutting this anaesthetic zone. Hence, if the root at L5 is affected, the requisite stimulus should be applied to the region served by L4 or S1. The nature of the requisite stimulus is such that a spatial and temporal summation process is bound to occur; this, coupled with the presence of a refractory period, suggests that the discharge responsible for the lightning pain comes from neurones in the posterior horn of the spinal cord. This discharge is rendered possible by the suppression, in a particular segment, of the inhibitory action exerted by fast-conducting myelinated fibres on the neurone pool in the posterior horn. The facilitatory action exerted by non-myelinated afferent fibres, by contrast, is not somatotopically organised to the same extent, with the result that the input reaching the spinal cord via the neighbouring roots is sufficient to raise the excitability of the neurones belonging to the deafferented segment to a critical level. This concept is consonant with the "gate control" theory propounded by MELZACK and WALL[10] and also tallies well with all the symptomatological characteristics of lightning pain.

If this model is applied to trigeminal neuralgia, it would seem that the lightning discharge typical of this pain syndrome originates in the neurones of the descending root nucleus, and that these neurones, while remaining subject to

318

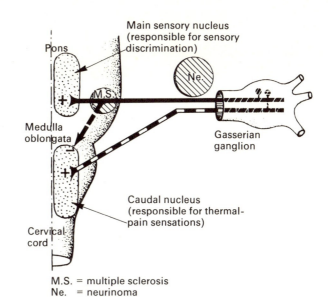

Fig. 2. Schematic representation of symptomatic trigeminal neuralgia. By reducing the speed of conduction of the myelinated fibres, the lesions upset the balance between the lemniscal and extra-lemniscal afferents to such an extent that at times a minimal afferent impulse induces a hypersynchronous discharge from the neurones in the descending root of the trigeminal nerve.

Main sensory nucleus (responsible for sensory discrimination)

Pons

Ne.

M.S.

Medulla oblongata

Gasserian ganglion

Caudal nucleus (responsible for thermal-pain sensations)

Cervical cord

M.S. = multiple sclerosis
Ne. = neurinoma

their specific afferents, escape for some reason or other from the inhibitory action of fast-conducting fibres. It is known that the myelinated fibres responsible for sensory discrimination in the facial region terminate in the main nucleus of the trigeminal nerve in the pons, but that, via collaterals, they exert an inhibitory action on the neurones of the descending root nucleus.

A series of observations which we were fortunate enough to make show that some neuralgias indicative of damage to the trigeminal nerve may simulate essential neuralgia so exactly that they even disappear in response to carbamazepine. Anatomical data relating to the occurrence of these pain syndromes in the course of multiple sclerosis suggest that the lesion responsible is situated in the pontine region, i.e. at the point where the fibres destined for the main sensory nucleus enter the pons (Figure 2). In cases where lightning pain is due to a neurinoma of the eighth cranial nerve or to Paget's disease, the precipitating factor is nerve-root compression. This compression, however, must be only of moderate degree and not so severe as to give rise to a detectable sensory deficit. The first effect of this sensory nerve compression is to reduce considerably the speed of conduction in those fibres that conduct fastest. The resultant temporal disorganisation of the afferent message is sufficient to upset the balance between the excitatory and inhibitory influences exerted on the neurones of the descending root nucleus. The mechanism of essential neuralgia might be similar. Electron-microscopic studies have revealed the presence of changes in certain myelin sheaths in the roots of the trigeminal nerve[6]. These changes might be due to mechanical causes, e.g. to the fact that in the course of ageing the nerve structures become subjected to compression of osteofibrous or vascular origin. One thing at all events is certain – namely, that these changes in the myelin sheaths are capable of interfering with the temporal organisation of the afferent message and of giving rise to increased excitability in the neurone pool of the spinal trigeminal nucleus.

Hence, trigeminal neuralgia does indeed deserve the appellation "epileptiform neuralgia" given it by KUGELBERG and LINDBLOM[9]. Paroxysmal activity of an epileptic type has been observed in the bulbothalamic pathways during stereotactic operations in patients suffering from neuralgia of the fifth cranial nerve. On an experimental level, the findings reported by ANDERSON et al.[2] are of great interest in this connection: in cats subjected to retrogasserian neurotomy these authors recorded neuronal hyperactivity of increasing intensity which was located in the spinal trigeminal nucleus and which reached its maximum one month after the operation. This hyperactivity is considerably increased by tactile stimulation of a cervical dermatome adjacent to the anaesthetic zone[8]. The inhibitory effect of carbamazepine on the excitatory synapses in this neurone pool has been demonstrated by FROMM and KILLIAN[5].

Based on symptomatological analyses and consonant with recently acquired knowledge in the field of physiology, the concept of "lightning pain" provides a pathophysiological interpretation for a symptom produced by widely differing causes. It also has the advantage of supplying an explanation for the at least relative effectiveness of hydantoins and of carbamazepine in this type of pain.

References

1 ALAJOUANINE, T., THUREL, R., BRUNELLI, A.: Les douleurs fulgurantes du tabes. Rev. neurol. *65*, 60 (1936)
2 ANDERSON, L.S., BLACK, R.G., ABRAHAM, J., WARD, A.A., Jr.: Neuronal hyperactivity in experimental trigeminal deafferentation. J. Neurosurg. *35*, 444 (1971)
3 CAMBIER, J., DEHEN, H.: Les douleurs fulgurantes. Etiologie et physiopathologie. Presse méd. *79*, 1419 (1971)
4 EKBOM, K.: Tegretol, a new therapy of tabetic lightning pains. Acta med. scand. *179*, 251 (1966)
5 FROMM, G.H., KILLIAN, J.M.: Effect of some anticonvulsant drugs on the spinal trigeminal nucleus. Neurology (Minneap.) *17*, 275 (1967)
6 KERR, F.W.L., MILLER, R.H.: The pathology of trigeminal neuralgia. Electron microscopic studies. Arch. Neurol. (Chic.) *15*, 308 (1966)
7 KILLIAN, J.M., FROMM, G.H.: Carbamazepine in the treatment of neuralgia. Arch. Neurol. (Chic.) *19*, 129 (1968)
8 KING, R.B., BARNETT, J.C.: Studies of trigeminal nerve potentials: overreaction to tactile facial stimulation in acute laboratory preparations. J. Neurosurg. *14*, 617 (1957)
9 KUGELBERG, E., LINDBLOM, U.: The mechanism of the pain in trigeminal neuralgia. J. Neurol. Neurosurg. Psychiat. *22*, 36 (1959)
10 MELZACK, R., WALL, P.D.: Pain mechanisms: a new theory. Science *150*, 971 (1965)

Current approaches to the treatment of trigeminal neuralgia

by M. Bonduelle*

Before presenting this paper of mine, I should like to say how very glad I am to see here among us today Dr. Blom, who was the first to use carbamazepine (®Tegretol) in the treatment of facial neuralgia.

A review of 100 cases

By way of introduction to the question of the treatment of essential trigeminal neuralgia, or tic douloureux, let me briefly review and bring up to date the results obtained in the 100 cases of my own on which I published a report in 1972[1].

These 100 cases have been followed up at regular intervals for several years, the oldest among them dating from the very first trials I conducted with carbamazepine, a drug whose introduction in 1962 can be said to have marked the beginning of a new era in the treatment of trigeminal neuralgia. In all these patients, medication with carbamazepine was initiated at a time when the drug had not yet found its way into everyday medical use and when every single case of facial neuralgia was automatically referred to a neurologist; nowadays, by a process of counterselection, a neurologist is called in only in those cases that have proved difficult to treat.

Evaluation of the results yielded by carbamazepine over a period of several years – as many as ten, in fact, in the oldest cases – has confirmed the first conclusions I had reached in 1963 and 1964[2,3]. In addition, it has provided a satisfactory answer to the question of the drug's long-term reliability – a question which could not of course be settled after I had been using carbamazepine for a mere six months or one year.

The overall results recorded in these 100 patients (68 women and 32 men), whose average age at the onset of the disease was 57 years, are shown in Table 1.

Table 1. Global assessment of the response to carbamazepine in 100 patients suffering from trigeminal neuralgia.	1972	1974
Very good and good	76	76
Moderately good	9	8
Failures	15	16

* Service de Neurologie, Hôpital Saint-Joseph, Paris, France.

The "very good and good" category comprises all cases in which the pain was completely or at least largely controlled (except perhaps for minor recurrences taking the form of a disagreeable sensation rather than of actual pain and occurring at the beginning of a meal, for example, or when the patient was washing) with average daily dosages of 800 mg. (range: 600–1,200 mg.). These dosages, taken in 3–6 fractional doses, were invariably well tolerated, although unpleasant side effects of a minor nature were encountered at the commencement of treatment. Side effects of this kind disappear spontaneously after a few days and might be avoided altogether by starting treatment with low doses and increasing them only gradually. This, however, is a procedure which the patient, anxious as he is to obtain relief from his pain, may well be reluctant to accept. In the 76 patients who responded well to the treatment, the side effects noted comprised: dizziness (18 cases), drowsiness (12 cases), and gastro-intestinal disturbances (12 cases).

In the eight patients assessed in 1974 as having shown only a "moderately good" response, signs of intolerance – i.e. drowsiness and dizziness – made it impossible to attain the requisite dosage level for one of the following two reasons:

1. *Low tolerance threshold*, i.e. the dosage could not be increased beyond a level of 200 mg. two or three times daily.
2. *High efficacy threshold*, i.e. satisfactory control of the neuralgia on a long-term basis or during acute exacerbations could not be achieved even at maximum dosage levels.

In the altogether 16 patients (15 in 1972 and an additional one since) in the "failures" category, signs of intolerance were even more marked and the degree of effectiveness was even more limited.

Only one out of these 100 patients failed to tolerate the drug at all, inasmuch as the eczema from which he had suffered in the past invariably recurred in response to medication with carbamazepine. The eczema would improve as soon as the drug was withdrawn, and it also showed a transient response when corticosteroids were administered in combination with carbamazepine; eventually, however, it would become worse again, with the result that treatment with carbamazepine finally had to be abandoned. In three other patients who developed eczema or an urticarial skin rash, medication with the drug did not need to be interrupted.

We have also had one further patient – not included in the present series – who was unable to tolerate carbamazepine at all. Every attempt at treatment, even with minimal doses, gave rise to severe urticarial reactions, accompanied by shivering and high fever. Supplementary administration of corticosteroids and also antihistamines had hardly any effect on these allergic manifestations. I might add in this connection that I have encountered only one instance of erythrodermia occurring in response to carbamazepine; the patient concerned was an epileptic, and the erythrodermia cleared following withdrawal of the drug.

322

In cases where treatment with carbamazepine has eventually to be discontinued, the reason usually is that side effects such as drowsiness, dizziness, and gastro-intestinal disturbances persist beyond the first few days of medication, thereby making it impossible to exceed a low or moderate dosage level (200 mg. two, three, or four times daily) and to reach the drug's efficacy threshold. This was in fact the case in five of the patients belonging to the present series. On the other hand, the majority (i.e. ten) of the failures were due to the fact that the drug proved insufficiently effective, even though it was well tolerated and could be administered in large doses of up to, for example, 200 mg. eight times daily. In all these cases, the drug had succeeded in controlling the pain to a satisfactory extent on a previous occasion.

The total of 16 patients in whom the drug proved a failure had therefore to be subjected later to the following methods of treatment:

1. Retrogasserian neurotomy (four cases).
2. Injection of alcohol into the gasserian ganglion (three cases).
3. Injection of alcohol, sometimes repeated, into a superficial branch of the trigeminal nerve (nine cases).

Principles of treatment

If the patient shows a good or very good response to carbamazepine, treatment does not seem to pose any problems at all. These are the cases in which a moderate and well-tolerated dose provides satisfactory control of pain and in which there is no need to try at all costs to obtain complete control by increasing the dosage.

Where retrogasserian neurotomy has been resorted to as a means of effecting a permanent cure, it is naturally impossible to study the spontaneous course of trigeminal neuralgia. It appears, however, in the light of the observations I have made over a period of several years since the introduction of carbamazepine into therapy, that the course of the disease may be marked by either of two phenomena, i.e. by acute exacerbations and by variations in the severity of the pain; this may apply not only, as is commonly said, to the first few months or years after the onset of the disease – during which the pain occurs in episodes of varying duration and severity, each episode being followed by a remission lasting several months or even years – but also to cases in which the pain persists for a long time.

By adapting the dosage of carbamazepine to the patient's requirements at any given moment, and by striving to administer no more than is absolutely necessary to attain satisfactory control of the pain, we can judge these fluctuations in severity, which are virtually typical of trigeminal neuralgia.

Complete remissions lasting several months are common, and in 14 of my patients, all suffering from moderately severe pain, the remission persisted for a considerable length of time – 18 months in one patient, two years in two others, three years in one, five years in one, and two to five years in the remaining nine, who, in fact were still in remission at the time of their last follow-up.

Considering that carbamazepine is undoubtedly effective and, as a rule, well tolerated, it is surprising to find that these qualities of the drug are not universally acknowledged and that some authors continue to place it on a par with the hydantoins, trichloro-ethylene (!), and vitamin B_{12}.

The success rate of 76% recorded in my own series of patients, coupled with the fact that all other authors who have published reports on the subject have observed similar success rates, should surely leave no room for doubt concerning the best approach to the treatment of trigeminal neuralgia. In all these 76 patients of mine the pain was kept permanently under control with carbamazepine; the drug did not lose its effectiveness in the course of time, and no other treatment was required. Some people, however, maintain that this conservative approach to therapy is not justified, because it means that – except possibly during remissions – the medication has to be continued indefinitely. At the International Symposium on Pain held in Paris in September 1973 (the proceedings of which have not been published) SWEET, for example, reported on a considerable number of patients (approximately 500, including apparently some with facial pain of varying origin) who had been subjected to surgery. He maintained that it was preferable to rid the patient of his pain once and for all by means of an operation.

For my own part, I would opt for drug treatment, because it is not only well tolerated in the great majority of cases, but also perfectly safe. Surgery, on the other hand, carries the penalty of permanent anaesthesia of one side of the face and, a point which is usually played down by neurosurgeons, it may also give rise to intolerable and intractable causalgia.

An attitude midway between these two extremes is adopted by some authors, including, for example, HEYCK[4], who tends to suggest that surgery should be resorted to in young or relatively young patients faced with the prospect of 10, 20, or even 30 years of drug treatment. On the other hand, he realises that a patient whose pain is well controlled by drugs will certainly be reluctant to agree to surgery.

To my way of thinking, the choice of treatment only becomes a problem in patients who show little or no response to carbamazepine. It may well be difficult or even impossible to add other drugs to the regimen in cases where carbamazepine is poorly or only moderately well tolerated, because neuroleptics are liable to aggravate drowsiness and dizziness, while the hydantoins aggravate, or even cause, dizziness.

In only three out of my 24 cases in which carbamazepine was either only fairly successful or of no avail at all did levomepromazine elicit some degree of response; in two of these patients its effect was sufficient to terminate an acute exacerbation, and in the other it produced a temporary improvement. As for the hydantoins, in only one case did they appear to bring about a transient improvement.

These two types of drug, i.e. levomepromazine and the hydantoins, have always struck me as being of very dubious value in the treatment of trigeminal neuralgia. By way of illustration, let me mention briefly the results I obtained with them in some cases treated prior to 1962.

Six out of 20 patients treated with hydantoins in a minimum dosage of 100 mg. three times daily were adjudged to have shown a partial and temporary improvement. Levomepromazine produced a partial and temporary improvement in 12 out of 20 cases, in three of which the response was assessed as both good and prompt.

When interpreting these results culled from case-record sheets, it is important to bear in mind that trigeminal neuralgia is a condition marked by exacerbations and spontaneous remissions. To be meaningful, therefore, the improvement in response to a drug must be immediate, as it is in the case of carbamazepine.

As regards surgery and the injection of alcohol, the following factors should be considered before resorting to either of these approaches:

1. The pain of trigeminal neuralgia occurs in a particular, frequently circumscribed region of the face; except in cases where the ophthalmic branch of the trigeminal nerve is affected, it seldom spreads secondarily to other areas.
2. The course of the disease is marked by acute exacerbations and remissions; even in cases where there has been permanent pain for many years, it is still possible that a lengthy remission may set in.
3. Finally, it must be remembered that retrogasserian neurotomy constitutes a permanent amputation.

Consequently, in acute exacerbations in which the pain can no longer be satisfactorily controlled by carbamazepine or in which the dosage cannot be increased to ensure such control, I prefer to gain time by resorting, for example, to combined drug therapy, even though I realise that this may have little or no additional effect. Another approach I adopt in these cases is to increase the dose of carbamazepine – sometimes to as much as 200 mg. ten or 12 times daily – in an attempt to reach a reasonable compromise between the benefit of reducing pain to a bearable level and the risk of provoking unpleasant side effects.

If the acute exacerbation fails to subside and further measures become necessary, I still do not perform a neurotomy or inject alcohol into the gasserian ganglion. Instead, I try first of all injecting alcohol into a superficial branch of the trigeminal nerve (almost always the infra-orbital branch). This is a minor intervention which is easy to carry out and does not have a traumatising effect. If it fails to elicit a satisfactory response, it in no way prejudices a subsequent decision to subject the patient to surgery. In all but one of the cases in which I have employed this type of injection to date, it has produced an adequate effect, even though the injection sometimes had to be repeated after a few months. In the one patient in whom the effect was not sufficient, alcohol had to be injected into the gasserian ganglion as well.

The injection of alcohol into a superficial branch of the trigeminal nerve is a procedure that is clearly indicated in cases where the pain is confined to the area served by the superficial branch in question. Experience has shown that it may still elicit a good response even if the pain extends beyond this area, inasmuch as the residual pain can then be controlled by means of drug treatment.

Only in cases where drug therapy has definitely proved of no avail is there, in my opinion, any justification for resorting to the injection of alcohol – either into the branches of the trigeminal nerve as they leave the skull or into the gasserian ganglion – or to surgery. If and when surgery does appear to be indicated, selective techniques should be employed which leave the intermediate branch intact and, at least in a certain number of cases, lead at the most only to a partial loss of sensitivity to touch.

References

1 BONDUELLE, M.: Révision de cent cas de névralgie du trijumeau (tic douloureux). Nouv. Presse méd. *1*, 2617 (1972)

2 BONDUELLE, M., HOUDART, R., BOUYGUES, P.: Traitement de la névralgie du trijumeau par un dérivé de l'iminostilbène: le G. 32.883. Rev. neurol. *108*, 61 (1963). This publication followed a preliminary communication at the IIIrd Congress of the Coll. int. neuro-psychopharmacol. (C.I.N.P.), Munich, 2nd–5th Sept. 1962

3 BONDUELLE, M., HOUDART, R., SIGWALD, J., BOUYGUES, P., LORMEAU, G.: Traitement médical efficace de la névralgie faciale par un dérivé de l'iminostilbène. Presse méd. *72*, 1905 (1964)

4 HEYCK, H.: Drug therapy of trigeminal pain. In Hassler, R., Walker, A. E. (Editors): Trigeminal neuralgia. Pathogenesis and pathophysiology, p. 115 (Thieme, Stuttgart/Saunders, Philadelphia 1970)

The physiopathogenesis of "idiopathic" trigeminal neuralgia and its bearing on the effect of carbamazepine in this indication

By L. Barraquer-Bordas*

"In this future progress, all have a part to play. Rutherford said, 'There are only two types of scientist: butterfly collectors and physicists'. I think this is a correct and a complimentary statement. The butterfly collector assembles the phenomena of the real world and only when his task is well developed can the physicist attempt to order and explain the phenomena ... Once the physicist has generated laws and theories, the butterfly collector takes on a second role to check to see if the laws apply in fact to the real world. In the challenge of pain, the clinician and basic scientist must play just such an interdependent role."[69]

Following the masterly review of the clinical neurophysiology of pain presented by Dr. Mumenthaler[60], as well as the excellent papers read by Dr. Cambier[19], on the physiopathogenesis of lightning pain, and by Dr. Bonduelle[14], on the effectiveness of carbamazepine (®Tegretol) in the treatment of trigeminal neuralgia, I should like to draw attention to the historical aspect of the observations and research which have provided us with a fairly good knowledge of the physiopathogenesis of this pain syndrome and have at the same time enabled us to understand to some extent why it should respond to carbamazepine. This specific, and usually effective, form of drug treatment for trigeminal neuralgia has now been available for some 15 years, and it would be impossible today to publish a paper, as Olivecrona[61] did in 1941, devoted solely to surgical methods of treating the condition. However brilliant or effective these methods may have been or may still be, the only reasons for resorting to them nowadays are either ignorance of the disorder or failure of drug therapy; in both instances, the surgical approach is based on purely empirical considerations. At present, as neurosurgeons themselves must realise, surgical treatment for trigeminal neuralgia, even when modern "conservative" techniques are employed, is the exception rather than the rule.

Successive stages of research into the aetiopathogenesis of "idiopathic" trigeminal neuralgia

A. First stage

1. Research was devoted initially to attempts at locating a well-defined, irritant lesion which some authors considered on more or less hypothetical grounds to be present in all cases.

---

* Servicio de Neurología, Hospital de la Santa Cruz y San Pablo, Facultad de Medicina, Universidad Autónoma, Barcelona, Spain.

2. The sites proposed for this "causal" lesion varied widely, depending on the author concerned.

3. No clear-cut differentiation was made between the presumed – and sometimes demonstrated – "aetiological cause" and the physiopathogenetic mechanism set in train by this cause. The physiopathogenetic mechanism itself continued to be regarded as part and parcel of the cause, and the possible existence of a chain of interrelated factors was, by and large, not even suspected.

B. Second stage

Subsequently, by contrast, research was directed towards finding a single physiopathogenetic mechanism which could not only account for the peculiarities of the clinical picture (extremely intense, paroxysmal, and recurrent pain, periods of remission, attacks triggered off by non-painful stimuli, refractory period following an attack, etc.), but also explain how this syndrome, usually thought of as being of indeterminate aetiology, can be induced by the same single physiopathogenetic mechanism in those rare but confirmed cases in which the neuralgia is of a symptomatic type – i.e. in which it is attributable to a clinically and anatomically identifiable factor. According to this line of reasoning, therefore, the occasional detection of a "causal lesion" does not imply that the fundamental mechanism of the neuralgic process has been elucidated.

The transition to present-day concepts

In a paper published in 1949[6] and dealing with the aetiopathogenesis of trigeminal neuralgia, I took as my starting point the questions raised by an observation recorded by CASTAÑER-VENDRELL and myself[20]. This observation related to a family in which, over a period of four generations, six members had suffered from tic douloureux. In the third generation, three out of nine brothers had displayed this clinical picture, and two of them had undergone retrogasserian neurotomy with successful results. The mode of inheritance appeared to be clearly of a dominant type, though with incomplete penetrance. At that time, a perusal of the literature disclosed only two similar family histories – one reported by HARRIS[32] and involving nine patients over three generations and the other by ALLAN[5] relating to three patients over three generations; in both these instances the mode of inheritance was likewise of the dominant type with apparently incomplete penetrance. Incidentally, it is worth noting that, in the family which we had described in our paper, the trigeminal neuralgia affected the same side of the face – the right side – in each of the six cases.

As regards the nature of the hereditary taint in our six patients, we suspected that it must have been due phenotypically to some, probably very slight, structural anomaly which modified the functional processes of the trigeminal sensory system, thus giving rise to the neuralgia.

328

An analysis of the available literature on tic douloureux disclosed at that time a number of findings and opinions of widely varying scope and importance. They comprised:

1. Assumptions which were more or less hypothetical and, in some respects, conflicting.

HARRIS[32], for example, held tenaciously to his idea that tic douloureux was an attenuated form of neuritis and usually of dental origin. Many years later, WARTENBERG[70] was still defending the concept of "neuralgic neuritis" and rejecting the notion that tic douloureux could be an authentic form of neuralgia. LERICHE[50] postulated the existence of cellular degeneration in the gasserian ganglion. OLIVECRONA[61], on the other hand, believed the cardinal factor to be traction on the nerve root caused by the fact that, owing to the shortening of the spinal column associated with the process of ageing, the neuraxis sinks lower in its osseous and dural bed.

2. Reports of concrete observations, some of them merely thought-provoking, and others presenting clear-cut and incontrovertible facts.

The interpretations placed by the investigators themselves on their observations, however, varied considerably. Some obviously looked upon their cases as exceptions, while others thought they had actually discovered the prevalent cause of trigeminal neuralgia.

According to TAPTAS[67], for instance, pathological changes in the internal carotid artery (aneurysms, thrombosis, dilatation, or elongation) might be important sources of trigeminal pain, inasmuch as they might cause irritation in or near the gasserian ganglion. TAPTAS described a typical case of tic douloureux said to have been triggered off by elongation of the carotid artery.

LOVE and WOLTMAN[53] reported two cases in which tumours of the gasserian region (an epidermoid in one case and a meningioma in the other) had given rise to paroxysmal lightning pain. In one of these patients there was even a trigger zone. The authors, however, considered such cases to be exceptions; and it is a fact that tumours in this region generally provoke pain which is not paroxysmal and is accompanied by an objective sensory deficit.

As regards the retrogasserian root, it used to be widely believed – to some extent, with good reason – that lesions in this area tended to produce sensory defects associated with little or no pain. KRAYENBÜHL[42], for instance, stated: "In Gasserian ganglion tumours continuous facial pain is the main symptom. In trigeminal root tumours facial pain is usually slight or absent and the clinical picture is one of cerebellopontine angle disorder." Nevertheless, ALAJOUANINE et al.[1] had previously reported a case of trigeminal neurinoma associated with lightning pains appearing against a background of continuous pain. Similar findings were also reported subsequently – for example, by HAMBY[31], who had observed four cases of cerebellopontine angle tumour with trigeminal neuralgia (epidermoid in two patients, arachnoiditis in one, and neurinoma of the acoustic nerve in one). The clinical picture consisted either of a single symptom or, at the most, of only a few symptoms. Particular interest was aroused by DANDY's contention[24] that the usual cause of trigeminal neuralgia was irritation of the root in the posterior fossa. DANDY claimed that, while in some cases (10.7% being the figure he quoted) a gross lesion (tumour, aneurysm, or angioma) could be detected in this area, in a much higher proportion of patients the clinical picture was due to compression and, possibly, indentation of the nerve either by an arterial branch (30.7% of cases) or by the petrosal vein (14%). Other authors have described cases of neuralgia associated with malformation of the bones at the base of the skull. It has, however, been demonstrated (cf. SUNDERLAND[66]) that contiguity between the trigeminal root and arterial branches does not necessarily lead to pain syndromes.

Concerning the intraparenchymal trajectory of the root, it is sufficient to point to the relative frequency with which trigeminal neuralgia – marked by paroxysms of lightning pain, presence of a trigger zone, etc. – occurs at some time during the course of multiple sclerosis.

In the light of anatomico-clinical studies performed in a series of cases, LEWY and GRANT[51] suggested that paroxysmal trigeminal neuralgia might have an even more central, supranuclear source – i.e. that it might be due to disease (probably chronic ischaemia) of certain zones in the thalamus.

When reviewing all these data in 1949, I concluded[6] that "idiopathic" trigeminal neuralgia would seem to reflect a physiopathogenetic change in a complex sensory system, inducing in that system a paroxysmal and recurrent tendency to excessive discharges and to a kind of synchronised summation. The important factor was not the topographical location of the supposed cause, but the mechanism by which this cause exerted its effect. In other words, I underlined the need to separate the peculiar physiopathogenetic process giving rise to the paroxysmal and recurrent painful discharge from the concrete irritant factor which might in certain cases set the process in motion.

The current status of research into trigeminal neuralgia

Since then more than 25 years have passed, and during this quarter of a century the conclusions which I reached merely intuitively in 1949 have become strengthened and substantiated, and have also undergone shifts in emphasis in a number of respects.

I propose to divide the last section of my talk into two parts, the second being devoted to a review of the current status of research into trigeminal neuralgia as it appears in the light of the recent International Symposium on Pain, the proceedings of which were edited by BONICA[17]. To start with, however, let me rapidly outline the progress that has been made in our knowledge of trigeminal neuralgia, a subject which has been dealt with at length in the three editions of my book *"Neurología fundamental"*[7] and in the monograph on pain which JANÉ-CARRENCÁ and I published in 1968[8].

It seems appropriate to begin by recalling two general theories connected with two aspects of the neurophysiology of pain, before going on to consider findings relating to the trigeminal system itself.

The first theory is that of WEDDELL[71] and his school[65] concerning the peripheral spatio-temporal constellation of impulses conditioned by the wide differences in the conduction velocity of various fibres (the velocity being proportional to the thickness of the fibres). According to WEDDELL, it is this complex constellation, and not the obligatory participation of allegedly specific fibres, that tends to govern the "pre-spinal origin" of somatic sensations.

The second theory is that of the "gate control" system propounded by MELZACK and WALL[57] and already referred to by Dr. MUMENTHALER and Dr. CAMBIER during this present symposium. I would merely recall here that, according to this theory, the small cells which inhibit Rolando's fasciculus play a decisive role in the ascending "transmission" of impulses connected with painful sensations. These cells are inhibited by thin peripheral fibres of type C, with the result that the pre-synaptic inhibition which they exert on the "transmitter cells", the origin of the "ascending action system", diminishes. By contrast, this inhibition is enhanced when the same small cells are bombarded chiefly with impulses from somewhat thicker fibres, thus closing the gate which controls the entry of pain. This theory had a tremendous impact when MELZACK and WALL first enunciated it ten years ago, and it has since occupied a leading place in studies relating to the genesis of a large number of pain phenomena, including the nuclear mechanism of "idiopathic" trigeminal neuralgia. Some authors, however, have attempted to introduce modifications of the gate control theory or have even adopted a frankly critical attitude towards it (e.g. MANFREDI[55]; DENNY-BROWN et al.[27]). A general review of opinions on this theory is to be found in the symposium proceedings edited by BONICA[17]. During the next few years the gate control theory will no doubt undergo further elaboration and adaptation.

As this theory implies, it has been demonstrated in the last 20 years that various sensory relays, including the sensory trigeminal nuclear complex, receive descending centrifugal cortical or reticular projections which activate or inhibit the filtration and "selection" of impulses. The central relays of this centrifugal control system are actuated by fast-conducting peripheral fibres.

As regards the trigeminal sensory system itself, the data acquired have come both from the field of the basic sciences and from that of clinical neurophysiology and neuropathology.

A. Neuro-anatomical and neurophysiological data
1. The organisation of the sensory trigeminal nuclear complex has been reviewed by KRUGER et al.[43-47], DARIAN-SMITH et al.[26], F. KERR[37], etc.; KRUGER and MICHEL[43-45] consider that thin fibres clearly predominate in the lower part of the descending root of the trigeminal nerve. According to these authors, the mandibular, maxillary, and ophthalmic regions are arrayed, not one above the other, as used to be thought, but in different columns belonging to one and the same rostrocaudal projection within the nucleus of the descending root.
2. The complexity of the projections ascending from the sensory trigeminal nuclear complex to the thalamus and cortex has been analysed by D. KERR et al.[36] and by HASSLER and WALKER[33].

331

3. The existence of the centrifugal control system just referred to has been confirmed.

B. Pathological data

1. KUGELBERG and LINDBLOM[48], in the light of findings obtained in electro-physiological experiments designed to analyse the characteristic signs and symptoms of patients with tic douloureux, argue that in this disorder there must be a repetitive discharge of a basically "epileptic" physiopathological mechanism – a conclusion, incidentally, which TROUSSEAU[68] had reached intuitively almost a century before.

2. Electron-microscopic studies conducted by F. KERR and MILLER[38] disclosed in the retrogasserian root the presence of a degenerative change in the myelin sheath, along with complex "proliferation", degenerative phenomena, etc., all of which were apparently due to ageing processes. Although, as F. KERR himself[37] suggested, these changes might perhaps give rise to "short-circuit" or "artificial synapse" phenomena, a more likely interpretation is that they induce in some way or other a distortion in the complex spatio-temporal constellation of the afferent impulses reaching the descending nuclear region of the trigeminal nerve, where the gate control system of MELZACK and WALL seems to be particularly unstable. It was along these lines that we worked out our synthesised approach in 1968[8].

Since then, additional data on the subject have been obtained as a result of more or less isolated studies, including especially those reported at the Freiburg Symposium of 1970[33] which was specifically devoted to the pathogenesis and physiopathology of trigeminal neuralgia.

Now I come to the last part of my paper, in which I should like to review briefly the most recent developments in this domain.

The sensory trigeminal nuclear system is so complex and variegated that, according to KRUGER and MOSSO[46], it has so far been possible to attribute concrete significance to only one part of it, i.e. to the caudal nucleus, whose cellular structure is similar to that of the neurones capping Rolando's fasciculus and giving rise to one of the fractions of the so-called spinothalamic tract.

On the one hand, ALBE-FESSARD et al.[2] have demonstrated that in monkeys there is a direct connection between the cells of the fifth Rexed lamina and the contralateral posteroventral nucleus of the thalamus. This pathway constitutes, in fact, the neo-spinothalamic tract, which is formed by myelinated, fast-conducting fibres. The peripheral field of its cells of origin is activated both by gentle stimuli and by non-intense noxious stimuli. In MOUNTCASTLE's nomenclature[59] this tract is classified as belonging to the "anterolateral system", in contradistinction to the posterior columns. But in the classification of ALBE-FESSARD et al.[2] this tract is a component of the "lemniscal system", since it joins Reil's ribbon (medial lemniscus) in the brainstem and projects to a specific thalamic nucleus, unlike the "extralemniscal systems" (such as the palaeo-spinothalamic or spino-reticulothalamic tracts, etc.) which project to a non-specific thalamonuclear system.

On the other hand, KITAHATA et al.[40] have identified, within the trigeminal nuclear system, a group of cells which are homologous with those of the fifth spinal lamina already referred to. This group of cells is excited by nociceptive cutaneous stimuli, and its identification might resolve some of the debate as to which cells – to use the nomenclature of MELZACK and WALL – are responsible for the "transmission" of pain sensations within the trigeminal system. Such groups of nerve cells are to be found in the magnocellularis zone of the most caudal portion of the caudal nucleus. KITAHATA et al. identified them in both physiological and histological studies. In addition, Mosso and KRUGER[58] have described (though without histological corroboration) the presence of nociceptive neuronal elements in the marginal zone of the caudal nucleus, i.e. in a site similar to that of the nociceptive cells which CHRISTENSEN and PERL[21] found in the first Rexed lamina in the lumbar dorsal horn. It should be pointed out, however, that KRUGER and Mosso took care in a later paper[46] to underline the value of the observations reported by KITAHATA et al.

Also worth noting is the fact that KING[39] demonstrated that the caudal nucleus exerts a tonic, hyperpolarising influence on primary, pre-terminal afferents of the trigeminal main sensory nucleus; according to this author, the nociceptive or non-nociceptive characteristics of the stimuli reaching the main sensory nucleus are modulated by the activity of the caudal nucleus. Applying current neurophysiological notions to the physiopathogenesis of "idiopathic" trigeminal neuralgia, CRUE and CARREGAL[22] summarise their views as follows: "It is our contention that pain is not a primary sensory modality, but that pain is a percept that probably begins in the central nervous system, in all likelihood in the region of layer 5 of the dorsal horn. Furthermore, repetitive postsynaptic neural firing centrally appears to be the logical explanation for temporal factors where pain sensation outlasts the initiating stimulus that precipitates it. Certainly in the chronic pain state, especially in the sudden, paroxysmal jabs in neuralgia, there now appears little doubt that there is an underlying uncontrolled central sensory epileptiform discharge." CRUE and CARREGAL also refer to the phenomenon of post-tetanic potentiation, a phenomenon which was considered by GRANIT[29] to play a fundamental role in the development of gamma spasticity. However, they doubt whether it is really involved in neuralgic pain, because it appears to be limited to the proprioceptive system.

Conclusion

In conclusion, I feel that at the present time a distinction should be drawn between the aetiology and the physiopathogenesis of "idiopathic" trigeminal neuralgia.

A. The aetiology of the disorder – i.e. the "cause" which gives rise to the pain process – may be very varied and of a purely fortuitous nature. It may take the form of a concrete, gross lesion acting either on the retrogasserian root (in the latter's extraparenchymal course or inside the brainstem itself, as in multiple sclerosis) or on other portions of the sensory trigeminal system such as the gasserian ganglion. Although the neuralgia appears to be idiopathic, it is in fact secondary. In many cases, its cause can be detected. In others, the causal factor may take the form of degenerative microlesions inside the trigeminal root, such as those which have been described by F. KERR[37]. Cases of this type would still fall under the heading "idiopathic or essential trigeminal neuralgia".

B. The really important point to bear in mind, however, is the existence of a physiopathogenetic process which accounts quite satisfactorily for the nature of the paroxysmal painful discharge and its characteristic features. This process takes place in the caudal part of the sensory trigeminal nuclear complex; moreover, it gives the peculiar pain syndrome its uniformity. To understand this process, we have to go back to the gate control system of MELZACK and WALL, a theory which has been amended and modified by recent neurophysiological findings. These findings shed great light on the role played by the neurones located in the fifth Rexed lamina, on the characteristics of their stimulation, and on the importance of their repetitive post-synaptic discharge. In other words, this process is a mechanism which, in a "basic" sense, may well be described as epileptiform. It is to be expected that studies in the years to come will elucidate more clearly its real nature. The hypothesis that, at least in some cases, dysfunction of the "centrifugal control system" mentioned above may play a part in the development of painful sensations cannot be rejected out of hand.

By virtue of its similarity to an epileptic discharge, this basic physiopathogenetic mechanism may also help us to understand why carbamazepine and also phenytoin sodium should exert a therapeutic effect in trigeminal neuralgia. However, although carbamazepine has proved to be an exceptionally good drug, a great deal of further research still remains to be done on its pharmacodynamics. Let us not forget that carbamazepine has shown itself to be effective not only in trigeminal neuralgia, but also, as demonstrated in other papers presented at this symposium, in various forms of epilepsy, in hemifacial spasm, and in the syndrome described by ISAACS[35] which is marked by neuromyotonia and continuous fascicular twitching of muscle fibres. In the latter condition carbamazepine appears to act at a very peripheral level, whereas in hemifacial spasm its mechanism of action is hard to define, despite the apparent similarity between this syndrome and trigeminal neuralgia. The physiopathogenesis of hemifacial spasm seems in fact to involve, not a central, nuclear mechanism, but ephaptic "artificial synapse" phenomena[30] (perhaps the basic mechanism in cases of so-called primary spasm) or, at least in the post-paralytic form, "misregeneration" or "misdirection" of nerve fibres.

The existence of so many different factors should encourage us to widen our investigations into the therapeutic effects of carbamazepine and thus to obtain new clinical data enabling us to undertake even more detailed neurophysiological and neuropharmacological studies. It is in this way that we can best reply to the challenge mentioned by WALL[69] in the passage I quoted at the beginning of this paper.

References

1 ALAJOUANINE, T., DE MARTEL, T., GUILLAUME, J.: Schwannome du trijumeau rétrogassérien. Ablation. Guérison. Rev. neurol. *37/II*, 89 (1930)

2 ALBE-FESSARD, D., LEVANTE, A., LAMOUR, Y.: Origin of spinothalamic and spino-reticular pathways in cats and monkeys, loc. cit.[17], p. 157

3 ALBE-FESSARD, D., LEVANTE, A., LAMOUR, Y.: Origin of spino-thalamic tract in monkeys. Brain Res. *65*, 503 (1974)

4 ALBE-FESSARD, D., TYC-DUMONT, S.: Fonctions somato-sensibles. In Kayser, C.: Physiologie, Vol. II: Système nerveux. Muscle, p. 429 (Flammarion, Paris 1969)

5 ALLAN, W.: Familial occurrence of tic douloureux. Arch. Neurol. Psychiat. (Chic.) *40*, 1019 (1938)

6 BARRAQUER-BORDAS, L.: Sobre la herencia y etiopatogenia del tic doloroso trigeminal. Arch. Neuro-psiquiat. (S. Paulo) *7*, 241 (1949)

7 BARRAQUER-BORDAS, L.: Neurología fundamental, 1st–3rd Ed. (Torray, Barcelona 1963, 1968, 1975)

8 BARRAQUER-BORDAS, L., JANÉ-CARRENCÁ, F.: El dolor. Anatomofisiología clínica y terapéutica farmacológica (Paz Montalvo, Madrid 1968)

9 BARRAQUER-BORDAS, J., PERES-SERRA, J., GRAU-VECIANA, J. M.: Efectos terapéuticos del Tegretol en síndromes álgicos diversos. Med. clín. (Barcelona) *45*, 409 (1965)

10 BARRAQUER-FERRE, L., BARRAQUER-BORDAS, L.: Neuralgia facial. Clín. y Lab. *31*, 81 (1946)

11 BESSOU, P., PERL, E.: Activation spécifique de fibres afférentes amyéliniques d'origine cutanée par des stimulus nocifs mécaniques ou thermiques chez le chat. J. Physiol. (Paris) *60*, Suppl. 1:218 (1968); abstract of paper

12 BESSOU, P., PERL, E. R.: Response of cutaneous sensory units with unmyelinated fibers to noxious stimuli. J. Neurophysiol. *32*, 1025 (1969)

13 BLOM, S.: Tic douloureux treated with new anticonvulsant. Experiences with G 32883. Arch. Neurol. (Chic.) *9*, 285 (1963)

14 BONDUELLE, M.: Current approaches to the treatment of trigeminal neuralgia. In Birkmayer, W. (Editor): Epileptic seizures – behaviour – pain, Int. Symp., St. Moritz 1975, p. 321 (Huber, Berne/Stuttgart/Vienna 1975)

15 BONDUELLE, M., BOUYGUES, P., SALLOU, C., GROBUIS, S.: Expérimentation clinique de l'anti-épileptique G. 32.883 (Tégrétol). Résultats portant sur 100 cas observés en trois ans. Rev. neurol. *110*, 209 (1964)

16 BONDUELLE, M., HOUDART, R., SIGWALD, J., BOUYGUES, P., LORMEAU, G.: Traitement médical efficace de la névralgie faciale par un dérivé de l'iminostilbène. Presse méd. *72*, 1905 (1964)

17 BONICA, J.J. (Editor): Advances in neurology, Vol. IV, Int. Symp. Pain (Raven Press, New York 1974)

18 BOWSHER, D.: Termination of the central pain pathway in man: the conscious appreciation of pain. Brain *80*, 606 (1957)

19 CAMBIER, J., DEHEN, H.: Trigeminal neuralgia in comparison with other forms of lightning pain, loc. cit.[14], p. 317

20 CASTAÑER-VENDRELL, E., BARRAQUER-BORDAS, L.: Six membres de la même famille avec tic douloureux du trijumeau. Mschr. Psychiat. Neurol. *118*, 77 (1949)

21 CHRISTENSEN, B. N., PERL, E. R.: Spinal neurons specifically excited by noxious or thermal stimuli: marginal zone of the dorsal horn. J. Neurophysiol. *33*, 293 (1970)

22 CRUE, B. L., Jr., CARREGAL, E. J. A.: Postsynaptic repetitive neuron discharge in neuralgic pain, loc. cit.[17], p. 643

23 DANDY, W. E.: The treatment of trigeminal neuralgia by the cerebellar route. Ann. Surg. *96*, 787 (1932)

24 DANDY, W. E.: Concerning the cause of trigeminal neuralgia. Amer. J. Surg. *24*, (N.S.), 447 (1934)

25 DANDY, W. E.: Intracranial arterial aneurysms (Ithaca 1944)

26 DARIAN-SMITH, I., MUTTON, P., PROCTOR, R.: Functional organization of tactile cutaneous afferents within the semilunar ganglion and trigeminal spinal tract of the cat. J. Neurophysiol. *28*, 682 (1965)

27 DENNY-BROWN, D., KIRK, E.J., YANAGISAWA, N.: The tract of Lissauer in relation to sensory transmission in the dorsal horn of spinal cord in the macaque monkey. J. comp. Neurol. *151*, 175 (1973)

28 DENNY-BROWN, D., YANAGISAWA, N.: The function of the descending root of the fifth nerve. Brain *96*, 783 (1973)

29 GRANIT, R.: Systems for control of movement. In: Ier Congr. int. Sci. neurol., p. 1 (Acta Medica Belgica, Brussels 1957)

30 GRANIT, R., LEKSELL, L., SKOGLUND, C.R.: Fibre interaction in injured or compressed region of nerve. Brain *67*, 125 (1944)

31 HAMBY, W.B.: Trigeminal neuralgia due to radicular lesions. Arch. Surg. *40*, 555 (1943)

32 HARRIS, W.: Bilateral trigeminal tic. Its association with heredity and disseminated sclerosis. Ann. Surg. *103*, 161 (1936)

33 HASSLER, R., WALKER, A.E. (Editors): Trigeminal neuralgia. Pathogenesis and pathophysiology (Thieme, Stuttgart/Saunders, Philadelphia 1970)

34 HAUGEN, F.P., MELZACK, R.: The effects of nitrous oxide on responses evoked in the brain stem by tooth stimulation. Anesthesiology *18*, 183 (1957)

35 ISAACS, H.: A syndrome of continuous muscle-fibre activity. J. Neurol. Neurosurg. Psychiat. *24*, 319 (1961)

36 KERR, D.I.B., HAUGEN, F.P., MELZACK, R.: Responses evoked in the brain stem by tooth stimulation. Amer. J. Physiol. *183*, 253 (1955)

37 KERR, F.W.L.: The divisional organization of afferent fibres of the trigeminal nerve. Brain *86*, 721 (1963)

38 KERR, F.W.L., MILLER, R.H.: The pathology of trigeminal neuralgia. Electron microscopic studies. Arch. Neurol. (Chic.) *15*, 308 (1966)

39 KING, R.B.: Interaction of noxious and non-noxious stimuli in primary sensory nuclei, loc. cit. [17], p. 659

40 KITAHATA, L.M., McALLISTER, R.G., TAUB, A.: Identification of central trigeminal nociceptors, loc. cit. [17], p. 83

41 KITAHATA, L.M., TAUB, A., KOSAKA, Y.: Lamina-specific suppression of dorsal-horn unit activity by ketamine hydrochloride. Anesthesiology *38*, 4 (1973)

42 KRAYENBÜHL, H.: Primary tumours of the root of the fifth cranial nerve: their distinction from tumours of the Gasserian ganglion. Brain *59*, 337 (1936)

43 KRUGER, L., MICHEL, F.: A single neuron analysis of buccal cavity representation in the sensory trigeminal complex of the cat. Arch. oral Biol. *7*, 491 (1962)

44 KRUGER, L., MICHEL, F.: A morphological and somatotopic analysis of single unit activity in the trigeminal sensory complex in the cat. Exp. Neurol. *5*, 139 (1962)

45 KRUGER, L., MICHEL, F.: Reinterpretation of the representation of pain based on physiological excitation of single neurons in the trigeminal sensory complex. Exp. Neurol. *5*, 157 (1962)

46 KRUGER, L., MOSSO, J.A.: An evaluation of duality in the trigeminal afferent system, loc. cit. [17], p. 73

47 KRUGER, L., SIMINOFF, R., WITKOVSKY, P.: Single neuron analysis of dorsal column nuclei and spinal nucleus of trigeminal in cat. J. Neurophysiol. *24*, 333 (1961)

48 KUGELBERG, E., LINDBLOM, U.: The mechanism of the pain in trigeminal neuralgia. J. Neurol. Neurosurg. Psychiat. *22*, 36 (1959)

49 LELE, P.P., WEDDELL, G.: The relationship between neurohistology and corneal sensibility. Brain *79*, 119 (1956)

50 LERICHE, R.: La cirugía del dolor. Versión esp.: Marín de Bernardo, J., Velilla Mateo, E. (Morata, Madrid 1942)

51 LEWY, F.H., GRANT, F.C.: Physiopathologic and pathoanatomic aspects of major trigeminal neuralgia. Arch. Neurol. Psychiat. (Chic.) *40*, 1126 (1938)

52 LEY, E., OBRADOR, S., URQUIZA, P.: Sobre los síndromes neurológicos que aparecen en las malformaciones de la base del cráneo y cerebelo-bulbares. Malformación de Arnold-Chiari. Rev. clín. esp. *32*, 21 (1949)

53 LOVE, J.G., WOLTMAN, H.W.: Trigeminal neuralgia and tumors of the gasserian ganglion. Proc. Mayo Clin. *17*, 490 (1942)

54 MANFREDI, M.: Differential block of conduction of larger fibers in peripheral nerve by direct current. Arch. ital. Biol. *108*, 52 (1970)

55 MANFREDI, M.: Modulation of sensory projections in anterolateral column of cat spinal cord by peripheral afferents of different size. Arch. ital. Biol. *108*, 72 (1970)

56 MELZACK, R.: Mechanisms of pathological pain. In Critchley, M., et al. (Editors): Scientific foundations of neurology, p. 153 (Heinemann, London 1972)

57 MELZACK, R., WALL, P.D.: Pain mechanisms: a new theory. Science *150*, 971 (1965)

58 MOSSO, J.A., KRUGER, L.: Spinal trigeminal neurons excited by noxious and thermal stimuli. Brain Res. *38*, 206 (1972)

59 MOUNTCASTLE, V.B., POWELL, T.P.S.: Neural mechanisms subserving cutaneous sensibility, with special reference to the role of afferent inhibition in sensory perception and discrimination. Bull. Johns Hopk. Hosp. *105*, 201 (1959)

60 MUMENTHALER, M.: The pathophysiology of pain, loc. cit. [14], p. 275

61 OLIVECRONA, H.: Die Trigeminusneuralgie und ihre Behandlung. Nervenarzt *14*, 49 (1941)

62 PERL, E.R.: Relation of cutaneous receptors to pain. In: Pain Symp., XXIVth Int. Congr. physiol. Sci., Washington, D.C. 1968. Proc. int. Un. physiol. Sci. *6*, 235 (1968)

63 PERL, E.R.: Myelinated afferent fibres innervating the primate skin and their response to noxious stimuli. J. Physiol. (Lond.) *197*, 593 (1968)

64 POGGIO, G.F., MOUNTCASTLE, V.B.: A study of the functional contributions of the lemniscal and spinothalamic systems to somatic sensibility. Central nervous mechanisms in pain. Bull. Johns Hopk. Hosp. *106*, 266 (1960)

65 SINCLAIR, D.C.: Cutaneous sensation and the doctrine of specific energy. Brain *78*, 584 (1955)

66 SUNDERLAND, S.: Neurovascular relations and anomalies at the base of the brain. J. Neurol. Neurosurg. Psychiat. *11*, 243 (1948)

67 TAPTAS, J.N.: Les dilatations et allongements de l'artère carotide interne. Etats fonctionnels et organiques. Rev. neurol. *80*, 338 (1948)

68 TROUSSEAU, A.: Clinique médicale de l'Hôtel-Dieu de Paris, Vol. II, p. 44 (Baillière et Fils, Paris/London/New York 1862)

69 WALL, P.D.: The future of attacks on pain, loc. cit. [17], p. 301

70 WARTENBERG, R.: Neuritis, sensory neuritis and neuralgia (Oxford University Press, New York 1958)

71 WEDDELL, A.G.M.: Observations on the anatomy of pain sensibility. In Keele, C.A., Smith, R. (Editors): The assessment of pain in man and animals, Proc. int. Symp., London 1961, p. 47 (Livingstone, Edinburgh/London 1962)

Patterns of psychomotor reactivity in relation to the analgesic effect of psycho-active drugs

by H. Reisner*

One distinctive feature of radicular pain syndromes in particular is the fact that, whereas some patients derive relief from their pain by keeping on the move, others find it preferable to remain as quiet and immobile as possible. This observation has been investigated by us in 77 patients – suffering from headache and nuchal pain, from shoulder-arm pain, or from pain in the lumbar region, hip, and leg – in tests in which their response to certain psycho-active drugs was systematically recorded.

In 39 of these 77 patients the pain was associated with enhanced motor function, its distribution being as follows: headache and nuchal pain (nine cases), shoulder-arm pain (14 cases), and lumbar, hip, and leg pain (16 cases). The remaining 38 patients exhibited reduced motor function; here, the pain was located in 15 cases in the head and nuchal region, in ten cases in the shoulder and arm, and in 13 chiefly in the hip and leg. These figures were obtained by arbitrarily selecting those patients in whom the psychomotor patterns of the pain syndromes representing each of the two extremes were particularly clear-cut.

By analogy with the classification adopted for depressive illness, including especially the distinction drawn between agitated and retarded forms of endogenous depression, I introduced the terms "agitated pain" and "retarded (or tensed) pain" for the two types of syndrome in question[3]: this appeared to be all the more justified since in many of these patients the pain was also accompanied by dysphoric mood disturbances with depressive overtones.

Classic examples of the two types of pain are very often to be found in cases of sciatica. Here, there are some patients who seek – and apparently do indeed obtain – relief from nocturnal exacerbations by getting out of bed and walking up and down for some considerable time. After the pain has eased, or perhaps even abated completely, they return to bed, but soon have to rise and move about again in order to relieve the pain once more. On the other hand, there is a second type of patient who avoids all movement and who either adopts in bed characteristic postures serving to relax the sciatic nerve, or else keeps his body immobilised in weird positions which seem to have little or nothing to do with relaxation of the affected nerves or nerve roots. The occurrence of these two extreme patterns of behaviour in the presence of pain frequently leads the inexperienced observer to conclude that the patient is hysterical. This conclusion would be correct only insofar as the psychomotor patterns in question can be regarded as an hysteriform, i. e. neurotic, reaction;

 * Neurologische Universitätsklinik, Vienna, Austria.

it would be utterly incorrect if the term "hysterical" were to be employed here in a pejorative connotation.

In both of the forms of radicular pain I have described, one is confronted with two possibilities: on the one hand, the pain may be of a primary type, i.e. caused usually by spinal lesions affecting the roots of the appurtenant sensory nerves; on the other hand, cases may occur in which the patient complains of pain of the same type and localisation, but in which the most prominent feature of the clinical picture is a depressive-dysphoric or possibly even a depressive-hypochondriacal mood disorder. In cases of this latter kind in which one has had an opportunity to keep the patient under medical observation over prolonged periods of his life, one finds that such predominantly depressive conditions will also already have given rise to the same symptoms during the initial phase of the disease occurring while the patient was still relatively young. What the patient was certainly suffering from at the time of this initial phase – and probably in subsequent phases as well – is not primary radicular irritation, but a secondary form of irritation due mainly to psychically induced muscular tension and resulting in symptoms which simulate or to some extent imitate those of a radicular syndrome. I refrain from describing these as "pseudo-radicular" symptoms, because, when a thorough neurological examination is performed, painful conditions of this type can always be distinguished from genuine radicular syndromes. Since they tend to be associated with depressive-dysphoric and hypochondriacal mood disorders, however, it is often very difficult in such cases to determine whether the pain of which the patient complains is simply a manifestation of his depression or whether the depression has been triggered off by the pain. Depending on which of these two possible explanations is correct, one can describe the patient as suffering either from agitated or retarded depression with secondary radicular pain or, alternatively, from primary agitated or retarded pain with secondary depression.

Diametrically opposed psychomotor patterns of the agitated or retarded type are also known to be encountered under other circumstances. The behaviour of humans in situations of catastrophe, for example, may be characterised at the one extreme by a senseless explosion of motor activity and frantic movement or, at the other extreme, by maximal inhibition of motor function taking the form of a "petrification reflex". The occurrence either of a hyperkinetic syndrome or of stupor in cases of catatonic schizophrenia provides a further example.

It is often also possible to draw a distinction between agitated and retarded types of pain in other painful conditions. It should be noted, however, that, even though there may be certain painful states which tend *per se* to involve pain of the first type and others pain of the second type, the difference between the two does not necessarily have anything to do with the aetiology of the pain as such. Some patients suffering from headache due to a cerebral tumour, for instance, may hold their heads perfectly still and remain motionless, whereas others contrive to endure the pain by constantly walking – or even running – to and fro. On the other hand, the agitated type of pain is

339

never encountered in genuine trigeminal neuralgia, and very rarely in the classic form of migraine. The pain experienced by patients with these two diseases is such that they invariably strive – preferably in the seclusion of a quiet darkened room – to immobilise either all the muscles of the face or those of the head and the entire body. In the case of toothache, by contrast, which is a symptomatic form of trigeminal neuralgia, both types of pain may be observed, and the same also applies to cervical migraine.

Having distinguished between the two different types of pain by reference to their psychomotor patterns, we felt that, by analogy with the approach adopted in the management of depressions, an attempt should now be made at treatment with certain appropriately selected psycho-active drugs. Here, it was found that agitated pain responded well to amitriptyline, i.e. to the same substance as is also known to yield good results in cases of agitated depression. In retarded pain, by contrast, imipramine and its derivatives elicited the desired response in far fewer cases, whereas better results were obtained with phenothiazines, chlordiazepoxide, and diazepam; in this retarded form of pain, amitriptyline and meprobamate very seldom produced any improvement. In retarded pain of radicular origin in particular, an important factor contributing towards relief of the pain seems to be, in addition to the psychotropic effect of the drug administered, its muscle-relaxing action, which serves to interrupt the vicious circle of pain – muscular contraction – ischaemia, thereby blocking neural irritation in the affected muscles; in this indication, therefore, it is psycho-active drugs with relatively strong muscle-relaxing properties that prove the most suitable.

An assessment of the efficacy of carbamazepine (®Tegretol) in the two types of pain I have described reveals that this drug is chiefly active against retarded pain in primary forms of neuralgia, but that it apparently also exerts a preventive effect in patients subject to migraine[5].

In genuine trigeminal neuralgia, as I have already emphasised, the pain is always of the retarded type. In neuralgia associated with herpes zoster, too, the pain is also often of this same type. In both of these conditions, carbamazepine is the drug of choice, whereas, in conformity with observations reported by Braunhofer and Zicha[1], we have found it less effective in radicular pain syndromes of the kind mentioned earlier in this paper, irrespective of whether or not these syndromes are accompanied by depressive-dysphoric symptoms. It would thus seem that the analgesic effect of psycho-active drugs must depend to quite a significant degree on whether the pain is due to the involvement of spinal or analogous intracranial ganglia or, alternatively, of sensory nerve roots.

Although it may sometimes happen that one and the same patient exhibits retarded pain at one stage in his life and agitated pain at another, as a rule in all painful conditions the psychomotor pattern of the individual's reaction to the pain remains the same. This consistent behaviour is by no means solely attributable to purely reflex mechanisms operating in the periphery, but also appears to be dependent – and probably decisively dependent – on the activity of certain structures within the brain which are bound up with the person's affectivity. While the processes involved no doubt primarily entail activation of certain segments in the limbic system, it is possible that, if one accepts HASSLER's theory[2] according to which the pallidal system contains an important centre of contact between psyche and muscles, activation of this pallidal centre may also play a role. To what extent the differing effects exerted by psycho-active drugs on agitated and retarded pain syndromes can be correlated with the sites of attack in structures of the limbic system that have been postulated for these drugs on the basis of pharmacological findings, is a question that has yet to be clarified.

References

1 BRAUNHOFER, J., ZICHA, L.: Eröffnet Tegretal neue Therapiemöglichkeiten bei bestimmten neurologischen und endokrinen Krankheitsbildern? Eine klinische elektroenzephalographische und dünnschichtchromatographische Studie. Med. Welt *17* (N.F.), 1875 (1966)
2 HASSLER, R.: Limbische und diencephale Systeme der Affektivität und Psychomotorik. In Hoff, H., et al. (Editors): Muskel und Psyche, Symp., Vienna 1963, p. 3 (Karger, Basle/New York 1964)
3 REISNER, H.: Psychopharmaka und Schmerzbekämpfung, loc. cit.[2], p. 116
4 REISNER, H.: Schmerz und Psychomotorik. In Janzen, R., et al. (Editors): Schmerz. Grundlagen – Pharmakologie – Therapie, p. 168 (Thieme, Stuttgart 1972)
5 ROMPEL, H., BAUERMEISTER, P.W.: Aetiology of migraine and prevention with carbamazepine (Tegretol): results of a double-blind, cross-over study. S. Afr. med. J. *44*, 75 (1970)

Primary hemifacial spasm and its treatment with carbamazepine

by P. Martinelli*

Primary hemifacial spasm constitutes a nosological entity characterised by the sudden occurrence, unheralded by prior signs or symptoms, of involuntary spasms of the muscles on one side of the face. The spasms can be described as either symptomatic or cryptogenic, depending on whether or not a causative lesion can be detected. They are encountered among adults, and they probably affect women more often than men[7]. The clinical picture begins as a rule with small contractions in the orbicular muscle of the eyelids, which are then followed by clonic and clonic-tonic spasms of all the muscles on one side of the face; in the fully developed attack, "paradoxical synergism" as described by BABINSKI[3] can be observed between the frontalis and the orbicular muscles of the eyelids. The paroxysm invariably assumes the same form in all patients, but the frequency of attacks may vary from case to case. Sometimes the clonic-tonic spasms succeed one another at very short intervals and are followed by post-paroxysmal hypotonia.

The attacks may be precipitated by voluntary movement or by an automatic or reflex movement; they may also develop spontaneously. They cannot be arrested by the use of will-power, nor do they stop during sleep. Between attacks the face is normal, although sometimes a slight residual tension of the muscles on the affected side of the face may be observed.

Electromyograms recorded simultaneously in several muscles of the face have proved to be of fundamental importance for an analysis of the signs and symptoms[16]. At rest, electromyography reveals the presence of isolated low-frequency potentials, series of potentials displaying a moderate frequency, or bursts of high-frequency potentials.

Voluntary movement, which in some cases assumes a clonic form, may be completely unrelated to the spasms, or else it may precipitate them. Sometimes the spasms may develop at the end of a voluntary movement. Often, there is a time lag of several hundred milliseconds between the end of the voluntary movement and the end of the spasms.

Hemifacial spasm is sometimes associated with slight signs of neurogenic atrophy or of misdirection of nerve fibres. Automatic or reflex activity may precipitate clonic-tonic spasms, but does not invariably do so.

It seems unlikely that the clinical picture of hemifacial spasm is of cortical[28], extrapyramidal[31], or reflex[7] origin, or that it is due to abnormal efferent impulses from the nucleus of the facial nerve. The most probable cause would appear to be a lesion of the nerve trunk[16].

 * Clinica delle Malattie Nervose e Mentali dell'Università, Bologna, Italy.

There are many possible ways in which the facial nerve may become subject to compression along its course[16]: ischaemia and resultant oedema, or simply a narrow foramen[37], for example, are liable to damage the nerve, even though the damage may be very slight and certainly not sufficient to prevent impulse conduction. The resultant condition may be described as a parabiosis[8], parabiosis being defined[34,35] as any change in a nerve due to chemical, mechanical, or toxic causes. The characteristic feature of a nerve in parabiosis is a spontaneous irritative activity[19,20] accompanied by the formation of an artificial synapse capable of transforming the single pre-synaptic potential into a series of post-synaptic impulses; this gives rise to a pseudo-reflex which may, in turn, produce a burst of impulses[8,19,20]. Mechanical lesions, however minor they may be, can produce cross-stimulation in neighbouring nerve fibres – so-called "cross-firing" – and thus activate all the fibres of a nerve[1,11,12]. An aetiopathogenetic mechanism based on the parabiosis theory might well account for the symptomatology of hemifacial spasm and, as ZÜLCH[37] has pointed out, also remove this condition from the cryptogenic category of diseases.

Primary hemifacial spasm must be distinguished from hemifacial spasms occurring as a sequel to facial paralysis. In the latter type of spasm the clinical signs and symptoms, electromyographic findings, and pathogenesis are completely different. The clinical manifestations comprise: permanent contraction of those facial muscles that were previously paralysed, accentuation of the cutaneous folds, narrowing of the palpebral fissure, and elevation of the corner of the mouth. Superimposed on this permanent state of contraction are rapid clonic spasms which invariably involve the same muscles in the same patient and are connected with blinking. Voluntary movement of one muscle gives rise to spasms in other facial muscles. These spasms, which the patient cannot suppress by an effort of will, constitute the typical associated movements that are an invariable feature of hemifacial spasm occurring as a sequel to facial paralysis; in cases where they affect all the facial muscles, they are referred to as mass movements. BABINSKI's "paradoxical synergism" may be present. Electromyographic examination confirms the presence of neurogenic atrophy and reveals regular, simultaneous activation of some, or all, facial muscles.

Post-paralytic hemifacial spasm is believed to be due to the misdirection of regenerated nerve fibres[9,10,14,17,21,22,36]. This theory would account for the clonic spasms produced by blinking, as well as for the associated or mass movements.

Possible explanations for the permanent muscular contraction include: absence of the point of insertion of the skin muscles in the bones of the face, irritation of motor fibres in a regeneration neuroma, or adverse neurotrophic effects on regenerating nerve fibres[2,5,16].

Treatment

For many years treatment for primary hemifacial spasm consisted in the use of non-specific methods directed at improving the nutritional status of the nerve, 343 at reducing oedema and excessive vasomotor reactions, at achieving muscle relaxation, at diminishing general nervous excitability, and at alleviating the psychological effects on the patient.

Surgical transection of the nerve, whether total or partial, injection of alcohol or infiltration of anaesthetics, crushing of the nerve, and decompression procedures leading to transient facial paralysis have all yielded results which are variable or not particularly satisfactory.

Of greater interest, it seems, is the possibility of inserting fragments of tantalum into the nerve, with the aim of preventing the discharges which give rise to the spasms[23].

The use of carbamazepine (®Tegretol) in the treatment of primary hemifacial spasm was prompted by the similarity between the paroxysmal motor activity observed in this form of spasm and the paroxysmal pain of trigeminal neuralgia, which is known to respond to carbamazepine. Both conditions – that is, trigeminal neuralgia and hemifacial spasm – are precipitated by a trigger mechanism.

Authors who have given carbamazepine a trial in the treatment of hemifacial spasm[17, 24, 27, 33] have reported the following findings:

1. The drug is effective in about two-thirds of cases, inasmuch as it reduces the intensity and the frequency of attacks. In some instances, it even causes the spasms to disappear altogether.
2. The duration of the disease seems to have a greater bearing on the likelihood of a response than the intensity of the spasms. In other words, the earlier treatment is instituted, the better the chances of success.
3. The most effective dose is between 600 and 1,200 mg. daily.
4. In certain cases, the drug may lose some of its effectiveness after a while, and the symptoms then reappear or become more pronounced. Raising the dose may have no effect in these cases.
5. Ineffectiveness of the drug may be due either to poor absorption or to the fact that the lesion responsible for the spasms is no longer amenable to therapy.
6. In a small number of patients, carbamazepine gives rise to side effects, such as drowsiness and dizziness, which are usually transitory.

We obtained similar results in five patients whom we treated with carbamazepine in a dosage of 600 mg. daily. Probably owing to the small number of patients involved, we have not noticed any loss of efficacy: irrespective of the degree of improvement achieved, the drug showed no diminution in its effectiveness over periods ranging from six to 20 months. The response obtained in one patient is illustrated by the electromyographic tracings reproduced in Figures 1 and 2.

One of the properties of carbamazepine is that it reduces the excitability of nerve or muscle fibres, probably by causing changes in membrane polarisation[13, 30]. Consequently, carbamazepine may be regarded as the drug of choice in the treatment of pathological conditions due to lesions in the extreme per-

P.E., 64 years old. Before carbamazepine.

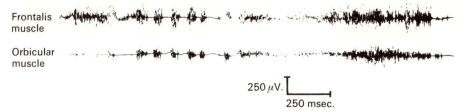

Frontalis
muscle

Orbicular
muscle

250 μV.

250 msec.

Fig. 1. Electromyograms of the frontalis and orbicular muscles of the eyelid prior to treatment with carbamazepine in a 64-year-old patient. Voluntary movement of the frontalis muscle invariably gives rise to spasm of the orbicular muscle, followed by bursts of clonic-tonic activity.

P.E., 64 years old. After carbamazepine.

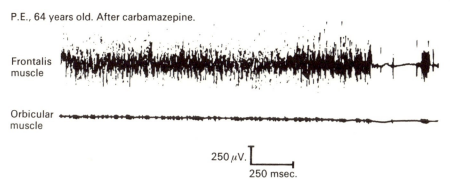

Frontalis
muscle

Orbicular
muscle

250 μV.

250 msec.

Fig. 2. Electromyograms of the frontalis and orbicular muscles of the eyelid in the same patient (cf. Figure 1) after six months of treatment with carbamazepine in a dosage of 600 mg. daily. Voluntary movement of the frontalis muscle is much freer and no longer triggers off spasms in the orbicular muscle, which merely displays very minor rhythmical bursts of activity.

ipheral portion of nerves or at the myoneural junction[15, 25, 32]. In such conditions, it sometimes elicits spectacular responses[4, 6, 26, 29].

To sum up, if one accepts the parabiosis theory as valid, and if parabiosis does in fact give rise to spontaneous stimulation and discharge of adjacent nerve fibres, then the effectiveness of carbamazepine in the treatment of primary hemifacial spasms must be attributed to the fact that the drug acts selectively on the mechanisms of the lesion.

References

1 ADRIAN, E.D.: The effects of injury on mammalian nerve fibres. Proc. roy. Soc. B *106*, 596 (1930)

2 ANDRÉ-THOMAS: Contribution à l'étude de l'anatomie pathologique de la paralysie faciale périphérique et de l'hémispasme facial. Rev. neurol. *15*, 1273 (1907)

3 BABINSKI, J.: Hémispasme facial périphérique. Rev. neurol. *13*, 443 (1905)

4 BADY, B., GIRARD, P., JALLADE, S., GAILLARD, L.: Une observation de pseudo-myotonie guérie par la carbamazépine. Lyon méd. *221*, 1431 (1969)

5 Bratzlavsky, M., Vander Eecken, H.: Postparalytic hemifacial spasm: pathogenetic problems. Electromyography *11*, 75 (1971)

6 Buscaino, G.A., Caruso, G., De Giacomo, P., Caliana, O., Ferrannini, E.: Patologia neuromuscolare insolita. Nota 1: reperti elettromiografici ed istoenzimatici muscolari in un soggetto con "sindrome di attività muscolare continua" ("neuromiotonia"). Acta neurol. (Naples) *25*, 206 (1970)

7 Ehni, G., Woltman, H.W.: Hemifacial spasm: review of one hundred and six cases. Arch. Neurol. Psychiat. (Chic.) *53*, 205 (1945)

8 Esslen, E.: Der Spasmus facialis – eine Parabioseerscheinung. Dtsch. Z. Nervenheilk. *176*, 149 (1957)

9 Esslen, E.: Electromyographic findings of two types of misdirection of regenerating axons. Electroenceph. clin. Neurophysiol. *12*, 738 (1960)

10 Esslen, E., Magun, R.: Electromyographic study of reinnervated muscle and of hemifacial spasm. Amer. J. phys. Med. *38*, 79 (1959)

11 Granit, R., Leksell, L., Skoglund, C.R.: Fibre interaction in injured or compressed region of nerve. Brain *67*, 125 (1944)

12 Hering, H., Scheid, P.: Kritische Bemerkungen zum Melkersson-Rosenthal-Syndrom als Teilbild des Morbus Besnier-Boeck-Schaumann. Arch. Derm. Syph. (Berl.) *197*, 344 (1954)

13 Hopf, H.C.: Anticonvulsant drugs and spike propagation of motor nerves and skeletal muscle. J. Neurol. Neurosurg. Psychiat. *36*, 574 (1973)

14 Howe, H.A., Tower, S.S., Duel, A.B.: Facial tic in relation to injury of the facial nerve. An experimental study. Arch. Neurol. Psychiat. (Chic.) *38*, 1190 (1937)

15 Isaacs, H.: A syndrome of continuous muscle-fibre activity. J. Neurol. Neurosurg. Psychiat. *24*, 319 (1961)

16 Jesel, M.: Hémispasme facial périphérique. Thesis, Strasbourg 1965

17 Jesel, M., Isch-Treussard, C.: Essai de traitement de l'hémispasme facial primitif par le Tégrétol (Geigy). Rev. Oto-neuro-ophtal. *39*, 130 (1967)

18 Jesel, M., Isch-Treussard, C., Isch, F.: Hémispasme facial postparalytique: secousse clonique hémifaciale et clignement, étude E.M.G.: Rev. neurol. *110*, 337 (1964)

19 Kugelberg, E.: Activation of human nerves by ischemia. Arch. Neurol. Psychiat. (Chic.) *60*, 140 (1948)

20 Kugelberg, E., Cobb, W.: Repetitive discharges in human motor nerve fibres during the post-ischaemic state. J. Neurol. Neurosurg. Psychiat. *14*, 88 (1951)

21 Lamy, H.: Note sur les contractions "synergiques paradoxales" observées à la suite de la paralysie faciale périphérique. Nouv. Iconogr. Salpêt. *18*, 424 (1905)

22 Lipschitz, R.: Beiträge zur Lehre von der Facialislähmung nebst Bemerkungen zur Frage der Nervenregeneration. Mschr. Psychiat. Neurol. *20*, 84 (1906)

23 Martin, H., Gignoux, B., Oudot, J.: Du traitement de l'hémispasme facial essentiel. J. Méd. Lyon *52*, 1483 (1971)

24 Maxion, H., Rosemann, G., Uebel, H.E.: Der Spasmus facialis. Klinischer Bericht über 25 Patienten. Nervenarzt *42*, 590 (1971)

25 Mertens, H.-G., Zschocke, S.: Neuromyotonie. Klin. Wschr. *43*, 917 (1965)

26 Papst, W.: Zur Differentialdiagnose der okulären Neuromyotonie. Ophthalmologica (Basle) *164*, 252 (1972)

27 Pechan, J.: Die Therapie des Hemispasmus facialis mit Tegretol. Med. Welt (Stuttg.) *23*, 384 (1972)

28 Roger, H., Gastaut, H., Roger, J.: Hémispasme facial d'allure essentielle. Electroencéphalogramme à type d'épilepsie myoclonique. Action de la triméthadione sur le spasme et les tracés E.E.G. Rev. neurol. *87*, 422 (1952)

29 Rohmer, F., Isch, F., Isch-Treussard, C., North, P.: Etude électro-clinique d'un cas de "neuro-myotonie" avec myokymies, réagissant favorablement à la carbamazépine. Rev. neurol. *125*, 239 (1971)

30 Schauf, C.L., Davis, F.A., Marder, J.: Effects of carbamazepine on the ionic conductances of Myxicola giant axons. J. Pharmacol. exp. Ther. *189*, 538 (1974)

31 Scheller, H.: Die Erkrankungen der peripheren Nerven. In Bergmann, G. von, et al.: Handbuch der inneren Medizin, 4th Ed., Vol. V/Part II: Neurologie, p. 1 (Springer, Berlin/Göttingen/Heidelberg 1953)

32 Sigwald, J., Guilleminault, C.: Syndromes de contracture permanente. Rev. Neurol. *124*, 191 (1971)

33 Weber, M., Brichet, B.: Traitement de l'hémispasme facial essentiel par le Tégrétol. Ann. méd. Nancy *11*, 1639 (1972)

34 Wedensky, N.E.: Die fundamentalen Eigenschaften des Nerven unter Einwirkung einiger Gifte. Pflügers Arch. ges. Physiol. *82*, 134 (1900)

35 Wedensky, N.E.: Die Erregung, Hemmung und Narkose. Pflügers Arch. ges. Physiol. *100*, 1 (1903)

36 Zülch, K.J.: Kann die Nachbehandlung während der Regeneration die Wiederherstellung der Leitungssysteme beeinflussen? Zbl. ges. Neurol. Psychiat. *133*, 146 (1955); abstract of paper

37 Zülch, K.J.: "Idiopathic" facial paresis. In Vinken, P.J., Bruyn, G.W. (Editors): Handbook of clinical neurology, Vol. VIII: Diseases of nerves, Part II, p. 241 (pp. 277–279) (North-Holland, Amsterdam/American Elsevier, New York 1970)

Discussion

M. Mumenthaler: There are a couple of questions that I should like to ask Dr. Bonduelle. The first concerns the side effects of carbamazepine (®Tegretol). In your paper, Dr. Bonduelle, you made a few brief references to dizziness, drowsiness, and gastro-intestinal upsets, but otherwise we haven't really heard much about the side effects of carbamazepine here today. Speaking from my own experience, I would say that dizziness rarely occurs as a side effect in our epileptics, most of whom belong to the younger age groups. But I do encounter this problem far more often in elderly patients – and these are the ones suffering from trigeminal neuralgia. Is it your impression, too, that side effects – which are occasionally so troublesome as to prevent the continuation of treatment – occur more frequently in older subjects?

Now for my second question. In cases where you interrupt treatment for trigeminal neuralgia when you have reason to believe that the patient has gone into a spontaneous remission, do you find – when you have to resume the medication because a relapse has occurred – that the drug proves just as effective as before, assuming of course that it had previously been effective?

M. Bonduelle: I'm afraid, Dr. Mumenthaler, that I can't supply a direct answer to your first question regarding the incidence of side effects in relation to age, because this is a point that has escaped my attention. What I can say, however, is that I have certainly noted a difference in the tolerability of carbamazepine in epileptics as compared with patients suffering from trigeminal neuralgia: the epileptics tolerate the drug better. As a rule, the epileptics require lower dosages than the patients with trigeminal neuralgia, in whom, of course, the method adopted if and when the neuralgia proves refractory is to increase the doses to the highest level that the patient can still tolerate. Whereas in cases of epilepsy one rarely has to exceed a dosage of 200 mg. five to six times daily, this very often becomes necessary in trigeminal neuralgia.

The second question you raised, Dr. Mumenthaler, concerned the interruption of treatment during remissions in patients with trigeminal neuralgia. In connection with these remissions, which had greatly intrigued me, I included in a paper published in 1972* the story of a particularly meticulous patient who noted down each day the dose of carbamazepine that he had taken. Thanks to this record, which he had been keeping for years, it was possible to follow the course of his illness very exactly. At one time, for example, his daily intake of tablets over successive periods lasting several days or weeks fluctuated as follows: 3, 2½, 6, 3, 2½, 1½, ½, etc. For three months he then managed without any tablets, after which he resumed the medication with doses which continued to vary. As illustrated by this case, it is the patient himself who adjusts the dosage to the intensity of the pain he experiences. The instructions he receives are that, when all pain has disappeared for several days, i.e. for about one week, he should start to reduce the daily dose by half a tablet a time and continue reducing it until the pain returns. It has been my experience that, in cases where the medication has been interrupted for several days, months, or even years, and then resumed in response to a renewed attack of trigeminal neuralgia, the drug's effectiveness in coping with a given intensity of pain remains the same as before.

S. Blom: I was very impressed by the results you reported today, Dr. Bonduelle, and also by the fact that, during his presentation, Dr. Cambier had the courage to write on the blackboard the words *"Ne touchez pas au trijumeau"*. I remember that in 1964 I tried to say something similar to a collection of between 100 and 200 American neurosurgeons, but they didn't seem to like it!

May I briefly explain why I started to give Tegretol a trial in trigeminal neuralgia in 1961. Between 1956 and 1959 I was working on the proprioceptive innervation of

---

* Bonduelle, M.: Révision de cent cas de névralgie du trijumeau (tic douloureux). Nouv. Presse méd. *1*, 2617 (1972)

the tongue. The tongue is innervated by a nerve which lacks a dorsal root, and I found that one important afferent inflow from the tongue must be transmitted via the lingual nerve. This led me to study the linguomandibular reflex, the linguohypoglossal reflex, and other trigeminal reflexes. Later, when I began working in clinical neurology, I soon learned that it was common to treat trigeminal neuralgia with diphenylhydantoin. I then undertook a series of animal experiments on the effect exerted by this substance on the linguomandibular reflex, and I found that it depressed this reflex rather strongly*. When the former GEIGY company asked me in 1961 to try their new drug, Tegretol, in epilepsy, I noticed that in the accompanying literature on the product there was a reference to the fact that it has a pronounced effect on the linguomandibular reflex. So nothing seemed to me more natural than to try it not only in epilepsy but above all in trigeminal neuralgia, and its effectiveness in this indication soon became obvious.

May I also ask Dr. CAMBIER a question. In the paper you presented, Dr. CAMBIER, you said that you had observed lightning pain "in the course of certain cases of diabetic neuropathy, in neuropathies associated with neoplasms, and in some degenerative neuropathies". I wonder whether, among these "degenerative neuropathies", you had any cases of amyloid neuropathy of the Portuguese type. We have a large number of such patients in the northern part of Sweden, and we have often noticed that the onset of their neurological symptoms is associated with lightning pains, which then subside later on. One remarkable thing about amyloid neuropathy is that, as DYCK and LAMBERT** in the U.S.A. have shown, the first nerve fibres to degenerate are the C fibres and that nevertheless lightning pains occur. Do you think, Dr. CAMBIER, that this is compatible with the gate control theory?

D. JANZ: The hypothesis that induced Dr. BLOM to give carbamazepine a trial in trigeminal neuralgia prompts me in turn to add a brief reference to another, apparently specific, effect which carbamazepine has been found to produce in patients with multiple sclerosis suffering from so-called "paroxysmal dysarthria and ataxia", a syndrome likewise affecting the tongue and mandible. This very rare condition, on which a number of reports were published several years ago***, was recently described again by my colleagues, Dr. WOLF and Dr. ASSMUS****. The patients experience – usually in the early stages of their multiple sclerosis – sudden attacks during which they have difficulty in speaking; they are no longer able to move their tongue and jaw, and they become ataxic. These disturbances, lasting only two to ten seconds, occur as many as 10–80 times a day. Judging from the fact that the E.E.G. shows no abnormalities, they certainly do not appear to be of an epileptic nature. In view

---

* BLOM, S.: Diphenylhydantoin and lidocaine in decerebrate cats. The effects on the linguomandibular reflex. Arch. Neurol. (Chic.) *8*, 506 (1963)
** DYCK, P.J., LAMBERT, E.H.: Dissociated sensation in amyloidosis. Arch. Neurol. (Chic.) *20*, 490 (1969)
*** ANDERMANN, F., COSGROVE, J.B.R., LLOYD-SMITH, D., WALTERS, A.M.: Paroxysmal dysarthria and ataxia in multiple sclerosis. A report of 2 unusual cases. Neurology (Minneap.) *9*, 211 (1959)
    ESPIR, M.L.E., MILLAC, P.: Treatment of paroxysmal disorders in multiple sclerosis with carbamazepine (Tegretol). J. Neurol. Neurosurg. Psychiat. *33*, 528 (1970)
    ESPIR, M.L.E., WALKER, M.E.: Carbamazepine in multiple sclerosis. Lancet 1967/I, 280; corresp.
    ESPIR, M.L.E., WATKINS, S.M., SMITH, H.V.: Paroxysmal dysarthria and other transient neurological disturbances in disseminated sclerosis. J. Neurol. Neurosurg. Psychiat. *29*, 323 (1966)
    HARRISON, M., McGILL, J.I.: Transient neurological disturbances in disseminated sclerosis: a case report. J. Neurol. Neurosurg. Psychiat. *32*, 230 (1969)
**** WOLF, P., ASSMUS, H.: Paroxysmale Dysarthrie und Ataxie. Ein pathognomonisches Anfallssyndrom bei multipler Sklerose. J. Neurol. (Berl.) *208*, 27 (1974)

of the good results that had been obtained with carbamazepine in trigeminal neuralgia, we decided also to give the drug a trial in these disorders, on the grounds that they are referable to the lower portion of the brainstem. Whereas diphenylhydantoin had elicited no response, we found that carbamazepine was able to eliminate this syndrome immediately.

J. CAMBIER: With reference to what you have just said, Dr. JANZ, you may perhaps have noticed that multiple sclerosis was included in Figure 2 of the paper I presented. This was intended as an allusion to the paroxysmal tonic manifestations of multiple sclerosis which you mentioned, and on which we published a report relating to ten cases in 1970*. Since then, the number of cases seen by us has risen to 15. These manifestations, which are not confined to dysarthria, often assume quite an extraordinary character. They are encountered in relatively benign forms of multiple sclerosis associated with few permanent neurological signs, the patient's disability arising from the fact that, when performing a volitional movement such as getting up from a chair or stretching his arm out of bed in the morning to switch off the alarm clock, he is liable to experience a sudden tonic spasm which cripples him for a brief moment. This phenomenon, which has probably been described long ago under the name of hemitetany and is indeed strictly confined to one side of the body, is triggered off by voluntary movements, is of extremely short duration, and, though sometimes taking the form of a purely motor disturbance, may also be accompanied by ipsilateral paraesthesia. In our experience, it may recur in some patients up to 50 times a day. It can very often be observed after the patient has been sitting in the waiting-room prior to a consultation, i.e. at the moment when one opens the surgery door to let him in. He is then paralysed on the spot and momentarily incapable of walking forward. A single daily tablet of carbamazepine is sufficient to eliminate this disorder, which, however, invariably reappears at once if the treatment is interrupted. Several years ago, a letter of ours appeared in the Lancet** in which we described a case of this kind after similar cases had been reported in the same journal by EKBOM and his colleagues***. We were able to follow up this patient from 1966 onwards and, after her death, to obtain anatomical evidence of the cause of the disturbances, which we published only recently****. The woman in question had been suffering from confirmed multiple sclerosis, the lesions being almost exclusively confined to the cervical part of the spinal cord; there were no plaques in the brainstem, and only one in the optic tract, but this was sufficient to confirm that the disease had indeed been multiple sclerosis. The epileptoid phenomenon to which I have been referring – and I deliberately use the term "epileptoid", because the disturbances really are tantamount to seizures – has a rather mysterious physiopathology. It is an, admittedly rare, feature of multiple sclerosis offering demonstrable proof of the extraordinary activity of carbamazepine.

There also exists another sign of multiple sclerosis, known as Lhermitte's sign, which is frequently encountered and easily observable, and in which carbamazepine also proves remarkably effective. In cases of multiple sclerosis, particularly in those where paraesthesia occurs as evidence that the dorsal columns are affected, sudden flexion

---

* CASTAIGNE, J., CAMBIER, J., MASSON, M., BRUNET, P., LECHEVALLIER, B., DELAPORTE, P., DEHEN, H.: Les manifestations motrices paroxystiques de la sclérose en plaques. Presse méd. *78*, 1921 (1970)
** CASTAIGNE, P., CAMBIER, J., BRUNET, P.: Spinal sensory-motor seizures. Lancet *1968/I*, 357; corresp.
*** EKBOM, K. A., WESTERBERG, C.-E., OSTERMAN, P. O.: Focal sensory-motor seizures of spinal origin. Lancet *1968/I*, 67
**** CASTAIGNE, P., CAMBIER, J., BARBIZET, J., BRUNET, P., POIRIER, J.: Crises sensitivo-motrices d'origine spinale au cours d'une sclérose en plaques à poussée aiguë terminale. Rev. neurol. *130*, 261 (1974)

of the neck provokes a shooting sensation, like an electric shock, running down the spine and into the legs. This phenomenon, Lhermitte's sign, is probably related to lightning pains insofar as it is followed by a refractory period: if one tries to elicit the sign several times in succession, it ceases to appear, and one has to wait a while before it can be obtained again. In all the patients for whom we have prescribed carbamazepine as treatment for Lhermitte's sign, it has disappeared in response to one or two tablets, but reappeared upon interruption of the medication.

I should now like to answer Dr. Blom's question. Amyloid neuropathies are rarely met with in France. I have, however, encountered one case, in which the disease was in an early stage and in which the lightning pains were alleviated by carbamazepine. I have also had considerable experience of diabetic neuropathies; here, lightning pains occur only in very minor forms exhibiting very few objective signs of neuropathy. But, from the standpoint of pathological anatomy, the underlying problem remains the same: the first axons to degenerate are those equipped with little myelin, whereas the first fibres subject to functional impairment are the rapidly conducting fibres. The first sign of a diabetic neuropathy – a sign that can be found in all diabetics if one searches carefully for it – is a slowing down of the conduction velocities. There must, I believe, be a stage in the evolution of the disease when the fibres containing little myelin in their sheaths have not yet undergone degeneration, whereas conduction in the rapidly conducting axons is already impaired, with the result that a physiopathological disorder then exists which may give rise to lightning pains. As the disease progresses, however, the poorly myelinated fibres degenerate, and the lightning pains consequently disappear.

P. Kielholz: I should like to make a few remarks on Dr. Reisner's paper. For many years now, we have very often been encountering pain as a feature of depressive syndromes. This pain occurs in three different forms: either as pain due to the excessive muscular tension associated with depression marked by anxiety, or as chronic painful conditions leading to exhaustion depression, or as prodromal pain in cases of endogenous depression. The indications for drug therapy in these three categories are, of course, exactly as outlined in your paper, Dr. Reisner. In other words, anxiolytic antidepressants are indicated in the anxious depressives, and drive-enhancing antidepressants in those suffering from retarded depression. We discovered that what, by analogy with your own terminology, might be referred to as "anxious pain" responded well to anxiolytic antidepressants, whereas "retarded pain" responded best to combinations of a major tranquilliser plus a drive-enhancing antidepressant. May I therefore ask whether you, Dr. Reisner, have also tried administering major tranquillisers together with drive-enhancing antidepressants as treatment for the types of pain that you have described as "retarded or tensed"?

G. Nissen: With reference to Dr. Reisner's paper, I'd like to add a couple of simple observations which we have made time and again in children. To begin with, it is well known that in healthy children the perception of pain is strongly dependent upon the momentary situation. This is apparent, for example, from the overshooting reactions which they exhibit in response to the pain caused by mild corporal punishment, and, conversely, from their relative insensitivity to such pain as they experience when having "fun and games", e.g. when fighting a "wrestling match" with their father.

In the case of feeble-minded children, on the other hand, we have repeatedly been struck by the fact that, when a doctor or a nurse has been assigned for the first time to a ward containing such children, he or she will after a while proffer the spontaneous comment that these children seem to be much less sensitive to pain than healthy children. They don't cry when they fall down, for example, or even when exposed to more painful stimuli.

Auto-aggressiveness is a manifestation frequently observed in severely imbecile children, who will often punch themselves in the face or literally bash their heads against a brick wall; despite the considerable pain which they must thus be inflicting upon themselves, quite some time elapses before they begin to scream or weep. In connection with this auto-aggressiveness, it has been our impression that the psyche, too, evidently plays a major role in the perception and interpretation of pain. These feeble-minded children are probably also lacking in ability to interpret pain. Incidentally, I should like to draw attention in this context to some very interesting investigations performed on young monkeys that had grown up in natural surroundings, or in surroundings in which they were exposed to relatively few stimuli; these animals differed very markedly from other monkeys in their reactions to pain – a finding which would seem to suggest the involvement of learning processes. A summary account of these studies is given by G. BENEDETTI in his book entitled "Psyche and Biology"*. I strongly suspect that similar arguments apply to the interactions between phantom-limb pain and personality structure.

H. REISNER: May I say how very pleased I am that Dr. KIELHOLZ was able to confirm my own experience with regard to depressions and pain. I am also grateful for his suggestion about giving major tranquillisers in combination with drive-enhancing antidepressants. I haven't tried this yet, and have only employed these two types of drug as monotherapy.
Dr. NISSEN brought up the question of differences in sensitivity to pain in children. I, too, believe that such differences exist in the pain threshold, particularly in children who have sustained damage to the brain, and I think that similar differences can also be observed in adults. A well-known example, dating back to the time when corporal punishment was still administered in the army, is that of those fortunate soldiers enviously referred to by their comrades as *prügelfaul*, i.e. who appeared largely impervious to pain. But this concept of differences in sensitivity to pain may prove very dangerous if and when it impinges upon the awareness of the public at large. I remember a court case a few years ago in Vienna – Dr. RETT will no doubt recall it too – at which an expert witness declared that one need have no scruples about beating an imbecile child, because such children are insensitive to pain!

M. BONDUELLE: Just a word in support of what Dr. MARTINELLI said in his paper about the effectiveness of carbamazepine in primary hemifacial spasm. I have some 20 patients in about half or two-thirds of whom carbamazepine has afforded a degree of relief that I would estimate at between 50 and 75%.

W. BIRKMAYER: Thank you, Dr. BONDUELLE. That, Ladies and Gentlemen, closes the topic of pain. To round off our symposium, I would like to suggest that Dr. BEIN, Dr. KIFFIN PENRY, and Dr. BONDUELLE should each give us a brief review of their impressions of the proceedings as a whole, after which I shall attempt to sum up.

 * BENEDETTI, G.: Psyche und Biologie (Hippocrates, Stuttgart 1973)

Concluding remarks

H. J. BEIN: Mr. Chairman, Ladies and Gentlemen, on various occasions in the course of this symposium, questions have been raised which involve fundamental aspects of pharmacology. With your permission, I should now like to try and comment on a few of these questions from the standpoint of a pharmacologist.

Pharmacology is a science in which the properties of active substances are analysed in various species and comparisons made between the effects of one substance and another. The choice of species is of relatively minor importance and is often dictated by practical considerations. The administration of an active substance invariably produces effects of one kind or another, and it is one of the pharmacologist's tasks to distinguish those findings that are relevant to the substance's activity from those that are non-specific. In the field of psychopharmacology, I have long been impressed by the fact that the breakthroughs achieved have originated, not from experimental research on animals, but from clinical research. This also applies to the treatment of epilepsy, inasmuch as research on the anti-epileptic activity of the bromides and of phenobarbitone was initiated by clinicians. The lesson to be learned from the pharmacology of psycho-active drugs is that one should not concentrate on the results of *individual* animal experiments but preferably study findings obtained in a variety of experimental models; in other words, one must establish a profile of the overall activity of a substance. This profile is frequently of more decisive significance than the effects which the substance produces in individual experimental procedures, particularly since in these individual tests substances belonging to a wide variety of therapeutic categories are very often found to exert the same effects. This also seems to be the case where anti-epileptic drugs are concerned. Inhibition of post-tetanic potentiation, for example, is by no means necessarily indicative of anti-epileptic activity; it is a marked feature of ®Lioresal (baclofen), for instance, although there is no clinical evidence that this preparation displays any particular anti-epileptic properties. Similarly, drug-induced seizures in animals can be counteracted by substances, such as major tranquillisers, which are not regarded as anti-epileptic agents in the strict sense of the term. In this connection, I should also like to draw attention to the fact that, according to findings obtained by Dr. KOELLA and his colleagues in a variety of test procedures, the anti-epileptic agents each exhibit differing activity profiles.

There are other respects, too, in which I perceive similarities between the psychoactive drugs as such and the anti-epileptic agents. Not every form of epilepsy will necessarily respond to the same preparation, and, even among patients suffering from clinically identical forms, there may be some who prove resistant to certain drugs but who do respond to other types of medication. In the case of diphenylhydantoin, it has been alleged that such resistance is not simply due to the fact that, in the patients in question, the active substance fails to reach therapeutically effective concentrations in the serum. We can therefore assume that epileptic disorders which run a similar clinical course may nevertheless differ in their response to a given drug. This would appear to suggest, firstly, that the various anti-epileptic agents must have differing mechanisms of action and, secondly, that even epileptic seizures which bear a close clinical resemblance to one another are liable to differ in their pathophysiology. We have also heard at this symposium that in refractory forms of epilepsy a combination of various anti-epileptic drugs is preferable to monotherapy. This, too, seems to indicate that these drugs differ in their mechanisms of action.

The situation I have been attempting to describe here strongly reminds me of the difficulties that still confronted us a few years ago with regard to the antidepressive drugs. Here, too, we were faced with an enigma: for some reason that defied rational explanation, the response of individual depressive patients to individual antidepressants – a response which is partly determined by genetic factors – had been found to differ, despite the fact that in what were regarded as relevant experimental procedures

353

these antidepressants exhibited a largely identical pattern of behaviour; moreover, as in the case of anti-epileptic drugs, combinations of antidepressants were then, and still are, being advocated for use in refractory forms of depression. It was only when it had been discovered that clinically identical depressions may be associated with differing biochemical disturbances, and when correlations had been established with experimental pharmacological findings, including especially those relating to biochemical changes, that new perspectives were opened up. In our research on epilepsy, we are evidently still lacking methods of analysis which would enable us to achieve finer clinical differentiations. In this connection, the heretical thought occurs to me that – because of the E.E.G., which plays such a dominant role in the diagnosis of epilepsy – we may possibly have been, and perhaps still are, unaware of any need to push ahead in the biochemical field.

If I understood Dr. PETSCHE correctly, he was unable – despite the remarkably sophisticated techniques he employed in his studies – to discern any difference in seizures elicited by penicillin as compared with pentetrazole. As a pharmacologist, I am also intrigued by the fact that the clinical improvement occurring in response to ®Tegretol (carbamazepine) is not always associated with a corresponding improvement in the E.E.G. findings. Speaking once again as a pharmacologist, I was also surprised that, when the pathophysiology of epileptic disorders was being discussed during this symposium, no mention was made of one very special category of seizures, namely, those due to withdrawal or overdosage of drugs – particularly of drugs which normally have an anticonvulsive effect, such as phenobarbitone. It has recently been reported that other psycho-active drugs, e.g. chlorpromazine and diazepam, may likewise exhibit this epileptogenic propensity*. Such findings may perhaps also be relevant to the observations made by Dr. KUHN with Tegretol in patients suffering from withdrawal symptoms following discontinuation of benzodiazepine medication.

Finally, I should like to point out that Tegretol is not the only anti-epileptic agent reported to exert a psychotropic effect in epilepsy as well as in other conditions. And it is therefore all the more galling for the pharmacologist to have to admit that no animal-experimental equivalent has yet been found. I can only hope that experimental research will benefit from the elaboration of finer techniques of clinical analysis, with the result that in due course it will then become possible to devise appropriate models.

J. KIFFIN PENRY: Mr. Chairman, Ladies and Gentlemen, may I begin by referring, not to the scientific side of this meeting, but to its organisational aspects. The conference room, the projection facilities, the acoustics, and the translations have all been excellent, and they have contributed a great deal to what I, at any rate, have been able to get out of this symposium. Having the manuscripts of the papers available in various languages has made a great deal of difference. To my way of thinking, there has only been one flaw, and that is that the participants have shown too many slides with too much material on them. This of course repeatedly happens at conferences all over the world. We travel thousands of miles and then present slides that cannot be read by the audience! However, this flaw can hardly be blamed on the organisers. On the contrary, I feel that Dr. ADAMS and the members of his staff certainly deserve a large measure of praise for making this meeting so successful.

In the course of the symposium a tremendous amount of scientific information has been presented. We have also heard a great deal about the conflicts between neurology and psychiatry, about the reluctance of neurologists and psychiatrists to work together at elucidating and treating the diseases of one and the same brain. It is, I feel, most important that representatives of the two disciplines should cooperate in the treatment not only of epilepsy, but also, to some extent, of behavioural disorders as well. Our

---

* TOONE, B.M., FENTON, G.W.: Epileptic seizures induced by psychotropic drugs. Electroenceph. clin. Neurophysiol. *37*, 326 (1974); abstract of paper

patients will certainly benefit if we all pool our efforts to arrive at an understanding of the same disease processes instead of arguing over our certificates or our tools.

Talks I have had with various participants at this meeting also suggest that a conflict exists between basic science and clinical science. For example, many clinicians become restless when listening to papers on the chemical structure of a drug, and they are apt to wonder what use this information is to them. On the other hand, the basic scientist working in his laboratory becomes equally restless when he has to listen to anecdotal reports on clinicians' experience with patients. It is, however, absolutely necessary that clinicians and basic scientists should take an interest in each other's field of study. This point was underlined by Dr. Petsche when he congratulated Dr. Mumenthaler on his brilliant review and said how astonishing it was that a clinician should have made such a penetrating study of neurophysiology. The art of medicine and the science of basic research must be brought together. As Dr. Birkmayer pointed out in the discussion following Dr. Heimann's paper, clinicians need more information from the basic scientists. They need to be told how to measure more accurately and how to be more objective. But these individual objective measurements must be placed into appropriate contexts, and this again confronts the clinician with a challenge. When I go into a pharmacology laboratory, for instance, and attempt to learn about gas-liquid chromatography, my aim is not to take over the pharmacologist's job, but simply to find out what he is doing, so that I can talk to him intelligently about his work. At the same time, I hope that he will get interested in what I am doing, thus helping as it were to bring science and art together.

This need for collaboration between clinicians and basic scientists was also very clearly illustrated in the excellent papers presented by Dr. Morselli and Dr. Oller Ferrer-Vidal on the problem of correlating the blood levels of carbamazepine with the drug's clinical effect. Dr. Dreyer pointed out that blood levels, though important, can also be misleading; and one certainly has to beware of drawing the wrong inferences from them. There is, in fact, still some scepticism about the use of blood levels as a means of improving the treatment offered to patients. Just how essential it is to monitor the blood levels, however, is illustrated only too well by the results of a study conducted by Cereghino et al.* in hospital patients, in whom the problem of compliance does not arise; here, it was found that, even though the patients received exactly the same dose in milligrammes per kilogramme over a period of 6–8 months, their blood levels differed by as much as 200%. An excellent paper dealing with this same problem has recently been published by Lund**, who carried out a three-year study in Stockholm. Other studies – by Sherwin et al.***, for example – have shown that as many as 30% of the patients who fail to respond to conventional dosage schedules could be controlled completely if recourse were had to blood-level determinations. After all, no internist would dare nowadays to try to manage diabetes mellitus without reference to the blood sugar, and yet in the treatment of epilepsy we still pay little attention to the blood levels of the drugs we use, simply because we don't understand the correlation between these levels and the drug's clinical effect. The challenge facing us today is to find ways and means of studying this correlation.

The final point I would like to comment on was one raised by Dr. Hagberg, among others, and it concerns the problem of epidemiology. We as physicians are so obsessed by our in-depth, interpersonal relationship with patients that we tend to forget that all epilepsy is not one, that each patient is different, that we need nosological

---

* Cereghino, J.J., Brock, J.T., Van Meter, J.C., Penry, J.K., Smith, L.D., White, B.G.: Carbamazepine for epilepsy. A controlled prospective evaluation. Neurology (Minneap.) *24*, 401 (1974)

** Lund, L.: Anticonvulsant effect of diphenylhydantoin relative to plasma levels. Arch. Neurol. (Chic.) *31*, 289 (1974)

*** Sherwin, A.L., Robb, J.P., Lechter, M.: Improved control of epilepsy by monitoring plasma ethosuximide. Arch. Neurol. (Chic.) *28*, 178 (1973)

classifications, and that we are not justified in using the word "epilepsy"* to describe a specific seizure**, which is a finite event in time. Similarly, we are having difficulty in putting our personal observations into an epidemiological context. This difficulty is due, not to differences in honesty, and not so much to differences in methodology – although these certainly exist – but rather to differences in terminology and in nosological classification.

M. BONDUELLE: Mr. Chairman, Ladies and Gentlemen, the most interesting aspects of this meeting have, I feel, already been clearly indicated by Dr. KIFFIN PENRY. As a research worker who is also concerned with basic neurological problems, he has stressed in particular the interest which the proceedings of the symposium have had for the biologists and pharmacologists among us. I think that at this gathering the basic scientists and the clinicians to whom he referred have indeed succeeded in establishing a dialogue – a dialogue which it is as a rule even more difficult to achieve than between neurologists and psychiatrists. Moreover, speaking as a clinician myself, I should like to emphasise how tremendously, in my opinion, this symposium has gained from the fact that speakers representing basic science have participated so actively in our deliberations on all three of the topics under discussion – epilepsy, behavioural disorders, and pain – on each of which I now wish to offer a few brief comments.

First of all, a word or two about epilepsy. I hope you will pardon me for recalling that it was at the Neuro-Psychopharmacology Congress held in Munich in 1962 that – along with Dr. LORGÉ***, whom I have had the pleasure of seeing again here at this symposium – I reported on the first results obtained with carbamazepine in the treatment of epilepsy****. The initial findings we put forward at that time have since been confirmed, also in the course of the present meeting. In this connection, I should like to add that I entirely agree with the conclusions reached by Dr. GRANT, particularly since they are exactly comparable with those that my colleagues and I published in 1962 and 1964*****. Dr. GRANT didn't include these publications in the list of references appended to his paper – presumably because they were so old that he was unaware of them, although they were in fact also referred to at a symposium which took place some years later in London******. At all events, the degree to which our views coincide is really remarkable.

For me personally, it is most gratifying to look back over the road we have travelled since our first report appeared in 1962, and to see how much progress has meanwhile been achieved. From the papers that have now been presented at this symposium, two things emerge which strike me as having a particularly interesting bearing on the treatment of epilepsy. Firstly, it has been confirmed that carbamazepine is a major anti-epileptic drug – a fact which I don't think anyone, or hardly anyone,

* MERLIS, J. K.: Proposal for an international classification of the epilepsies. Epilepsia (Amst.) *11*, 114 (1970)
** GASTAUT, H.: Clinical and electroencephalographical classification of epileptic seizures. Epilepsia (Amst.) *11*, 102 (1970)
*** LORGÉ, M.: Über ein neuartiges Antiepilepticum der Iminostilbenreihe (G. 32883). In Bradley, P. B., et al. (Editors): Neuro-Psychopharmacology, Vol. III, Proc. IIIrd Meet. Coll. int. neuro-psychopharmacol. (C.I.N.P.), Munich 1962, p. 299 (Elsevier, Amsterdam/London/New York 1964)
**** BONDUELLE, M., BOUYGUES, P., SALLOU, C., CHEMALY, R.: Bilan de l'expérimentation clinique de l'anti-épileptique G. 32883 (5-carbamoyl-5-H-dibenzo-b,f,azépine). Résultats de 89 observations, loc. cit., p. 312
***** BONDUELLE, M., BOUYGUES, P., SALLOU, C., GROBUIS, S.: Expérimentation clinique de l'anti-épileptique G. 32.883 (Tégrétol). Résultats portant sur 100 cas observés en trois ans. Rev. neurol. *110*, 209 (1964)
****** BONDUELLE, M.: My study of Tegretol in the treatment of epilepsy. In Wink, C. A. S. (Editor): Tegretol in epilepsy, Rep. int. clin. Symp., London 1972, p. 80 (Nicholls, Manchester 1972)

doubted from the very beginning. Not only has the value of carbamazepine as an anti-epileptic been demonstrated on a large scale, but in certain forms of epilepsy this drug would also seem to be the best treatment currently available. Secondly, what I likewise find very remarkable is the evident trend towards the use of carbamazepine as monotherapy.

Incidentally, from the proceedings of this symposium it is also apparent that the indications for carbamazepine in epilepsy have now become more clearly delineated, and there is reason to hope that the introduction of techniques for monitoring the blood levels – techniques which were sorely lacking at the time we first began studying carbamazepine – will enable us to handle the drug even more effectively.

The second theme of our symposium, i.e. behavioural disorders, is one to which numerous studies have been devoted and one that has given rise to a great deal of debate. With regard to the importance of carbamazepine in the treatment of such disorders, I would remind you that its psychotropic activity was another of its properties which received due emphasis in the very first papers published on the drug. This psychotropic effect has been discussed at length at the present meeting, and we have seen that it can also be exploited for the correction of behavioural disorders not only in epileptic but also in non-epileptic patients.

Finally, just one critical comment on the way in which our third topic – pain – has been dealt with. Although we have been offered what I consider to be a satisfactory explanation of the mechanisms underlying pain, I feel it rather a pity that no attempt was made to tackle the question as to the mechanism of action by which carbamazepine relieves pain.

Very briefly summarised, these, then, were my impressions of the symposium, and I hope that what I have said also reflects the opinions of all those present here.

In closing, I should like to congratulate CIBA-GEIGY on this very successful meeting and to express our thanks for the generous hospitality we have enjoyed here. I should also like to compliment and thank Dr. ADAMS, under whose watchful eye this gathering has been so brilliantly organised and who has put himself to so much trouble on behalf of us all. I likewise wish to congratulate all the members of the CIBA-GEIGY staff who have contributed to the success of the symposium and to thank them for their kindness and courtesy. With his customary eloquence, Dr. BIRKMAYER will, I am sure, contrive to say all this better than I can. What he won't do, however, is to spare a word of thanks for the Chairman! Allow me therefore to express our gratitude to him for having instigated and inspired this symposium and for having chaired the meeting with such vigilance, energy, and unfailing youthfulness.

W. BIRKMAYER: Ladies and Gentlemen, it is by no means easy to find suitable words with which to round off our symposium, because everything worth saying seems already to have been said in the course of the proceedings. I therefore propose to confine myself to giving you a relatively brief summary of my own personal impressions.

The various topics featured in the programme have been exhaustively discussed, and we have succeeded, I think, in providing both the clinician and the general practitioner not only with an informative review of epilepsy, of behavioural disturbances in non-epileptic children and adolescents, and of pain syndromes of a neuralgic type, but also with guidelines which should prove of benefit to all those engaged in the treatment of these three groups of disorders.

Without wishing in any way to question the value of the other presentations we have heard, I should like to single out for special mention the papers delivered by Dr. PETSCHE and Dr. MUMENTHALER. There can be no doubt that the scientific background data contained in these two papers helped considerably to ensure a high standard of debate in the ensuing discussions.

It is interesting to note that medicine, too, has its catchwords, many of which remain in vogue for only a short time. I suspect that one such catchword may be "pharmacokinetics". It is not, believe me, that I have anything against pharmacokinetics, but I merely wish to point out that one should beware of exaggerating the importance of pharmacokinetic findings. As the meticulous and elegant studies reported by several participants at this symposium have confirmed once again, detailed investigations into a drug's metabolism, with particular reference to its metabolites and their effects, are certainly deserving of our full attention, because an excessively rapid rate of degradation may result in ineffectiveness or in too short a duration of action, and a metabolite may possibly give rise to side effects. Nevertheless, there are some substances – such as ®Symmetrel (amantadine) for example – which might be said to have no pharmacokinetics insofar as they are excreted in unchanged form.

In those parts of our proceedings which were devoted to questions of treatment, one of our concerns was to re-examine with a critical eye the position occupied at present by one particular drug, i.e. Tegretol, which has already been in use for many years. From the autoradiogram of the mouse that Dr. FAIGLE showed us, it was clear that carbamazepine also penetrates into the brain, and this is an essential point, because it is in the brain that we want the substance to exert its effect. In the light of my long years of experience as a neurologist, I would say that Tegretol constitutes a welcome addition to the armamentarium of modern anticonvulsive agents, and that it definitely marks a step forward from the days when the barbiturates were virtually all we had at our disposal for the treatment of epilepsy. During our symposium, however, several speakers have drawn attention to the fact not only that Tegretol can be regarded as an anticonvulsant endowed with psychotropic properties, but also that it is capable of eliciting a beneficial response in neuralgia – especially trigeminal neuralgia – and in behavioural disturbances in non-epileptic children and adolescents. But Tegretol is not effective in all cases; it has its quota of failures, and it possesses side effects of which one must be aware.

In our three half-day sessions we have successfully tackled a vast programme, and I think we can safely claim that the mental energy we have expended has proved worthwhile and that we have made useful contributions to three topics which are of considerable practical importance. We have undoubtedly been aided and abetted in our task by the fact that we were able to hold our symposium in such delightful surroundings, that the technical facilities, including the simultaneous translations, were so excellent, and that the whole meeting was organised in an exemplary fashion. For all this we owe a sincere vote of thanks to the symposium's sponsors – that is, to CIBA-GEIGY – and to all the members of the company's staff who have worked so hard behind the scenes.

To you, too, Ladies and Gentlemen, who have participated in the proceedings either as presenters of papers or as contributors to the discussions, I likewise offer my warmest thanks. Each and every one of you has played his part in making this symposium the success that I am sure you will agree it has been.

R. OBERHOLZER: Mr. Chairman, Ladies and Gentlemen, the topics dealt with in the course of this symposium have also offered an opportunity. for discussing one of CIBA-GEIGY's pharmaceutical products and for re-examining its main indications. This is an opportunity for which we are most grateful, because we have always striven to establish and maintain close contacts with clinicians and practising physicians, upon whom we are dependent for that steady flow of information which serves to provide a sound basis for the use of our drugs.

The necessity for critical appraisal is not confined solely to newly introduced preparations; on the contrary, products that are already well established – such as Tegretol, about which we have been hearing so much during these last two days – also need to be reassessed from time to time, so that such uncertainties as may have existed from the very beginning or have emerged meanwhile can be clarified in the light of new facts and findings and the drug's indications either expanded accordingly or, if necessary, narrowed down. Where clarifications of this kind are called for, a symposium like the present one, at which so many eminently qualified specialists have been gathered together, undoubtedly constitutes a forum whose judgments carry weight, especially when – as in this instance – the drug in question has been discussed within the context of a broad field of topics calculated to highlight those aspects that are of direct relevance and importance both from the practical as well as from the scientific standpoint.

I am particularly gratified that in his concluding remarks our Chairman vouchsafed the opinion that the symposium had proved a success, since this was the verdict of a man who by virtue of his vast and varied experience is most certainly competent to assess the value of a medical meeting. That it is above all to you, Ladies and Gentlemen, that we owe the success of this gathering, deserves, I feel, to be repeated. At the same time, however, I would emphasise once again what a great debt of gratitude we all owe to Dr. BIRKMAYER, who, "*fortiter in re, suaviter in modo*", has conducted the proceedings to such a highly satisfactory conclusion.

Index

369

Psycho-active drugs, analgesic effect correlated with psychomotor reactivity 338–341
– –, combination with anti-epileptic drugs 88
– –, cross-sectional versus longitudinal studies 224
– –, epileptogenic propensity 354
– –, influence of personality type on response to 217, 218, 220, 224, 225
– –, – – pretreatment status on response to 218, 225, 256
– –, – – situational factors on response to 218, 221, 224, 225
– –, peripheral sites of attack 314, 316
– –, pharmacology 353, 354
– –, pharmacopsychological studies with 217–226, 227
– –, predictability of response 223–225
– –, response to, and level of arousal 219, 220, 224, 225
Psychological performance and level of arousal 218–220, 224, 227, 228
Psychomotor patterns in pain syndromes 338–341
Psychopharmacological studies, see Pharmacopsychological studies
Psychoses, chronic, in epilepsy 178, 192
–, episodic, in epilepsy 176, 178, 181, 182, 184, 192, 193
–, paranoid, in epilepsy 179, 180
–, productive, in epilepsy 175–179, 182, 184
–, schizophrenia-like, in epilepsy 177, 178, 191, 192
Psychosis, epileptic, use of carbamazepine 206
Psychotic disorders, effect of dipropyl-acetate 82, 96
– symptoms, use of carbamazepine 96, 269
– syndrome due to carbamazepine 99
Psychotropic effect of carbamazepine 50, 96, 110, 195, 199–204, 205–208, 227, 228, 253–257, 259–263, 266, 268–270, 273, 357
Purkinje cell discharge, effect of carbamazepine 41
Pyridoxine, see Vitamin B$_6$
Pyritinol, use in behavioural disorders in children 238, 239

Radicotomy 299, 303, 317, 318
–, lightning pain following 317, 318
Radiculotomy 298, 316

Rage reaction in cats, effect of carbamazepine 44, 46, 50
Reactions, acute exogenous, in epilepsy 175, 176, 180, 181, 184
Receptors, sensory, function of 279, 280
–, –, specificity of 277–282, 285
–, –, structure of 277, 281, 282
Ritalin, see Methylphenidate
Rivotril, see Clonazepam
Rolandic discharges, see Epilepsy, benign, of childhood

Scalp, E.E.G. recordings from 12
Sclerosis, tuberous, as a possible cause of infantile spasms 63
–, –, – – – – – neonatal convulsions 63
Seizure discharges, electrically induced 16, 23
– –, laminar analysis 22–25, 27
– –, morphological units involved 12, 25
– –, ouabain-induced 21
– –, penicillin-induced 13–16, 19, 23, 41
– –, pentetrazole-induced 13, 16, 23
– –, spatio-temporal organisation 19, 20
– –, synchronisation 12, 19, 21–23, 25, 27
Seizures, cerebro-organic, use of carbamazepine 205
–, complex partial, use of carbamazepine 87, 166, 168
–, electrically induced, effect of carbamazepine 33–40, 45
–, generalised tonic-clonic, use of dipropylacetate 87
–, paroxysmal motor, use of carbamazepine 304
–, partial motor, use of carbamazepine 89, 166, 168
–, primarily generalised 21, 62
–, – –, use of carbamazepine 90, 112, 113, 166, 168
–, role of cerebral cortex in 20–22
–, secondarily generalised 51, 62
–, – –, use of carbamazepine 90, 112, 113, 166, 168
–, tonic 64
–, types correlated with age in children 52
Self-sustained activity in E.E.G. 12, 17
Situational factors, influence on response to psycho-active drugs 218, 221, 224, 225
Skin reactions due to carbamazepine 98, 101–103, 107, 109, 118, 246, 256, 267, 322
Sleep disturbances due to carbamazepine 109

371